Therapeutic Strategies

PROSTATE CANCER

Therapeutic Strategies

PROSTATE CANCER

Edited by

Mark R. Feneley
Heather A. Payne

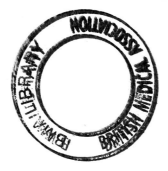

CLINICAL PUBLISHING

OXFORD

Clinical Publishing
an imprint of Atlas Medical Publishing Ltd

Oxford Centre for Innovation
Mill Street, Oxford OX2 0JX, UK
Tel: +44 1865 811116
Fax: +44 1865 251550
Email: info@clinicalpublishing.co.uk
Web: www.clinicalpublishing.co.uk

Distributed in USA and Canada by:

Clinical Publishing
30 Amberwood Parkway
Ashland OH 44805 USA

Tel: 800-247-6553 (toll free within U.S. and Canada)
Fax: 419-281-6883
Email: order@bookmasters.com

Distributed in UK and Rest of World by:
Marston Book Services Ltd
PO Box 269
Abingdon
Oxon OX14 4YN UK

Tel: +44 1235 465500
Fax: +44 1235 465555
Email: trade.orders@marston.co.uk

© Atlas Medical Publishing Ltd 2007

First published 2007

A catalogue record for this book is available from the British Library

ISBN-13 978 1 904392 88 0
ISBN-10 1 904392 88 1

The publisher makes no representation, express or implied, that the dosages in this book are correct. Readers must therefore always check the product information and clinical procedures with the most up-to-date published product information and data sheets provided by the manufacturers and the most recent codes of conduct and safety regulations. The authors and the publisher do not accept any liability for any errors in the text or for the misuse or misapplication of material in this work

Typeset by Prepress Projects Ltd, Perth, UK
Printed by Biddles Ltd, King's Lynn, Norfolk

Contents

Editors

MARK R. FENELEY, MD MA FRCS FRCSUrol, Consultant Urologist, Institute of Urology, University College London, London, UK

HEATHER A. PAYNE, MBBS FRCP RRCR, Consultant Oncologist, Meyestein, Institute of Urology, University College London, London, UK

Contributors

PETER C. ALBERTSEN, MD, Division of Urology, University of Connecticut Health Center, Farmington, Connecticut, USA

OMAR AL-SALIHI, BSc MBBS MRCP FRCR, Consultant Oncologist, University College London Hospital, London, UK

ANDREW J. ARMSTRONG, MDScM, Duke Comprehensive Cancer Center, Department of Medicine, Division of Medical Oncology, Duke University Medical Center, Durham, North Carolina, USA

DENISE C. BABINEAU, PhD, Assistant Staff, Department of Quantitative Health Sciences, Cleveland Clinic Foundation, Cleveland, Ohio, USA

DAVID G. BOSTWICK, MD MBA FCAP, CEO, President, Medical Director, Bostwick Laboratories, Glen Allen, Virginia, USA

JAMES D. BROOKS, MD, Associate Professor, Department of Urology, Stanford University School of Medicine, Stanford, California, USA

ARTHUR L. BURNETT, MD, Department of Urology, Johns Hopkins Hospital, Baltimore, Maryland, USA

MICHAEL A. CARDUCCI, MD ScM, Associate Professor of Oncology and Urology, Sidney Kimmel Comprehensive Cancer Center, Johns Hopkins School of Medicine, Baltimore, Maryland, USA

STEVEN L. CHANG, MD, Department of Urology, Stanford University School of Medicine, Stanford, California, USA

KIM N. CHI, MD FRCP[C], Assistant Professor, Department of Medicine, Division of Medical Oncology, University of British Columbia, Medical Director-Vancouver Centre Clinical Trials Unit, BC Cancer Agency, Vancouver, British Columbia, Canada

CHRISTOPHER FARNHAM, MB BS BSc FRCP, Consultant in Palliative Care, St John's Hospice, Hospital of St John and St Elizabeth, London, UK

Mark R. Feneley, MD(Cantab) FRCS(Eng) FRCS(Urol), Senior Lecturer in Urological Oncological Surgery, University College London, London, UK

Adrian C. Gardner, FRCS, Specialist Registrar in Orthopaedics and Trauma, Royal Orthopaedic Hospital NHS Trust, Birmingham, UK

Robert H. Getzenberg, PhD, Director of Urology Research, Professor, Urology and Oncology, The Brady Urological Institute, Johns Hopkins Hospital, Baltimore, Maryland, USA

David Gillat, ChM FRCS, Consultant Urologist, The Cotswold Centre, Southmead, Bristol, UK

Martin E. Gleave, MD FRCS[C], Professor, Department of Urological Sciences, University of British Columbia, Director of Research, The Prostate Centre, Vancouver General Hospital, Vancouver, British Columbia, Canada

Michael W. Kattan, PhD, Chairman, Department of Quantitative Health Sciences, Cleveland Clinic Foundation, Cleveland, Ohio, USA

Bruce R. Kava, MD, Department of Urology, University of Miami Miller School of Medicine, Miami, Florida, USA

Vincent Khoo, MBBS FRACR FRCR MD, Consultant and Honorary Senior Lecturer in Clinical Oncology, Department of Radiotherapy and Oncology, Royal Marsden Hospital & Institute of Cancer Research, London, UK

Roger S. Kirby, MA MD FRCS (Urol), The Prostate Centre, London, UK

Laurence Klotz, MD FRCSC, Chief, Division of Urology, Sunnybrook and Women's College Health Sciences Centre, Toronto, Ontario, Canada

Eddy S. Leman, PhD, The Brady Urological Institute, Johns Hopkins Hospital, Baltimore, Maryland, USA

Faye Lim, MB BS BSc MRCP, Specialist Registrar in Oncology, University College London Hospital, London, UK

Sarah Marietti, MD, Division of Urology, University of Connecticut Health Center, Farmington, Connecticut, USA

Isabelle Meiers, MD, Bostwick Laboratories, Regents Park, London, UK

Anita Mitra, MBBS MRCP FRCR, Clinical Research Fellow, Institute of Cancer Research, Sutton, UK

Don Newling, MBBChir. FRCS, Medical Director (Oncology), AstraZeneca, Alderley Park, Macclesfield, UK

Alan M. Nieder, MD, Department of Urology, University of Miami Miller School of Medicine, Miami, Florida, USA

Joe O'Sullivan, MD FRCPI FFRRCSI, Consultant/Senior Lecturer in Oncology, The Northern Ireland Cancer Centre, Centre for Cancer Research and Cell Biology, Queen's University Belfast, Belfast City Hospital, Belfast, UK

HEATHER A. PAYNE, MB BS FRCP RRCR, Consultant Oncologist, Meyerstein, Institute of Urology, University College London, London, UK

COLIN PURCELL, MB MRCP, Specialist Registrar in Medical Oncology, The Northern Ireland Cancer Centre, Centre for Cancer Research and Cell Biology, Queen's University Belfast, Belfast City Hospital, Belfast, UK

MARK S. SOLOWAY, MD, Professor and Chairman, Department of Urology, University of Miami Miller School of Medicine, Miami, Florida, USA

ALISTAIR J. STIRLING, FRCS, Consultant Spinal Surgeon, Royal Orthopaedic Hospital NHS Trust, Birmingham, UK

ROGER M. TILMAN, FRCS, Consultant Orthopaedic Oncologist, Royal Orthopaedic Hospital NHS Trust, Birmingham, UK

Section I

Prevention and diagnosis

1

Nutrition, lifestyle interventions and prevention

Steven L. Chang, James D. Brooks

INTRODUCTION

Over the past 50 years, the perception of prostate cancer in the USA has undergone radical change in the medical community. In the 1950s, the diagnosis of prostate cancer carried with it a high association with morbidity and mortality; patients commonly presented with metastatic disease and 75% of all treated patients died within 3 years [1]. In contrast, the past 25 years have seen the advent of widespread prostate cancer screening with prostate-specific antigen (PSA) as well as optimized surgical, radiotherapeutic and pharmacological treatments. Since the mid-1990s, the overall 5-year survival rate for men in the USA diagnosed with prostate cancer has exceeded 98% [2]. As a result, prostate cancer is currently viewed as an eminently treatable disease given proper screening and management.

Despite the significant improvement in the *diagnosis* and *treatment* of patients with prostate cancer, there has been relatively little success in the *prevention* of this malignancy. Consequently, prostate cancer stands as the most common non-cutaneous malignancy in the USA with an estimated 234460 new cases in 2006 [3]. The slow progress in preventing prostate cancer results from, for the most part, the ongoing struggle by researchers to identify the factors that affect the development of prostate cancer.

While the details of prostate carcinogenesis remain elusive, studies on the epidemiology of prostate cancer have yielded the greatest amount of information regarding potential risk factors as well as preventative agents. To date, the most well-established prostate cancer risk factors include age, family history and race. While such endogenous risk factors are immutable, recent epidemiological studies have strongly suggested that exogenous risk factors, including environmental exposure as well as lifestyle, may also significantly influence the development of prostate cancer [4, 5]. Therefore, while genetic factors predispose an individual to prostate cancer, environmental triggers are also probably necessary for the manifestation of this malignancy. Furthermore, prostate cancer develops slowly, taking years or decades to become clinically manifest, leaving abundant time for preventative intervention strategies. This chapter summarizes the available data on nutrition and lifestyle interventions in the prevention of prostate cancer.

NUTRITION

Over the past several decades, there has been dramatic progress in the understanding of the molecular processes underlying carcinogenesis (Figure 1.1). More recently, it has become

Steven L. Chang, MD, Department of Urology, Stanford University School of Medicine, Stanford, California, USA
James D. Brooks, MD, Associate Professor, Department of Urology, Stanford University School of Medicine, Stanford, California, USA

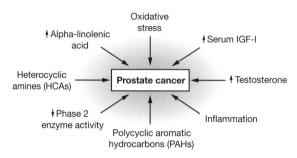

Figure 1.1   Putative mechanisms of prostate carcinogenesis. IGF-1, insulin-like growth factor-1.

clear that dietary factors are able to modulate the events preceding tumorigenesis. As a result, there is considerable interest in determining what nutritional components might modify the risk of prostate cancer. Migratory and epidemiological studies have implicated a 'Western diet', characterized by a high intake of red meat, dairy produce and animal fat, in the development of prostate malignancy (Figure 1.2) [4, 6, 7]. As helpful as these studies have been in elucidating the relationship between diet and prostate cancer, they must be interpreted with caution. Even a statistically significant correlation between an exposure and prostate carcinogenesis does not prove causation; contributing or confounding factors may also be present but not taken into account. As a result, the influence of nutrition on prostate cancer development is currently an area of intense investigation with ongoing epidemiological studies, randomized prospective controlled clinical trials and molecular research in the laboratory.

POTENTIAL PROSTATE CANCER RISK FACTORS

DAIRY PRODUCE

The Dietary Guidelines for Americans 2005 recommend increasing intake of dairy produce to reduce the risk of colon cancer, insulin resistance and osteoporosis [8]. The consumption of dairy produce, however, has been frequently associated with an elevated risk of developing prostate cancer. In 9 of 11 prospective case–control studies, there was a positive association between high dairy produce intake and development of prostate malignancy, although the reported increased risk was relatively modest [9–17]. Moreover, Chan *et al.* have reported a particularly strong correlation in advanced or metastatic prostate cancers, suggesting a role for dairy products not only in the development of prostate malignancy but also in the progression of disease [18]. The underlying mechanism linking dairy produce to prostate cancer remains unclear at this time, although there is growing evidence that fat, calcium and vitamin D may play important roles.

FAT

The high fat content in dairy produce has been proposed as a potential causative agent in developing prostate cancer. The implication of dietary fat as a modifiable risk factor, in both dairy as well as meat products, initially grew out of early epidemiological studies that observed a positive association between per capita intake of fat and prostate cancer mortality [19, 20]. More recently, animal studies have demonstrated a reduced growth rate of LNCaP cells in animals fed a diet low in fat compared with animals fed a high-fat diet [21, 22]. One proposed mechanism linking dietary fat and prostate malignancy is the production of reactive oxygen species during dietary fat metabolism. The resulting oxidative stress damages DNA through intercalation, increasing the risk for prostate cancer [23]. Other investiga-

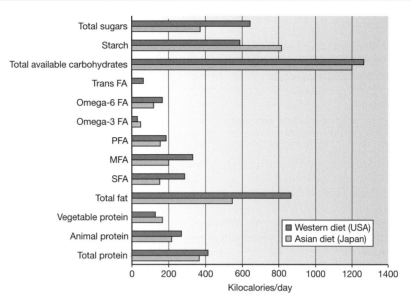

Figure 1.2 Comparison of Western and Asian dietary patterns. FA, fatty acids; PFA, polyunsaturated fatty acids; MFA, monounsaturated fatty acids; SFA, saturated fatty acids. (From Zhou BF, Stamler J, Dennis B *et al*. Nutrient intakes of middle-aged men and women in China, Japan, United Kingdom, and USA in the late 1990s: the INTERMAP study. *J Hum Hypertens* 2003; 17:623–630.)

tors have suggested that high dietary fat intake may increase the serum level of insulin-like growth factor (IGF)-I and concomitantly decrease the serum level of various insulin-like growth factor-binding proteins (IGFBP) [24]. The decrease in IGFBP levels is believed to down-regulate the expression of p53 and p21 proteins, leading to an inhibition of apoptosis and a proliferation of prostate cancer cell lines [25]. A third hypothesis is that a high-fat diet results in an elevation in the level of intraprostatic testosterone, altering the androgen milieu and thus predisposing to prostate carcinogenesis [26, 27].

Most epidemiological studies demonstrate an association between high dietary fat consumption and an increased risk of prostate cancer [28, 29]. Nevertheless, some [10, 30] have demonstrated no relationship between fat intake and prostate cancer, including the Netherlands Cohort Study, which prospectively followed over 58 000 men [11]. Further confounding the issue, Tseng and colleagues found that consumption of low-fat milk was significantly associated with prostate cancer risk, implicating dairy produce as a more important risk modifier than fat [16, 31].

In an attempt to clarify the relationship between dietary fat and prostate cancer, researchers have investigated the carcinogenic potential of specific types of fats, focusing mainly on linolenic acid and alpha-linolenic acid. In three studies, alpha-linolenic acid was shown to have a positive association with prostate cancer development [30, 32, 33], while a negative correlation was observed with an increased linolenic to alpha-linolenic acid ratio [30, 32]. However, two prospective cohort studies were inconclusive regarding the role of alpha-linolenic acid in prostate cancer development [11, 29]. Therefore, although a comprehensive review of the literature offers compelling evidence that decreasing dietary fat intake decreases the risk for developing prostate cancer [34], it is important to note that most of these studies are observational, rather than interventional, and the available laboratory data are inconsistent. The current evidence strongly suggests that decreasing intake of dietary fat may reduce the risk of prostate carcinogenesis although the exact dietary intake quantity remains to be determined. Further evaluation and investigation is still needed to better define the relationship between fat intake and prostate cancer.

CALCIUM/VITAMIN D

Calcium, through its interaction with vitamin D, is another component of dairy products that has been postulated to promote prostate carcinogenesis. The initial interest in calcium and vitamin D followed observations by Schwartz and Hulka of increased prostate cancer incidence in populations with vitamin D deficiency: (1) men living in the northern USA with less sun exposure [necessary to convert inactive vitamin D to active vitamin D (calcitriol)], and (2) men with increased skin pigmentation (e.g. African-Americans) [35]. Calcitriol has been associated with inhibited prostate tumour development and progression although the underlying mechanisms are unclear [36, 37]. Thus, consumption of calcium has been proposed to increase prostate cancer risk by suppressing vitamin D production via depressed parathyroid hormone levels [38].

Two prospective studies have demonstrated an increased risk of developing prostate cancer related to high calcium intake [15, 39]. In the Health Professionals Follow-up Study, among men who consumed more than 2000 mg of calcium per day the incidence of metastatic prostate cancer was increased fivefold compared with men who ingested less than 500 mg of calcium per day [39]. With moderate amounts (< 2000 mg) of calcium consumption, however, two other prospective studies (including a randomized clinical trial) revealed no association between calcium intake and prostate malignancy [11, 40]. Moreover, analysis of secondary endpoints from a randomized study evaluating the use of calcium supplements and colorectal cancer did not show any increased incidence of prostate cancer and actually suggested a possible protective effect [40]. As a result, studies linking high intake of dietary or supplemental calcium with an increased risk of prostate cancer [15, 38, 41] should be interpreted with caution, and additional well-controlled studies are needed to better delineate calcium as a risk factor when consumed in both moderate and high dosages. Based on available data, limiting daily calcium intake to less than 2000 mg may be beneficial for the prevention of prostate cancer.

MEAT

Consumption of meat, particularly red meat, has been proposed as a modifiable prostate cancer risk factor although findings from epidemiological studies have been mixed [4]. While several large cohort studies have shown no association [11, 42, 43], equally large studies report a positive association between a large dietary intake of meat and increased risk of prostate cancer, including the Physicians Health Study [relative risk (RR) = 2.5, 95% confidence interval 0.9–6.7] [44], the Health Professionals Follow-up Study (RR = 2.64, 95% confidence interval 1.21–5.77) [29] and a case–control study conducted in Uruguay [odds ratio (OR) = 2.0, 95% confidence interval 1.1–3.8] [45]. The mechanism by which meat may increase the risk of developing prostate cancer is currently under active investigation. The association might simply be due to the concomitant increase in dietary fat intake, although other potential carcinogens are consumed with meat, such as heterocyclic amines and zinc. Additionally, diets high in meat are frequently low in plant foods including fruits and vegetables, beans and whole grains; thus, these diets may be low in anti-carcinogenic components such as micronutrients and phyto-oestrogens (see below).

HETEROCYCLIC AMINES

One possible reason for the association between dietary meat intake with prostate cancer is that well-cooked meat, as a result of grilling and pan-frying above 180°C for long periods, contains abundant heterocyclic amines (HCAs) [46]. HCAs have been associated with development of gastric, colorectal, pancreatic and breast cancers in humans [47–49]. In animal studies, the presence of HCAs increases gene mutation frequency and promotes tumour formation in the prostate of rats [50, 51]. In a prospective cohort study Cross et al. found that high consumption (i.e. 10 g per day) of very well-done meat was associated with a 42% increased risk of prostate cancer [52]. While these recent data are intriguing, hard evidence linking HCAs and prostate cancer is limited, and other studies report no association [53]. Well-designed, prospective trials are needed to further define the role of HCAs in prostate cancer development.

ZINC

Consumption of meat, particularly red meat, could elevate the risk of prostate cancer by concomitantly increasing the intake of zinc, an essential component of testosterone synthesis. Ecological studies have shown higher prostate cancer mortality rates in countries with higher per capita zinc intake [54, 55]. Zinc is concentrated in the prostate and, under normal physiological states, zinc levels in the prostate are approximately 10-fold higher than in other soft tissues [56]. Moreover, zinc plays a role in maintaining the balance of testosterone and dihydrotestosterone within prostate cells *in vitro* [57]. However, the importance of zinc in prostate carcinogenesis and the possible mechanisms by which it acts remain poorly defined.

Clinical studies on zinc and prostate cancer have thus far been equivocal. A recent study by Leitzmann *et al.* reported that men who consumed high doses of supplemental zinc (i.e. over 100 mg/day) had a 2.29-fold increased risk of developing advanced prostate cancer and men who took lower dosages of supplemental zinc for long periods of time (i.e. over 10 years) had a 2.37-fold increased risk [58]. While these data based on supplemental zinc appear compelling, zinc obtained from dietary sources has not been shown to confer an increased chance of prostate malignancy [59]. To further complicate this issue, well-designed case–control studies have demonstrated a possible protective effect of dietary zinc [60] and zinc supplements [61] with respect to prostate cancer. Whether or not zinc plays a role in the apparent association between meat consumption and prostate carcinogenesis remains unclear.

POTENTIAL PROSTATE CANCER PREVENTATIVE AGENTS

The incidence of prostate cancer is highest in Western nations, while the lowest rates are found in Asian nations. Based on epidemiological and migratory studies, a wide variety of dietary components of the 'Asian diet' have been proposed to confer protection against prostate carcinogenesis (Figure 1.2). Considerable basic, epidemiological and clinical research is under way to test whether some foods might reduce the risk of developing prostate cancer.

PHYTO-OESTROGENS

Phyto-oestrogens are biologically active plant substances that have chemical structures similar to physiological oestrogens. These compounds have been identified in grains, herbs, fruits and, most notably, in soy products. Following digestion, phyto-oestrogens are able to bind to oestrogen receptors and weakly exert both oestrogenic as well as anti-oestrogenic effects [62, 63]. As a result, phyto-oestrogens have been thought to affect hormone-responsive carcinomas including breast, ovarian and endometrial cancers [64–67]. Because of the well-recognized effects of androgens and oestrogens on prostate cancer, it is possible the lower incidence of prostate cancer in Asian populations might be related to the relatively higher consumption of phyto-oestrogen-rich soy products [68].

Isoflavones, including genistein and daidzein, are the most well-studied phyto-oestrogens. They are found in large quantities in soybeans and soy products and at lower levels in kidney beans, chickpeas and lentils. The 'Asian diet' consists of approximately 10 times the quantity of isoflavonoid phyto-oestrogens compared with the average American diet [69].

In 1989, Severson *et al.* were the first to report that soy products might protect against the development of prostate cancer [10]. This prospective study involving 8000 Hawaiian men of Japanese descent demonstrated a decreased risk of prostate cancer in those who consumed tofu at least five times a week compared with those who had lower intakes of tofu (RR = 0.35, 95% confidence interval 0.08–1.43); however, the study did not control for other dietary differences between the groups. Several subsequent studies have also supported the association of consumption of soy products with a lower risk of prostate cancer including a large-scale epidemiological study involving 59 countries [70, 71].

Isoflavonoid phyto-oestrogens, including genistein and daidzein, inhibit the growth of prostate cancer cell lines, both androgen dependent and independent [72–76]. Animal studies have also consistently shown a protective effect of phyto-oestrogens in both prostate cancer development [77–80] and progression [81]. However, Naik *et al.* reported that a diet rich in genistein failed to inhibit the growth of hormone-refractory cell lines in rats, suggesting that phyto-oestrogens may be protective only in cases of androgen-dependent prostate cancer [72]. Based on these studies and others, it has been postulated that the possible protective effects of phyto-oestrogens are related to inhibition of the 5-alpha-reductase enzyme and a consequent alteration in androgen signalling [82, 83], decrease in angiogenesis due to lowering of serum levels of IGF-I [84], induction of apoptosis [85, 86] or reduction of oxidative damage through free radical scavenging and anti-oxidation [87–89]. It is most likely that phyto-oestrogens exert direct and indirect effects that act through several pathways to suppress prostate carcinogenesis. While efforts to investigate the entire family of phyto-oestrogens are ongoing [90], the available laboratory data at this time appear to support the epidemiological findings that increased intake of phyto-oestrogens may prevent prostate carcinogenesis.

While there is compelling evidence that strongly suggests that phyto-oestrogens decrease the risk of prostate cancer, the excitement surrounding phyto-oestrogens as a protective agent has been tempered by some epidemiological studies on soy consumption and prostate cancer risk that failed to achieve statistical significance [91–93]. Some studies have showed no association [94, 95], and others an inverse association [96]. Therefore, at this time, phyto-oestrogens, especially soy products, represent excellent *candidate* prostate cancer preventative agents, awaiting large, randomized clinical trials to determine their true clinical efficacy.

LYCOPENE

Increasing evidence suggests that lycopene, a phytochemical found in tomatoes and other red fruits, may reduce the occurrence of prostate cancer. Lycopene is the most common carotenoid found in the human body and a potent antioxidant. Interest in lycopene as a potential protective agent for prostate carcinogenesis grew from multiple epidemiological studies [60, 97–103], particularly a large cohort study that followed 14 000 Seventh Day Adventist men [42] and the Health Professionals Follow-up Study [98]. Both studies showed that the incidence of prostate cancer was significantly lower in men with a higher consumption of tomato products. However, a meta-analysis evaluating 10 cohort and 11 case–control studies concluded that the protective effect of lycopene on prostate cancer appears to be relatively modest and limited to men who consume large amounts of tomatoes (i.e. 10 servings per week) [104].

To overcome the limitations of food intake surveys, several studies have sought to correlate serum lycopene levels with prostate cancer incidence rates. Unfortunately, the findings from these association studies have been inconsistent. Of the nine studies that assessed blood lycopene concentrations, five reported a significantly lower plasma concentration of lycopene in men with prostate cancer than in matched controls [105–109] while the other four found no association [95, 110–113].

Laboratory studies have bolstered evidence that lycopene interferes with prostate carcinogenesis. Bowen *et al.* performed a randomized placebo-controlled study on 32 men with localized prostate cancer and found decreased levels of DNA damage in prostate tissue among subjects who ingested 30 mg of lycopene per day for 3 weeks prior to prostatectomy compared with control subjects [114]. Lycopene will inhibit the growth of prostate cancer cells *in vitro* [115] although only at supraphysiological concentrations [116] or in conjunction with vitamin E [117]. Lycopene also protects against oxidative damage [118–121] and reduces serum levels of IGF-I [122, 123], both hypothesized to be key features of prostate carcinogenesis. While lycopene could act through these and other biological effects, their relevance to prostate carcinogenesis in man will require considerable investigation.

CRUCIFEROUS VEGETABLES

Consumption of cruciferous vegetables (Table 1.1) has been linked to a decreased risk of prostate cancer in several epidemiological studies [101, 124–126]. The anticarcinogenic properties of these vegetables have been attributed to isothiocyanates, in particular sulforaphane. During the process of mastication, isothiocyanates are generated following the breakdown of glucoraphanin, a naturally occurring compound in plant cell walls. Zhang *et al.* isolated sulforaphane from broccoli based on its ability to activate carcinogen detoxification (phase 2) enzymes [127]. Sulforaphane induces phase 2 enzyme activity in prostate cells *in vitro* and *in vivo*, which could protect against DNA damage [128–130]. Sulforaphane can also inhibit extracellular signal-regulated kinases, suppress NF-κB [131], block cellular proliferation through cell cycle inhibition [132] and induce apoptosis [132, 133].

Epidemiological studies, however, have not consistently demonstrated an association between cruciferae and the risk of prostate cancer. Several studies have reported no association [99, 111, 134, 135], including the Health Professionals Follow-up Study cohort, which followed almost 48 000 men for 6 years [98]. The inconsistent findings between studies have been attributed to a combination of heterogeneity among the study cohorts, failure to control for potential confounders such as fat consumption, and measures of vegetable intake that were not comprehensive [136]. Several recent population-based studies have demonstrated a statistically significant reduced risk of prostate cancer in men who consume relatively large quantities of cruciferous vegetables [101, 102, 137–139]. While additional epidemiological and mechanistic studies as well as intervention trials are needed to assess the potential of cruci-

Table 1.1   Cruciferous vegetables

Arugula
Bok choy
Broccoli
Brussels sprouts
Cabbage
Cauliflower
Collard greens
Daikon radish
Kale
Kohlrabi
Mustard greens
Napa (Chinese cabbage)
Rutabaga
Turnips
Watercress

ferous vegetables to reduce prostate cancer risk, sulforaphane and other isothiocyanates are lead compounds for prostate cancer prevention.

VITAMIN E

Vitamin E is a family of essential, fat-soluble vitamin compounds that are found in green leafy vegetables, nuts, vegetable oils and fortified cereals. The most abundant and active form of vitamin E is α-tocopherol. This vitamin has been proposed to be a preventative agent in the development of prostate cancer due to its known ability to scavenge free radicals and act as a potent antioxidant at the level of membrane phospholipids [140].

In vitro and *in vivo* studies have shown that vitamin E may alter prostate tumorigenesis through several mechanisms. Sigounas *et al.* showed that α-tocopherol causes a dose-dependent inhibition of prostate cancer cell proliferation (CRL-1740) through induction of apoptosis [141]. Subsequent experiments demonstrated that vitamin E triggered apoptosis in LNCaP and PC-3 prostate cancer cell lines [142, 143]. α-Tocopherol will also produce cell cycle arrest at G1 [144] and can act as a weak antiandrogen [145].

Interest in vitamin E as a prostate cancer preventative agent arose from analysis of secondary endpoints in two intervention trials targeting lung cancer. The Alpha-Tocopherol, Beta-Carotene Cancer Prevention Trial (ATBC) was a randomized, double-blind, placebo-controlled trial that followed over 29 000 Finnish men for at least 5 years [146]. Although the ATBC was closed early because of a statistically significant increase in lung cancer among beta-carotene-treated subjects, a 32% lower incidence of prostate cancer diagnoses was noted among men who received 50 mg of α-tocopherol supplementation daily (95% confidence interval 0.12–0.47) as well as a 40% reduction in prostate cancer mortality. The Beta-Carotene and Retinol Efficacy Trial (CARET) also demonstrated a statistically significant inverse relationship between serum α-tocopherol levels and the risk of prostate cancer [147]. Based on the surprising findings of these two large clinical trials, the preventative value of vitamin E in prostate cancer as well as a possible synergistic effect with selenium is currently being evaluated in the Selenium and Vitamin E Cancer Prevention Trial (SELECT). This National Cancer Institute-sponsored randomized, double-blinded study is now following over 32 000 men randomized to receive either vitamin E, selenium, both vitamin E and selenium, or a placebo, with final results expected in 2013 [148].

However, not all available data support the use of supplemental vitamin E to prevent the development of prostate cancer. No association between supplemental vitamin E and prostate cancer was found in the Physicians Health Study [149] or the Prostate, Lung, Colorectal and Ovarian Cancer Screening Trial [150]. In addition, the potential protective effects of vitamin E for prostate cancer might be limited to current or recent smokers [149]. Furthermore, recent data have questioned the safety of high doses of vitamin E. A recent meta-analysis has found an increase in all-cause mortality in 9 of 11 trials evaluating high-dose vitamin E (> 400 IU/day) [151, 152]. Owing to the potential health risks as well as the inconsistent epidemiological data, supplemental vitamin E should be used with caution.

SELENIUM

A large body of data implicates selenium, an essential trace element, as a prostate cancer preventative agent. Selenium is found in nuts, fruits and vegetables as well as in over-the-counter supplements and multivitamins. The typical American dietary intake of selenium ranges from 80 to 165 µg/day [153]. Once ingested, it is widely distributed throughout the body tissues, including the prostate [154], and then incorporated into antioxidant enzyme systems [155]. *In vitro* and *in vivo* studies suggest that the anticarcinogenic properties of selenium may be due to several possible mechanisms including cell cycle arrest of prostate cancer cells [156, 157], apoptosis [158] or the disruption of androgen receptor signalling [157].

Like vitamin E, interest in selenium as a prostate cancer preventative agent originated from an intervention trial evaluating its role in another malignancy. The Nutritional Prevention of Cancer (NPC) trial was a randomized clinical trial to determine the effect of selenium on non-melanoma skin cancer, and included 974 men [159]. In their initial report in 1996 and a follow-up study in 2003, investigators reported a statistically significant reduction in the incidence of prostate cancer at 7.4 years in men who ingested $200 \mu g$ of selenium daily compared with control subjects (RR 0.51, 95% confidence interval 0.29–0.87) [160]. Prior to the NPC trial, the data relating selenium to prostate cancer had been inconsistent [161, 162]. However, because of the encouraging conclusions drawn from the secondary analysis of the NPC trial as well as several epidemiological studies, selenium is now being evaluated in the SELECT trial alongside vitamin E as possible preventative agents in prostate cancer [163].

FISH

Cross-national comparisons have shown an inverse relationship between per capita consumption of fish and the incidence of prostate cancer [70, 164]. These observations have prompted more detailed evaluations of the effect fish intake might have on prostate cancer development. A Swedish prospective cohort study with 30-year follow-up found that the incidence of prostate cancer was two- to threefold higher in men who seldom consumed fish than in men who consumed fish moderately often (RR = 2.3, 95% confidence interval 1.2–4.5) [165]. In the Health Professionals Follow-up Study, men with a high consumption of fish (> 3 times/week) were less likely to develop prostate cancer, and this association was strongest for metastatic prostate cancer (RR 0.56, 95% confidence interval 0.37–0.86) [166]. Again, the findings of these two large studies have been contradicted by other large epidemiological studies that report no association between consumption of fish and prostate cancer [11, 44, 167].

Basic investigations have added to the case favouring fish consumption and fish oils as protective agents. Omega-3 fatty acids, unique nutritional components of various fish including salmon, sardines, mackerel, tuna and anchovies, are thought to be the important biologically active agents in prostate cancer prevention. Rose and Connelly demonstrated a statistically significant ($P < 0.001$) inhibition in the growth of the PC-3 prostate cancer cell line by docosahexaenoic acid (DHA) and eicosapentaenoic acid (EPA), two forms of omega-3 fatty acids, although the DU-145 prostate cancer cell line was not susceptible [168]. Later studies confirmed growth inhibition in other model systems [169, 170]. Interestingly, DU-145 prostate cancer cells transplanted into nude mice did display inhibition of growth in animals fed diets rich in DHA and EPA [171–173]. Omega-3 fatty acids will modulate IGF-1 levels [174, 175], alter arachidonic acid metabolism [176, 177], change intraprostatic androgen levels [178, 179] and activate peroxisome proliferator-activated receptors [180].

Despite these promising findings, the effectiveness of omega-3 fatty acids remains controversial and much more work needs to be done. Three prospective case–control studies found no association between serum levels of omega-3 fatty acids and prostate cancer [30, 44, 181]. In fact, it remains unclear whether omega-3 fatty acids or some other component of fish intake are responsible for the reduction in the risk of prostate cancer seen in some epidemiological studies [182]. Until further studies to better define the role of fish intake and prostate cancer are available, it is advisable to follow the guidelines of the American Heart Association for adults to consume at least two servings of fish weekly for maintenance of good cardiovascular health, with the possibility that this diet might also reduce the risk of prostate cancer [183].

LIFESTYLE

Smoking, physical activity and obesity have all been shown to modulate the endocrine system. As prostate cancer is endocrine dependent, these potentially modifiable lifestyle risk factors have been investigated for connections to prostate cancer.

Smoking

While smoking has been established as an important risk factor for other genitourinary malignancies including bladder cancer [184] and renal cell carcinoma [185], the effects of cigarette smoking on prostate cancer are unclear. Cigarette smoking has been proposed to increase prostate cancer risk by altering circulating steroid hormone levels or through exposure to carcinogens. Cigarette smoking is associated with increased serum levels of bioavailable testosterone and lower levels of bioavailable oestrogen, producing a hormonal milieu favourable for prostate cancer development [186, 187]. Additionally, cigarettes contain substantial quantities of cadmium [188] and polycyclic aromatic hydrocarbons (PAHs), substances that have been implicated in prostate carcinogenesis [189, 190].

Somewhat surprisingly, a relationship between cigarette smoking and prostate cancer has been found in only a handful of epidemiological studies. In particular, statistically significant positive correlations were documented in large cohort studies involving Swedish construction workers (RR = 1.3) [191], men in rural Iowa (RR = 2.9, 95% confidence interval 1.3–6.7) [192], male members of a health plan in California (RR = 1.9, 95% confidence interval 1.2–3.1) [193] and male residents of northwestern Washington state (OR = 1.4, 95% confidence interval 1.0–2.0) [194]. Importantly, a dose–response relationship has also been demonstrated: in the Swedish study, former smokers had a relative risk of 1.09 while current smokers of at least 15 cigarettes a day for at least 30 years had a relative risk of 1.3 [191]. A similar dose–response relationship was reported in the Iowa [193] and northwestern Washington state cohorts [194]. Furthermore, cigarette smoking has been associated with more aggressive prostate cancer. The Health Professionals Follow-up Study found a higher risk of metastatic prostate cancers (RR = 1.81, 95% confidence interval 1.05–3.11) as well as prostate cancer death (RR = 2.06, 95% confidence interval 1.08–3.9) in men with at least a 15 pack-year history over the preceding 10-year period [195].

Despite these persuasive findings, the link between cigarette smoking and prostate cancer is far from established. Overall, 10 of 16 population-based studies have observed no association between current or previous cigarette smoking and an increased incidence of prostate cancer [9, 10, 28, 42, 195–200], although some of these studies have been criticized for methodological shortcomings. These include inadequate control for confounders as well as surveillance and attribution bias [201]. Furthermore, recent studies have suggested that the carcinogenic potential of cigarette smoking is largely influenced by the ability of men to detoxify carcinogens from cigarettes. There is growing evidence that polymorphisms in the genes involved in metabolism of PAHs, cadmium or other substances might significantly modify the risk of prostate cancer in men exposed to cigarette smoke [202, 203]. While further population-based and laboratory studies are still needed, the emerging data are highly suggestive that cigarette smoking may be a modifiable risk factor for prostate carcinogenesis.

Physical Activity and Obesity

Physical activity and avoidance of obesity have long been associated with improved overall health. Besides helping to prevent cardiovascular disease and promote psychological well-being, exercise and maintenance of normal body weight are becoming increasingly recognized as factors in the prevention of carcinoma, particularly colon and breast cancer [204–206]. In the case of prostate cancer prevention, however, the roles of exercise and obesity remain unclear.

Several biological effects of physical activity and obesity have been proposed to influence prostate cancer risk. Both physical activity and weight changes have been shown to affect endogenous hormone metabolism. Physically inactive and obese patients have increased rates of insulin resistance [207, 208], increased IGF-I levels [209], decreased IGFBP-3 levels [210] and higher levels of bioavailable androgens due to stimulation of gonadal and adrenal androgen synthesis and decreased levels of circulating sex hormone-binding globulin (SHBG) [211]. All of these hormonal alterations have been associated with an increased risk of prostate carcinogenesis [212–214].

Despite the presumed protective effects of physical activity and avoidance of obesity based on the hormonal alterations described above, the epidemiological data have been mixed. In fact, a comprehensive review by Freidenreich and Orenstein classified physical activity as only a 'probable' preventative factor for prostate cancer. To date, at least 16 studies have demonstrated a decreased incidence of prostate cancer in men who report increased physical activity although the average risk reduction of prostate cancer was moderate at best (10–30%) and statistical significance was achieved in only 11 studies [197, 215–229]. No association between prostate cancer risk and physical activity has been found in at least nine studies [230–237]. Surprisingly, four studies found an increased risk of prostate cancer in men with higher levels of physical activity[162, 192, 238, 239]. Methodological differences between these studies may account, at least in part, for the contradictory findings. For instance, several studies focused on 'recent physical activity' rather than lifelong physical activity. Given the long latency of prostate cancer, exposure to exercise long before diagnosis might be critically important.

The relationship between obesity and prostate cancer also remains unclear. Several large epidemiological studies have concluded that increasing body size or body mass index (BMI) is associated with a greater risk of developing prostate cancer. In a large Norwegian study involving over 25 000 men, Veierod et $al.$ showed a statistically significant positive association with BMI and prostate cancer development (BMI > 27.6 kg/m^2, RR = 2.2, 95% confidence interval 1.1–4.7) [28]. Similar positive, albeit modest, findings were reported in a large Swedish cohort (> 82 kg, RR = 1.16, 95% confidence interval 1.03–1.31) [240], a second Norwegian cohort (BMI≥30 kg/m^2, RR = 1.09, 95% confidence interval 1.04–1.15) [241] and an American cohort (BMI > 26.6 kg/m^2, RR = 2.1, 95% confidence interval 1.1–4.3) [236]. In contrast, other large cohort studies have shown no association between body size or BMI and prostate cancer [233, 242–246]. An inverse relationship between body size and prostate cancer has also been reported [247]. The contradictory data obtained from these studies make it difficult to draw even general conclusions regarding the effect of obesity on prostate cancer.

Although the link between obesity and prostate cancer remains unclear, several studies have reported intriguing subgroup analyses. Recent studies have reported a higher biochemical failure rate following radical prostatectomy in obese men, suggesting that excess body weight may be associated with a more aggressive form of prostate cancer [248, 249]. Giovannucci et $al.$ have proposed that obesity may be protective for early-onset cases based on data from the Health Professionals Follow-up Study [250]. Although this study found no overall association between BMI and prostate cancer, subgroup analysis revealed a decreased risk of prostate cancer associated with increased BMI only in men with a family history of prostate cancer and those under the age of 60 years. Thus, Giovannucci et $al.$ argued that the tumours in younger men and those secondary to genetic predisposition might be driven preferentially by increased androgens. Because obesity is associated with decreased serum testosterone and elevation of serum oestrogen levels, the hormonal alterations secondary to excess weight may be protective in this subset of men.

Although the available data are equivocal, increasing physical activity and decreasing excess weight remain extremely appealing preventative factors as they potentially reduce the risk of not only prostate cancer but also other chronic diseases without any of the adverse effects associated with chemopreventative agents. The American Cancer Society currently recommends a minimum of 30 min of moderate to vigorous exercise each day on 5 days or more a week and maintenance of BMI between 18.5 kg/m^2 and 25.0 kg/m^2 [251].

CONCLUSIONS

Prostate cancer is a particularly attractive target for prevention strategies because of the long latency between premalignant lesions and clinically evident tumours. Although the evidence for dietary and lifestyle alterations is incomplete, the reported associations between nutrition, lifestyle and prostate cancer development are highly encouraging and will fuel continued vigorous scientific efforts to develop preventative strategies. Hopefully, progress in prostate cancer prevention over the next 50 years will match the successes accumulated over the past 50 years in the diagnosis and management of this disease.

REFERENCES

1. Cancer of the prostate. *The Lancet* 1959; 273:398–399.
2. *SEER Cancer Statistics Review*, 1975–2003. National Cancer Institute, Bethesda, 2005.
3. *Cancer Facts & Figures – 2006*. American Cancer Society (ACS), 2006.
4. Kolonel LN, Altshuler D, Henderson BE. The multiethnic cohort study: exploring genes, lifestyle and cancer risk. *Natl Rev Cancer* 2004; 4:519–527.
5. Moradi T, Delfino RJ, Bergstrom SR, Yu ES, Adami HO, Yuen J. Cancer risk among Scandinavian immigrants in the US and Scandinavian residents compared with US whites, 1973–89. *Eur J Cancer Prev* 1998; 7:117–125.
6. Denis L, Morton MS, Griffiths K. Diet and its preventive role in prostatic disease. *Eur Urol* 1999; 35:377–387.
7. Dagnelie PC, Schuurman AG, Goldbohm RA, Van den Brandt PA. Diet, anthropometric measures and prostate cancer risk: a review of prospective cohort and intervention studies. *BJU Int* 2004; 93:1139–1150.
8. Nicklas TA, Weaver C, Britten P, Stitzel KF. The 2005 Dietary Guidelines Advisory Committee: developing a key message. *J Am Diet Assoc* 2005; 105:1418–1424.
9. Le Marchand L, Kolonel LN, Wilkens LR, Myers BC, Hirohata T. Animal fat consumption and prostate cancer: a prospective study in Hawaii. *Epidemiology* 1994; 5:276–282.
10. Severson RK, Nomura AM, Grove JS, Stemmermann GN. A prospective study of demographics, diet, and prostate cancer among men of Japanese ancestry in Hawaii. *Cancer Res* 1989; 49:1857–1860.
11. Schuurman AG, van den Brandt PA, Dorant E, Goldbohm RA. Animal products, calcium and protein and prostate cancer risk in The Netherlands Cohort Study. *Br J Cancer* 1999; 80:1107–1113.
12. Chan JM, Pietinen P, Virtanen M *et al.* Diet and prostate cancer risk in a cohort of smokers, with a specific focus on calcium and phosphorus (Finland). *Cancer Causes Control* 2000; 11:859–867.
13. Michaud DS, Augustsson K, Rimm EB, Stampfer MJ, Willet WC, Giovannucci E. A prospective study on intake of animal products and risk of prostate cancer. *Cancer Causes Control* 2001; 12:557–567.
14. Chan JM, Stampfer MJ, Ma J, Gann PH, Gaziano JM, Giovannucci EL. Dairy products, calcium, and prostate cancer risk in the Physicians Health Study. *Am J Clin Nutr* 2001; 74:549–554.
15. Rodriguez C, McCullough ML, Mondul AM *et al.* Calcium, dairy products, and risk of prostate cancer in a prospective cohort of United States men. *Cancer Epidemiol Biomarkers Prev* 2003; 12:597–603.
16. Tseng M, Breslow RA, Graubard BI, Ziegler RG. Dairy, calcium, and vitamin D intakes and prostate cancer risk in the National Health and Nutrition Examination Epidemiologic Follow-up Study cohort. *Am J Clin Nutr* 2005; 81:1147–1154.
17. Kesse E, Bertrais S, Astorg P *et al.* Dairy products, calcium and phosphorus intake, and the risk of prostate cancer: results of the French prospective SU.VI.MAX (Supplementation en Vitamines et Mineraux Antioxydants) study. *Br J Nutr* 2006; 95:539–545.
18. Chan JM, Giovannucci E, Andersson SO, Yuen J, Adami HO, Wolk A. Dairy products, calcium, phosphorous, vitamin D, and risk of prostate cancer (Sweden). *Cancer Causes Control* 1998; 9:559–566.
19. Armstrong B, Doll R. Environmental factors and cancer incidence and mortality in different countries, with special reference to dietary practices. *Int J Cancer* 1975; 15:617–631.
20. Howell MA. Factor analysis of international cancer mortality data and per capita food consumption. *Br J Cancer* 1974; 29:328–336.

21. Wang Y, Corr JG, Thaler HT, Tao Y, Fair WR, Heston WD. Decreased growth of established human prostate LNCaP tumors in nude mice fed a low-fat diet. *J Natl Cancer Inst* 1995; 87:1456–1462.

22. Ngo TH, Barnard RJ, Anton T *et al.* Effect of isocaloric low-fat diet on prostate cancer xenograft progression to androgen independence. *Cancer Res* 2004; 64:1252–1254.

23. Fleshner NE, Kucuk O. Antioxidant dietary supplements: Rationale and current status as chemopreventive agents for prostate cancer. *Urology* 2001; 57:90–94.

24. Barnard RJ, Aronson WJ. Preclinical models relevant to diet, exercise, and cancer risk. *Recent Results Cancer Res* 2005; 166:47–61.

25. Leung PS, Aronson WJ, Ngo TH, Golding LA, Barnard RJ. Exercise alters the IGF axis in vivo and increases p53 protein in prostate tumor cells in vitro. *J Appl Physiol* 2004; 96:450–454.

26. Howie BJ, Shultz TD. Dietary and hormonal interrelationships among vegetarian Seventh-Day Adventists and nonvegetarian men. *Am J Clin Nutr* 1985; 42:127–134.

27. Bishop DT, Meikle AW, Slattery ML, Stringham JD, Ford MH, West DW. The effect of nutritional factors on sex hormone levels in male twins. *Genet Epidemiol* 1988; 5:43–59.

28. Veierod MB, Laake P, Thelle DS. Dietary fat intake and risk of prostate cancer: a prospective study of 25,708 Norwegian men. *Int J Cancer* 1997; 73:634–638.

29. Giovannucci E, Rimm EB, Colditz GA *et al.* A prospective study of dietary fat and risk of prostate cancer. *J Natl Cancer Inst* 1993; 85:1571–1579.

30. Harvei S, Bjerve KS, Tretli S, Jellum E, Robsahm TE, Vatten L. Prediagnostic level of fatty acids in serum phospholipids: omega-3 and omega-6 fatty acids and the risk of prostate cancer. *Int J Cancer* 1997; 71:545–551.

31. Grant WB. A multicountry ecologic study of risk and risk reduction factors for prostate cancer mortality. *Eur Urol* 2004; 45:271–279.

32. De Stefani E, Deneo–Pellegrini H, Boffetta P, Ronco A, Mendilaharsu M. Alpha-linolenic acid and risk of prostate cancer: a case–control study in Uruguay. *Cancer Epidemiol Biomarkers Prev* 2000; 9:335–338.

33. Leitzmann MF, Stampfer MJ, Michaud DS *et al.* Dietary intake of n-3 and n-6 fatty acids and the risk of prostate cancer. *Am J Clin Nutr* 2004; 80:204–216.

34. Fleshner N, Bagnell PS, Klotz L, Venkateswaran V. Dietary fat and prostate cancer. *J Urol* 2004; 171:S19–24.

35. Schwartz GG, Hulka BS. Is vitamin D deficiency a risk factor for prostate cancer? (Hypothesis). *Anticancer Res* 1990; 10:1307–1311.

36. Lokeshwar BL, Schwartz GG, Selzer MG *et al.* Inhibition of prostate cancer metastasis in vivo: a comparison of 1,23-dihydroxyvitamin D (calcitriol) and EB1089. *Cancer Epidemiol Biomarkers Prev* 1999; 8:241–248.

37. Nonn L, Peng L, Feldman D, Peehl DM. Inhibition of p38 by vitamin D reduces interleukin-6 production in normal prostate cells via mitogen-activated protein kinase phosphatase 5: implications for prostate cancer prevention by vitamin D. *Cancer Res* 2006; 66:4516–4524.

38. Chan JM, Giovannucci EL. Dairy products, calcium, and vitamin D and risk of prostate cancer. *Epidemiol Rev* 2001; 23:87–92.

39. Giovannucci E, Rimm EB, Wolk A *et al.* Calcium and fructose intake in relation to risk of prostate cancer. *Cancer Res* 1998; 58:442–447.

40. Baron JA, Beach M, Wallace K *et al.* Risk of prostate cancer in a randomized clinical trial of calcium supplementation. *Cancer Epidemiol Biomarkers Prev* 2005; 14:586–589.

41. Kristal AR, Cohen JH, Qu P, Stanford JL. Associations of energy, fat, calcium, and vitamin D with prostate cancer risk. *Cancer Epidemiol Biomarkers Prev* 2002; 11:719–725.

42. Mills PK, Beeson WL, Phillips RL, Fraser GE. Cohort study of diet, lifestyle, and prostate cancer in Adventist men. *Cancer* 1989; 64:598–604.

43. Hsing AW, McLaughlin JK, Schuman LM *et al.* Diet, tobacco use, and fatal prostate cancer: results from the Lutheran Brotherhood Cohort Study. *Cancer Res* 1990; 50:6836–6840.

44. Gann PH, Hennekens CH, Sacks FM, Grodstein F, Giovannucci EL, Stampfer MJ. Prospective study of plasma fatty acids and risk of prostate cancer. *J Natl Cancer Inst* 1994; 86:281–286.

45. Deneo-Pellegrini H, De Stefani E, Ronco A, Mendilaharsu M. Foods, nutrients and prostate cancer: a case–control study in Uruguay. *Br J Cancer* 1999; 80:591–597.

46. Wogan GN, Hecht SS, Felton JS, Conney AH, Loeb LA. Environmental and chemical carcinogenesis. *Semin Cancer Biol* 2004; 14:473–486.

47. Sugimura T, Terada M. Experimental chemical carcinogenesis in the stomach and colon. *Jpn J Clin Oncol* 1998; 28:163–167.

48. Mitra AK, Faruque FS, Avis AL. Breast cancer and environmental risks: where is the link? *J Environ Health* 2004; 66:24–32, 40

49. Anderson KE, Kadlubar FF, Kulldorff M *et al.* Dietary intake of heterocyclic amines and benzo(a)pyrene: associations with pancreatic cancer. *Cancer Epidemiol Biomarkers Prev* 2005; 14:2261–2265.

50. Shirai T, Sano M, Tamano S *et al.* The prostate: a target for carcinogenicity of 2-amino-1-methyl-6-phenylimidazo[4,5-b]pyridine (PhIP) derived from cooked foods. *Cancer Res* 1997; 57:195–198.

51. Stuart GR, Holcroft J, de Boer JG, Glickman BW. Prostate mutations in rats induced by the suspected human carcinogen 2-amino-1-methyl-6-phenylimidazo[4,5-b]pyridine. *Cancer Res* 2000; 60:266–268.

52. Cross AJ, Peters U, Kirsh VA *et al.* A prospective study of meat and meat mutagens and prostate cancer risk. *Cancer Res* 2005; 65:11779–11784.

53. Norrish AE, Ferguson LR, Knize MG, Felton JS, Sharpe SJ, Jackson RT. Heterocyclic amine content of cooked meat and risk of prostate cancer. *J Natl Cancer Inst* 1999; 91:2038–2044.

54. Biesalski HK. Meat and cancer: meat as a component of a healthy diet. *Eur J Clin Nutr* 2002; 56 Suppl. 1:S2–11.

55. Schrauzer GN, White DA, Schneider CJ. Cancer mortality correlation studies. IV: associations with dietary intakes and blood levels of certain trace elements, notably Se-antagonists. *Bioinorg Chem* 1977; 7:35–56.

56. Kerr WK, Keresteci AG, Mayoh H. The distribution of zinc within the human prostate. *Cancer* 1960; 13:550–554.

57. Leake A, Chisholm GD, Habib FK. The effect of zinc on the 5 alpha-reduction of testosterone by the hyperplastic human prostate gland. *J Steroid Biochem* 1984; 20:651–655.

58. Leitzmann MF, Stampfer MJ, Wu K, Colditz GA, Willett WC, Giovannucci EL. Zinc supplement use and risk of prostate cancer. *J Natl Cancer Inst* 2003; 95:1004–1007.

59. Platz EA, Helzlsouer KJ. Selenium, zinc, and prostate cancer. *Epidemiol Rev* 2001; 23:93–101.

60. Key TJ, Silcocks PB, Davey GK, Appleby PN, Bishop DT. A case–control study of diet and prostate cancer. *Br J Cancer* 1997; 76:678–687.

61. Kristal AR, Stanford JL, Cohen JH, Wicklund K, Patterson RE. Vitamin and mineral supplement use is associated with reduced risk of prostate cancer. *Cancer Epidemiol Biomarkers Prev* 1999; 8:887–892.

62. Bingham SA, Atkinson C, Liggins J, Bluck L, Coward A. Phyto-oestrogens: where are we now? *Br J Nutr* 1998; 79:393–406.

63. Setchell KD. Soy isoflavones — benefits and risks from nature's selective estrogen receptor modulators (SERMs). *J Am Coll Nutr* 2001; 20:354S–362S; discussion 381S–383S.

64. Gikas PD, Mokbel K. Phytoestrogens and the risk of breast cancer: a review of the literature. *Int J Fertil Womens Med* 2005; 50:250–258.

65. Wietrzyk J, Grynkiewicz G, Opolski A. Phytoestrogens in cancer prevention and therapy — mechanisms of their biological activity. *Anticancer Res* 2005; 25:2357–2366.

66. Gercel–Taylor C, Feitelson AK, Taylor DD. Inhibitory effect of genistein and daidzein on ovarian cancer cell growth. *Anticancer Res* 2004; 24:795–800.

67. Konstantakopoulos N, Montgomery KG, Chamberlain N *et al.* Changes in gene expressions elicited by physiological concentrations of genistein on human endometrial cancer cells. *Mol Carcinog* 2006.

68. Messina MJ. Legumes and soybeans: overview of their nutritional profiles and health effects. *Am J Clin Nutr* 1999; 70:439S–450S.

69. Messina M, Barnes S. The role of soy products in reducing risk of cancer. *J Natl Cancer Inst* 1991; 83:541–546.

70. Hebert JR, Hurley TG, Olendzki BC, Teas J, Ma Y, Hampl JS. Nutritional and socioeconomic factors in relation to prostate cancer mortality: a cross-national study. *J Natl Cancer Inst* 1998; 90:1637–1647.

71. Lee MM, Gomez SL, Chang JS, Wey M, Wang RT, Hsing AW. Soy and isoflavone consumption in relation to prostate cancer risk in China. *Cancer Epidemiol Biomarkers Prev* 2003; 12:665–668.

72. Naik HR, Lehr JE, Pienta KJ. An in vitro and in vivo study of antitumor effects of genistein on hormone refractory prostate cancer. *Anticancer Res* 1994; 14:2617–2619.

73. Rokhlin OW, Cohen MB. Differential sensitivity of human prostatic cancer cell lines to the effects of protein kinase and phosphatase inhibitors. *Cancer Lett* 1995; 98:103–110.

74. Peterson G, Barnes S. Genistein and biochanin A inhibit the growth of human prostate cancer cells but not epidermal growth factor receptor tyrosine autophosphorylation. *Prostate* 1993; 22:335–345.

75. Davis JN, Muqim N, Bhuiyan M, Kucuk O, Pienta KJ, Sarkar FH. Inhibition of prostate specific antigen expression by genistein in prostate cancer cells. *Int J Oncol* 2000; 16:1091–1097.

76. Santibanez JF, Navarro A, Martinez J. Genistein inhibits proliferation and in vitro invasive potential of human prostatic cancer cell lines. *Anticancer Res* 1997; 17:1199–1204.

77. Onozawa M, Kawamori T, Baba M *et al.* Effects of a soybean isoflavone mixture on carcinogenesis in prostate and seminal vesicles of F344 rats. *Jpn J Cancer Res* 1999; 90:393–398.

78. Pollard M, Wolter W. Prevention of spontaneous prostate-related cancer in Lobund–Wistar rats by a soy protein isolate/isoflavone diet. *Prostate* 2000; 45:101–105.

79. Mentor–Marcel R, Lamartiniere CA, Eltoum IE, Greenberg NM, Elgavish A. Genistein in the diet reduces the incidence of poorly differentiated prostatic adenocarcinoma in transgenic mice (TRAMP). *Cancer Res* 2001; 61:6777–6782.

80. Kato K, Takahashi S, Cui L *et al.* Suppressive effects of dietary genistein and daidzin on rat prostate carcinogenesis. *Jpn J Cancer Res* 2000; 91:786–791.

81. Bylund A, Saarinen N, Zhang JX *et al.* Anticancer effects of a plant lignan 7-hydroxymatairesinol on a prostate cancer model in vivo. *Exp Biol Med (Maywood)* 2005; 230:217–223.

82. Weber KS, Jacobson NA, Setchell KD, Lephart ED. Brain aromatase and 5alpha-reductase, regulatory behaviors and testosterone levels in adult rats on phytoestrogen diets. *Proc Soc Exp Biol Med* 1999; 221:131–135.

83. Evans BA, Griffiths K, Morton MS. Inhibition of 5 alpha-reductase in genital skin fibroblasts and prostate tissue by dietary lignans and isoflavonoids. *J Endocrinol* 1995; 147:295–302.

84. Zhou JR, Gugger ET, Tanaka T, Guo Y, Blackburn GL, Clinton SK. Soybean phytochemicals inhibit the growth of transplantable human prostate carcinoma and tumor angiogenesis in mice. *J Nutr* 1999; 129:1628–1635.

85. Magee PJ, Rowland IR. Phyto-oestrogens, their mechanism of action: current evidence for a role in breast and prostate cancer. *Br J Nutr* 2004; 91:513–531.

86. Shenouda NS, Zhou C, Browning JD *et al.* Phytoestrogens in common herbs regulate prostate cancer cell growth in vitro. *Nutr Cancer* 2004; 49:200–208.

87. Wei H, Wei L, Frenkel K, Bowen R, Barnes S. Inhibition of tumor promoter-induced hydrogen peroxide formation in vitro and in vivo by genistein. *Nutr Cancer* 1993; 20:1–12.

88. Adlercreutz H. Phyto-oestrogens and cancer. *Lancet Oncol* 2002; 3:364–373.

89. Djuric Z, Chen G, Doerge DR, Heilbrun LK, Kucuk O. Effect of soy isoflavone supplementation on markers of oxidative stress in men and women. *Cancer Lett* 2001; 172:1–6.

90. Lin X, Switzer BR, Demark-Wahnefried W. Effect of mammalian lignans on the growth of prostate cancer cell lines. *Anticancer Res* 2001; 21:3995–3999.

91. Jacobsen BK, Knutsen SF, Fraser GE. Does high soy milk intake reduce prostate cancer incidence? The Adventist Health Study (United States). *Cancer Causes Control* 1998; 9:553–557.

92. Persky V, Van Horn L. Epidemiology of soy and cancer: perspectives and directions. *J Nutr* 1995; 125:709S–712S.

93. Sonoda T, Nagata Y, Mori M *et al.* A case–control study of diet and prostate cancer in Japan: possible protective effect of traditional Japanese diet. *Cancer Sci* 2004; 95:238–242.

94. Stattin P, Adlercreutz H, Tenkanen L *et al.* Circulating enterolactone and prostate cancer risk: a Nordic nested case–control study. *Int J Cancer* 2002; 99:124–129.

95. Nomura AM, Hankin JH, Lee J, Stemmermann GN. Cohort study of tofu intake and prostate cancer: no apparent association. *Cancer Epidemiol Biomarkers Prev* 2004; 13:2277–2279.

96. Strom SS, Yamamura Y, Duphorne CM *et al.* Phytoestrogen intake and prostate cancer: a case–control study using a new database. *Nutr Cancer* 1999; 33:20–25.

97. Giovannucci E, Rimm EB, Liu Y, Stampfer MJ, Willett WC. A prospective study of tomato products, lycopene, and prostate cancer risk. *J Natl Cancer Inst* 2002; 94:391–398.

98. Giovannucci E, Ascherio A, Rimm EB, Stampfer MJ, Colditz GA, Willett WC. Intake of carotenoids and retinol in relation to risk of prostate cancer. *J Natl Cancer Inst* 1995; 87:1767–1776.

99. Le Marchand L, Hankin JH, Kolonel LN, Wilkens LR. Vegetable and fruit consumption in relation to prostate cancer risk in Hawaii: a reevaluation of the effect of dietary beta-carotene. *Am J Epidemiol* 1991; 133:215–219.

100. Hayes RB, Ziegler RG, Gridley G *et al.* Dietary factors and risks for prostate cancer among blacks and whites in the United States. *Cancer Epidemiol Biomarkers Prev* 1999; 8:25–34.

101. Cohen JH, Kristal AR, Stanford JL. Fruit and vegetable intakes and prostate cancer risk. *J Natl Cancer Inst* 2000; 92:61–68.

102. Kolonel LN, Hankin JH, Whittemore AS *et al.* Vegetables, fruits, legumes and prostate cancer: a multiethnic case–control study. *Cancer Epidemiol Biomarkers Prev* 2000; 9:795–804.

103. Schuurman AG, Goldbohm RA, Dorant E, van den Brandt PA. Vegetable and fruit consumption and prostate cancer risk: a cohort study in The Netherlands. *Cancer Epidemiol Biomarkers Prev* 1998; 7:673–680.

104. Etminan M, Takkouche B, Caamano–Isorna F. The role of tomato products and lycopene in the prevention of prostate cancer: a meta-analysis of observational studies. *Cancer Epidemiol Biomarkers Prev* 2004; 13:340–345.

105. Gann PH, Ma J, Giovannucci E *et al.* Lower prostate cancer risk in men with elevated plasma lycopene levels: results of a prospective analysis. *Cancer Res* 1999; 59:1225–1230.

106. Lu QY, Hung JC, Heber D *et al.* Inverse associations between plasma lycopene and other carotenoids and prostate cancer. *Cancer Epidemiol Biomarkers Prev* 2001; 10:749–756.

107. Rao AV, Fleshner N, Agarwal S. Serum and tissue lycopene and biomarkers of oxidation in prostate cancer patients: a case–control study. *Nutr Cancer* 1999; 33:159–164.

108. Vogt TM, Mayne ST, Graubard BI *et al.* Serum lycopene, other serum carotenoids, and risk of prostate cancer in US Blacks and Whites. *Am J Epidemiol* 2002; 155:1023–1032.

109. Wu K, Erdman JWJ, Schwartz SJ *et al.* Plasma and dietary carotenoids, and the risk of prostate cancer: a nested case–control study. *Cancer Epidemiol Biomarkers Prev* 2004; 13:260–269.

110. Chang S, Erdman JWJ, Clinton SK *et al.* Relationship between plasma carotenoids and prostate cancer. *Nutr Cancer* 2005; 53:127–134.

111. Hsing AW, Comstock GW, Abbey H, Polk BF. Serologic precursors of cancer. Retinol, carotenoids, and tocopherol and risk of prostate cancer. *J Natl Cancer Inst* 1990; 82:941–946.

112. Huang HY, Alberg AJ, Norkus EP, Hoffman SC, Comstock GW, Helzlsouer KJ. Prospective study of antioxidant micronutrients in the blood and the risk of developing prostate cancer. *Am J Epidemiol* 2003; 157:335–344.

113. Zhou JR, Mukherjee P, Gugger ET, Tanaka T, Blackburn GL, Clinton SK. Inhibition of murine bladder tumorigenesis by soy isoflavones via alterations in the cell cycle, apoptosis, and angiogenesis. *Cancer Res* 1998; 58:5231–5238.

114. Bowen P, Chen L, Stacewicz–Sapuntzakis M *et al.* Tomato sauce supplementation and prostate cancer: lycopene accumulation and modulation of biomarkers of carcinogenesis. *Exp Biol Med (Maywood)* 2002; 227:886–893.

115. Hall AK. Liarozole amplifies retinoid-induced apoptosis in human prostate cancer cells. *Anticancer Drugs* 1996; 7:312–320.

116. Kotake–Nara E, Kushiro M, Zhang H, Sugawara T, Miyashita K, Nagao A. Carotenoids affect proliferation of human prostate cancer cells. *J Nutr* 2001; 131:3303–3306.

117. Pastori M, Pfander H, Boscoboinik D, Azzi A. Lycopene in association with alpha-tocopherol inhibits at physiological concentrations proliferation of prostate carcinoma cells. *Biochem Biophys Res Commun* 1998; 250:582–585.

118. Cantrell A, McGarvey DJ, Truscott TG, Rancan F, Bohm F. Singlet oxygen quenching by dietary carotenoids in a model membrane environment. *Arch Biochem Biophys* 2003; 412:47–54.

119. Stahl W, Junghans A, de Boer B, Driomina ES, Briviba K, Sies H. Carotenoid mixtures protect multilamellar liposomes against oxidative damage: synergistic effects of lycopene and lutein. *FEBS Lett* 1998; 427:305–308.

120. Matos HR, Capelozzi VL, Gomes OF, Mascio PD, Medeiros MH. Lycopene inhibits DNA damage and liver necrosis in rats treated with ferric nitrilotriacetate. *Arch Biochem Biophys* 2001; 396:171–177.

121. Matos HR, Marques SA, Gomes OF *et al.* Lycopene and beta–carotene protect in vivo iron-induced oxidative stress damage in rat prostate. *Braz J Med Biol Res* 2006; 39:203–210.

122. Siler U, Barella L, Spitzer V *et al.* Lycopene and vitamin E interfere with autocrine/paracrine loops in the Dunning prostate cancer model. *FASEB J* 2004; 18:1019–1021.

123. Mucci LA, Tamimi R, Lagiou P *et al.* Are dietary influences on the risk of prostate cancer mediated through the insulin-like growth factor system? *BJU Int* 2001; 87:814–820.

124. Ambrosone CB, McCann SE, Freudenheim JL, Marshall JR, Zhang Y, Shields PG. Breast cancer risk in premenopausal women is inversely associated with consumption of broccoli, a source of isothiocyanates, but is not modified by GST genotype. *J Nutr* 2004; 134:1134–1138.

125. Zhang SM, Hunter DJ, Rosner BA *et al.* Intakes of fruits, vegetables, and related nutrients and the risk of non-Hodgkin's lymphoma among women. *Cancer Epidemiol Biomarkers Prev* 2000; 9:477–485.

126. Verhoeven DT, Goldbohm RA, van Poppel G, Verhagen H, van den Brandt PA. Epidemiological studies on brassica vegetables and cancer risk. *Cancer Epidemiol Biomarkers Prev* 1996; 5:733–748.

127. Zhang Y, Talalay P, Cho CG, Posner GH. A major inducer of anticarcinogenic protective enzymes from broccoli: isolation and elucidation of structure. *Proc Natl Acad Sci USA* 1992; 89:2399–2403.

128. Brooks JD, Paton VG, Vidanes G. Potent induction of phase 2 enzymes in human prostate cells by sulforaphane. *Cancer Epidemiol Biomarkers Prev* 2001; 10:949–954.

129. Jones SB, Brooks JD. Modest induction of phase 2 enzyme activity in the F-344 rat prostate. *BMC Cancer* 2006; 6:62.

130. Verhoeven DT, Verhagen H, Goldbohm RA, van den Brandt PA, van Poppel G. A review of mechanisms underlying anticarcinogenicity by brassica vegetables. *Chem Biol Interact* 1997; 103:79–129.

131. Xu C, Shen G, Chen C, Gelinas C, Kong AN. Suppression of NF-kappaB and NF-kappaB-regulated gene expression by sulforaphane and PEITC through IkappaBalpha, IKK pathway in human prostate cancer PC-3 cells. *Oncogene* 2005; 24:4486–4495.

132. Singh SV, Herman-Antosiewicz A, Singh AV *et al.* Sulforaphane-induced G2/M phase cell cycle arrest involves checkpoint kinase 2-mediated phosphorylation of cell division cycle 25C. *J Biol Chem* 2004; 279:25813–25822.

133. Choi S, Singh SV. Bax and Bak are required for apoptosis induction by sulforaphane, a cruciferous vegetable-derived cancer chemopreventive agent. *Cancer Res* 2005; 65:2035–2043.

134. Graham S, Haughey B, Marshall J *et al.* Diet in the epidemiology of carcinoma of the prostate gland. *J Natl Cancer Inst* 1983; 70:687–692.

135. Villeneuve PJ, Johnson KC, Kreiger N, Mao Y. Risk factors for prostate cancer: results from the Canadian National Enhanced Cancer Surveillance System. The Canadian Cancer Registries Epidemiology Research Group. *Cancer Causes Control*.1999; 10:355–367.

136. Kristal AR, Lampe JW. Brassica vegetables and prostate cancer risk: a review of the epidemiological evidence. *Nutr Cancer* 2002; 42:1–9.

137. Jain MG, Hislop GT, Howe GR, Ghadirian P. Plant foods, antioxidants, and prostate cancer risk: findings from case–control studies in Canada. *Nutr Cancer* 1999; 34:173–184.

138. Sunny L. A low fat diet rich in fruits and vegetables may reduce the risk of developing prostate cancer. *Asian Pac J Cancer Prev* 2005; 6:490–496.

139. Joseph MA, Moysich KB, Freudenheim JL *et al.* Cruciferous vegetables, genetic polymorphisms in glutathione S-transferases M1 and T1, and prostate cancer risk. *Nutr Cancer* 2004; 50:206–213.

140. McCall MR, Frei B. Can antioxidant vitamins materially reduce oxidative damage in humans? *Free Radic Biol Med* 1999; 26:1034–1053.

141. Sigounas G, Anagnostou A, Steiner M. dl-alpha-tocopherol induces apoptosis in erythroleukemia, prostate, and breast cancer cells. *Nutr Cancer* 1997; 28:30–35.

142. Israel K, Yu W, Sanders BG, Kline K. Vitamin E succinate induces apoptosis in human prostate cancer cells: role for Fas in vitamin E succinate-triggered apoptosis. *Nutr Cancer* 2000; 36:90–100.

143. Malafa MP, Fokum FD, Andoh J *et al.* Vitamin E succinate suppresses prostate tumor growth by inducing apoptosis. *Int J Cancer* 2006; 118:2441–2447.

144. Ni J, Chen M, Zhang Y, Li R, Huang J, Yeh S. Vitamin E succinate inhibits human prostate cancer cell growth via modulating cell cycle regulatory machinery. *Biochem Biophys Res Commun* 2003; 300:357–363.

145. Thompson TA, Wilding G. Androgen antagonist activity by the antioxidant moiety of vitamin E, 2,2,5,7,8-pentamethyl-6-chromanol in human prostate carcinoma cells. *Mol Cancer Ther* 2003; 2:797–803.

146. Heinonen OP, Albanes D, Virtamo J *et al.* Prostate cancer and supplementation with alpha-tocopherol and beta-carotene: incidence and mortality in a controlled trial. *J Natl Cancer Inst* 1998; 90:440–446.

147. Goodman GE, Schaffer S, Omenn GS, Chen C, King I. The association between lung and prostate cancer risk, and serum micronutrients: results and lessons learned from beta-carotene and retinol efficacy trial. *Cancer Epidemiol Biomarkers Prev* 2003; 12:518–12526.

148. Klein EA, Lippman SM, Thompson IM *et al.* The selenium and vitamin E cancer prevention trial. *World J Urol* 2003; 21:21–27.

149. Chan JM, Stampfer MJ, Ma J, Rimm EB, Willett WC, Giovannucci EL. Supplemental vitamin E intake and prostate cancer risk in a large cohort of men in the United States. *Cancer Epidemiol Biomarkers Prev* 1999; 8:893–899.

150. Kirsh VA, Hayes RB, Mayne ST *et al.* Supplemental and dietary vitamin E, beta-carotene, and vitamin C intakes and prostate cancer risk. *J Natl Cancer Inst* 2006; 98:245–254.

151. Miller ER 3rd, Pastor-Barriuso R, Dalal D, Riemersma RA, Appel LJ, Guallar E. Meta-analysis: high-dosage vitamin E supplementation may increase all-cause mortality. *Ann Intern Med* 2005; 142:37–46.

152. Lonn E, Bosch J, Yusuf S *et al.* Effects of long–term vitamin E supplementation on cardiovascular events and cancer: a randomized controlled trial. *JAMA* 2005; 293:1338–1347.

153. Schrauzer GN. Selenomethionine: a review of its nutritional significance, metabolism and toxicity. *J Nutr* 2000; 130:1653–1656.

154. Sabichi AL, Lee JJ, Taylor RJ *et al.* Selenium accumulation in prostate tissue during a randomized, controlled short-term trial of l-selenomethionine: a Southwest Oncology Group Study. *Clin Cancer Res* 2006; 12:2178–2184.

155. Ip C, Thompson HJ, Zhu Z, Ganther HE. In vitro and in vivo studies of methylseleninic acid: evidence that a monomethylated selenium metabolite is critical for cancer chemoprevention. *Cancer Res* 2000; 60:2882–2886.

156. Zhu Z, Jiang W, Ganther HE, Thompson HJ. Mechanisms of cell cycle arrest by methylseleninic acid. *Cancer Res* 2002; 62:156–164.

157. Zhao H, Whitfield ML, Xu T, Botstein D, Brooks JD. Diverse effects of methylseleninic acid on the transcriptional programme of human prostate cancer cells. *Mol Biol Cell* 2004; 15:506–519.

158. Yamaguchi K, Uzzo RG, Pimkina J *et al.* Methylseleninic acid sensitizes prostate cancer cells to TRAIL-mediated apoptosis. *Oncogene* 2005; 24:5868–5877.

159. Clark LC, Combs GFJ, Turnbull BW *et al.* Effects of selenium supplementation for cancer prevention in patients with carcinoma of the skin. A randomized controlled trial. Nutritional Prevention of Cancer Study Group. *JAMA* 1996; 276:1957–1963.

160. Duffield-Lillico AJ, Dalkin BL, Reid ME *et al.* Selenium supplementation, baseline plasma selenium status and incidence of prostate cancer: an analysis of the complete treatment period of the Nutritional Prevention of Cancer Trial. *BJU Int* 2003; 91:608–612.

161. Criqui MH, Bangdiwala S, Goodman DS *et al.* Selenium, retinol, retinol-binding protein, and uric acid. Associations with cancer mortality in a population-based prospective case–control study. *Ann Epidemiol* 1991; 1:385–393.

162. West DW, Slattery ML, Robison LM, French TK, Mahoney AW. Adult dietary intake and prostate cancer risk in Utah: a case–control study with special emphasis on aggressive tumors. *Cancer Causes Control* 1991; 2:85–94.

163. Lippman SM, Goodman PJ, Klein EA *et al.* Designing the Selenium and Vitamin E Cancer Prevention Trial (SELECT). *J Natl Cancer Inst* 2005; 97:94–102.

164. Kobayashi M, Sasaki S, Hamada GS, Tsugane S. Serum n-3 fatty acids, fish consumption and cancer mortality in six Japanese populations in Japan and Brazil. *Jpn J Cancer Res* 1999; 90:914–921.

165. Terry P, Lichtenstein P, Feychting M, Ahlbom A, Wolk A. Fatty fish consumption and risk of prostate cancer [letter]. *Lancet* 2001; 357(9270):1764–1766.

166. Augustsson K, Michaud DS, Rimm EB *et al.* A prospective study of intake of fish and marine fatty acids and prostate cancer. *Cancer Epidemiol Biomarkers Prev* 2003; 12:64–67.

167. Schuurman AG, van den Brandt PA, Dorant E, Brants HA, Goldbohm RA. Association of energy and fat intake with prostate carcinoma risk: results from The Netherlands Cohort Study. *Cancer* 1999; 86:1019–1027.

168. Rose DP, Connolly JM. Effects of fatty acids and eicosanoid synthesis inhibitors on the growth of two human prostate cancer cell lines. *Prostate* 1991; 18:243–254.

169. Pandalai PK, Pilat MJ, Yamazaki K, Naik H, Pienta KJ. The effects of omega-3 and omega-6 fatty acids on in vitro prostate cancer growth. *Anticancer Res* 1996; 16:815–820.

170. Chung BH, Mitchell SH, Zhang JS, Young CY. Effects of docosahexaenoic acid and eicosapentaenoic acid on androgen-mediated cell growth and gene expression in LNCaP prostate cancer cells. *Carcinogenesis* 2001; 22:1201–1206.

171. Rose DP, Cohen LA. Effects of dietary menhaden oil and retinyl acetate on the growth of DU 145 human prostatic adenocarcinoma cells transplanted into athymic nude mice. *Carcinogenesis* 1988; 9:603–605.

172. Karmali RA, Reichel P, Cohen LA *et al.* The effects of dietary omega-3 fatty acids on the DU-145 transplantable human prostatic tumor. *Anticancer Res* 1987; 7:1173–1179.

173. Connolly JM, Coleman M, Rose DP. Effects of dietary fatty acids on DU145 human prostate cancer cell growth in athymic nude mice. *Nutr Cancer* 1997; 29:114–119.

174. Holmes MD, Pollak MN, Willett WC, Hankinson SE. Dietary correlates of plasma insulin-like growth factor I and insulin-like growth factor binding protein 3 concentrations. *Cancer Epidemiol Biomarkers Prev* 2002;11:852–861.

175. Probst–Hensch NM, Wang H, Goh VH, Seow A, Lee HP, Yu MC. Determinants of circulating insulin-like growth factor I and insulin-like growth factor binding protein 3 concentrations in a cohort of Singapore men and women. *Cancer Epidemiol Biomarkers Prev* 2003; 12:739–746.

176. Chaudry AA, Wahle KW, McClinton S, Moffat LE. Arachidonic acid metabolism in benign and malignant prostatic tissue in vitro: effects of fatty acids and cyclooxygenase inhibitors. *Int J Cancer* 1994; 57:176–180.
177. Ringbom T, Huss U, Stenholm A *et al.* Cox-2 inhibitory effects of naturally occurring and modified fatty acids. *J Nat Prod* 2001; 64:745–749.
178. Pham H, Ziboh VA. 5 alpha-reductase-catalyzed conversion of testosterone to dihydrotestosterone is increased in prostatic adenocarcinoma cells: suppression by 15-lipoxygenase metabolites of gamma-linolenic and eicosapentaenoic acids. *J Steroid Biochem Mol Biol* 2002; 82:393–400.
179. Liang T, Liao S. Inhibition of steroid 5 alpha-reductase by specific aliphatic unsaturated fatty acids. *Biochem J* 1992; 285:557–562.
180. Chambrier C, Bastard JP, Rieusset J *et al.* Eicosapentaenoic acid induces mRNA expression of peroxisome proliferators-activated receptor gamma. *Obes Res* 2002; 10:518–525.
181. Mannisto S, Pietinen P, Virtanen MJ *et al.* Fatty acids and risk of prostate cancer in a nested case–control study in male smokers. *Cancer Epidemiol Biomarkers Prev* 2003; 12:1422–1428.
182. Astorg P. Dietary N-6 and N-3 polyunsaturated fatty acids and prostate cancer risk: a review of epidemiological and experimental evidence. *Cancer Causes Control* 2004; 15:367–386.
183. Krauss RM, Eckel RH, Howard B *et al.* Revision 2000: a statement for healthcare professionals from the Nutrition Committee of the American Heart Association. *J Nutr* 2001; 131:132–146.
184. Pelucchi C, Bosetti C, Negri E, Malvezzi M, La Vecchia C. Mechanisms of Disease: the epidemiology of bladder cancer. *Nat Clin Pract Urol* 2006; 3:327–340.
185. Yuan JM, Castelao JE, Gago-Dominguez M, Yu MC, Ross RK. Tobacco use in relation to renal cell carcinoma. *Cancer Epidemiol Biomarkers Prev* 1998; 7:429–433.
186. Ferrini RL, Barrett-Connor E. Sex hormones and age: a cross-sectional study of testosterone and estradiol and their bioavailable fractions in community-dwelling men. *Am J Epidemiol* 1998; 147:750–754.
187. Dai WS, Gutai JP, Kuller LH, Cauley JA. Cigarette smoking and serum sex hormones in men. *Am J Epidemiol* 1988; 128:796–805.
188. Kalcher K, Kern W, Pietsch R. Cadmium and lead in the smoke of a filter cigarette. *Sci Total Environ* 1993; 128:21–35.
189. Sahmoun AE, Case LD, Jackson SA, Schwartz GG. Cadmium and prostate cancer: a critical epidemiologic analysis. *Cancer Invest* 2005; 23:256–263.
190. Rybicki BA, Nock NL, Savera AT, Tang D, Rundle A. Polycyclic aromatic hydrocarbon-DNA adduct formation in prostate carcinogenesis. *Cancer Lett* 2005.
191. Adami HO, Bergstrom R, Engholm G *et al.* A prospective study of smoking and risk of prostate cancer. *Int J Cancer* 1996; 67:764–768.
192. Cerhan JR, Torner JC, Lynch CF *et al.* Association of smoking, body mass, and physical activity with risk of prostate cancer in the Iowa 65+ Rural Health Study (United States). *Cancer Causes Control* 1997; 8:229–238.
193. Hiatt RA, Armstrong MA, Klatsky AL, Sidney S. Alcohol consumption, smoking, and other risk factors and prostate cancer in a large health plan cohort in California (United States). *Cancer Causes Control* 1994; 5:66–72.
194. Plaskon LA, Penson DF, Vaughan TL, Stanford JL. Cigarette smoking and risk of prostate cancer in middle-aged men. *Cancer Epidemiol Biomarkers Prev* 2003; 12:604–609.
195. Giovannucci E, Rimm EB, Ascherio A *et al.* Smoking and risk of total and fatal prostate cancer in United States health professionals. *Cancer Epidemiol Biomarkers Prev* 1999; 8:277–282.
196. Thompson MM, Garland C, Barrett-Connor E, Khaw KT, Friedlander NJ, Wingard DL. Heart disease risk factors, diabetes, and prostatic cancer in an adult community. *Am J Epidemiol* 1989; 129:511–517.
197. Thune I, Lund E. Physical activity and the risk of prostate and testicular cancer: a cohort study of 53,000 Norwegian men. *Cancer Causes Control* 1994; 5:549–556.
198. Gronberg H, Damber L, Damber JE. Total food consumption and body mass index in relation to prostate cancer risk: a case–control study in Sweden with prospectively collected exposure data. *J Urol* 1996; 155:969–974.
199. Engeland A, Andersen A, Haldorsen T, Tretli S. Smoking habits and risk of cancers other than lung cancer: 28 years' follow-up of 26,000 Norwegian men and women. *Cancer Causes Control* 1996; 7:497–506.
200. Heikkila R, Aho K, Heliovaara M *et al.* Serum testosterone and sex hormone-binding globulin concentrations and the risk of prostate carcinoma: a longitudinal study. *Cancer* 1999; 86:312–315.
201. Hickey K, Do KA, Green A. Smoking and prostate cancer. *Epidemiol Rev* 2001; 23:115–125.

202. Caceres DD, Iturrieta J, Acevedo C, Huidobro C, Varela N, Quinones L. Relationship among metabolizing genes, smoking and alcohol used as modifier factors on prostate cancer risk: exploring some gene–gene and gene–environment interactions. *Eur J Epidemiol* 2005; 20:79–88.
203. Yang J, Wu HF, Zhang W *et al.* Polymorphisms of metabolic enzyme genes, living habits and prostate cancer susceptibility. *Front Biosci* 2006; 11:2052–2060.
204. Williams MT, Hord NG. The role of dietary factors in cancer prevention: beyond fruits and vegetables. *Nutr Clin Pract* 2005; 20:451–459.
205. Friedenreich CM, Orenstein MR. Physical activity and cancer prevention: etiologic evidence and biological mechanisms. *J Nutr* 2002; 132:3456S–3464S.
206. McTiernan A. Obesity and cancer: the risks, science, and potential management strategies. *Oncology (Williston Park)* 2005; 19:871–81; discussion 881–2, 885–6.
207. Goodpaster BH, Kelley DE, Wing RR, Meier A, Thaete FL. Effects of weight loss on regional fat distribution and insulin sensitivity in obesity. *Diabetes* 1999; 48:839–847.
208. Kelley DE, Goodpaster BH. Effects of physical activity on insulin action and glucose tolerance in obesity. *Med Sci Sports Exerc* 1999; 31:S619–23.
209. Morimoto LM, Newcomb PA, White E, Bigler J, Potter JD. Variation in plasma insulin-like growth factor-1 and insulin-like growth factor binding protein-3: personal and lifestyle factors (United States). *Cancer Causes Control* 2005; 16:917–927.
210. Haydon AM, Macinnis RJ, English DR, Morris H, Giles GG. Physical activity, insulin-like growth factor 1, insulin-like growth factor binding protein 3, and survival from colorectal cancer. *Gut* 2006; 55:689–694.
211. Kaaks R, Lukanova A. Effects of weight control and physical activity in cancer prevention: role of endogenous hormone metabolism. *Ann NY Acad Sci* 2002; 963:268–281.
212. Stattin P, Bylund A, Rinaldi S *et al.* Plasma insulin-like growth factor-I, insulin-like growth factor-binding proteins, and prostate cancer risk: a prospective study. *J Natl Cancer Inst* 2000; 92:1910–1917.
213. Harman SM, Metter EJ, Blackman MR, Landis PK, Carter HB. Serum levels of insulin-like growth factor I (IGF-I), IGF-II, IGF-binding protein-3, and prostate-specific antigen as predictors of clinical prostate cancer. *J Clin Endocrinol Metab* 2000; 85:4258–4265.
214. Gann PH, Hennekens CH, Ma J, Longcope C, Stampfer MJ. Prospective study of sex hormone levels and risk of prostate cancer. *J Natl Cancer Inst* 1996; 88:1118–1126.
215. Friedenreich CM, McGregor SE, Courneya KS, Angyalfi SJ, Elliott FG. Case–control study of lifetime total physical activity and prostate cancer risk. *Am J Epidemiol* 2004; 159:740–749.
216. Vena JE, Graham S, Zielezny M, Brasure J, Swanson MK. Occupational exercise and risk of cancer. *Am J Clin Nutr* 1987; 45:318–327.
217. Yu H, Harris RE, Wynder EL. Case–control study of prostate cancer and socioeconomic factors. *Prostate* 1988; 13:317–325.
218. Albanes D, Blair A, Taylor PR. Physical activity and risk of cancer in the NHANES I population. *Am J Public Health* 1989; 79:744–750.
219. Brownson RC, Chang JC, Davis JR, Smith CA. Physical activity on the job and cancer in Missouri. *Am J Public Health* 1991; 81:639–642.
220. Lee IM, Paffenbarger RSJ, Hsieh CC. Physical activity and risk of prostatic cancer among college alumni. *Am J Epidemiol* 1992; 135:169–179.
221. Paffenbarger RSJ, Lee IM, Wing AL. The influence of physical activity on the incidence of site-specific cancers in college alumni. *Adv Exp Med Biol* 1992; 322:7–15.
222. Hsing AW, McLaughlin JK, Zheng W, Gao YT, Blot WJ. Occupation, physical activity, and risk of prostate cancer in Shanghai, People's Republic of China. *Cancer Causes Control* 1994; 5:136–140.
223. Steenland K, Nowlin S, Palu S. Cancer incidence in the National Health and Nutrition Survey I. Follow-up data: diabetes, cholesterol, pulse and physical activity. *Cancer Epidemiol Biomarkers Prev* 1995; 4:807–811.
224. Oliveria SA, Kohl HWr, Trichopoulos D, Blair SN. The association between cardiorespiratory fitness and prostate cancer. *Med Sci Sports Exerc* 1996; 28:97–104.
225. Hartman TJ, Albanes D, Rautalahti M *et al.* Physical activity and prostate cancer in the Alpha-Tocopherol, Beta-Carotene (ATBC) Cancer Prevention Study (Finland). *Cancer Causes Control* 1998; 9:11–18.
226. Giovannucci E, Leitzmann M, Spiegelman D *et al.* A prospective study of physical activity and prostate cancer in male health professionals. *Cancer Res* 1998; 58:5117–5122.

227. Clarke G, Whittemore AS. Prostate cancer risk in relation to anthropometry and physical activity: the National Health and Nutrition Examination Survey I Epidemiological Follow-Up Study. *Cancer Epidemiol Biomarkers Prev* 2000; 9:875–881.

228. Wannamethee SG, Shaper AG, Walker M. Physical activity and risk of cancer in middle-aged men. *Br J Cancer* 2001; 85:1311–1316.

229. Norman A, Moradi T, Gridley G *et al.* Occupational physical activity and risk for prostate cancer in a nationwide cohort study in Sweden. *Br J Cancer* 2002; 86:70–75.

230. Severson RK, Nomura AM, Grove JS, Stemmermann GN. A prospective analysis of physical activity and cancer. *Am J Epidemiol* 1989; 130:522–529.

231. Le Marchand L, Kolonel LN, Yoshizawa CN. Lifetime occupational physical activity and prostate cancer risk. *Am J Epidemiol* 1991; 133:103–111.

232. Dosemeci M, Hayes RB, Vetter R *et al.* Occupational physical activity, socioeconomic status, and risks of 15 cancer sites in Turkey. *Cancer Causes Control* 1993; 4:313–321.

233. Whittemore AS, Kolonel LN, Wu AH *et al.* Prostate cancer in relation to diet, physical activity, and body size in blacks, whites, and Asians in the United States and Canada. *J Natl Cancer Inst* 1995; 87:652–661.

234. Pukkala E, Kaprio J, Koskenvuo M, Kujala U, Sarna S. Cancer incidence among Finnish world class male athletes. *Int J Sports Med* 2000; 21:216–220.

235. Liu S, Lee IM, Linson P, Ajani U, Buring JE, Hennekens CH. A prospective study of physical activity and risk of prostate cancer in US physicians. *Int J Epidemiol* 2000; 29:29–35.

236. Putnam SD, Cerhan JR, Parker AS *et al.* Lifestyle and anthropometric risk factors for prostate cancer in a cohort of Iowa men. *Ann Epidemiol* 2000; 10:361–369.

237. Lacey JVJ, Deng J, Dosemeci M *et al.* Prostate cancer, benign prostatic hyperplasia and physical activity in Shanghai, China. *Int J Epidemiol* 2001; 30:341–349.

238. Polednak AP. College athletics, body size, and cancer mortality. *Cancer* 1976; 38:382–387.

239. Sung JF, Lin RS, Pu YS, Chen YC, Chang HC, Lai MK. Risk factors for prostate carcinoma in Taiwan: a case–control study in a Chinese population. *Cancer* 1999; 86:484–491.

240. Andersson SO, Wolk A, Bergstrom R *et al.* Body size and prostate cancer: a 20-year follow-up study among 135006 Swedish construction workers. *J Natl Cancer Inst* 1997; 89:385–389.

241. Engeland A, Tretli S, Bjorge T. Height, body mass index, and prostate cancer: a follow-up of 950000 Norwegian men. *Br J Cancer* 2003; 89:1237–1242.

242. Nilsen TI, Vatten LJ. Anthropometry and prostate cancer risk: a prospective study of 22,248 Norwegian men. *Cancer Causes Control* 1999; 10:269–275.

243. Nomura A, Heilbrun LK, Stemmermann GN. Body mass index as a predictor of cancer in men. *J Natl Cancer Inst* 1985; 74:319–323.

244. Schuurman AG, Goldbohm RA, Dorant E, van den Brandt PA. Anthropometry in relation to prostate cancer risk in the Netherlands Cohort Study. *Am J Epidemiol* 2000; 151:541–549.

245. Hubbard JS, Rohrmann S, Landis PK *et al.* Association of prostate cancer risk with insulin, glucose, and anthropometry in the Baltimore longitudinal study of aging. *Urology* 2004; 63:253–258.

246. Friedenreich CM, McGregor SE, Courneya KS, Angyalfi SJ, Elliott FG. Case–control study of anthropometric measures and prostate cancer risk. *Int J Cancer* 2004; 110:278–283.

247. Porter MP, Stanford JL. Obesity and the risk of prostate cancer. *Prostate* 2005; 62:316–321.

248. Freedland SJ, Aronson WJ, Kane CJ *et al.* Impact of obesity on biochemical control after radical prostatectomy for clinically localized prostate cancer: a report by the Shared Equal Access Regional Cancer Hospital database study group. *J Clin Oncol* 2004; 22:446–453.

249. Amling CL, Riffenburgh RH, Sun L *et al.* Pathologic variables and recurrence rates as related to obesity and race in men with prostate cancer undergoing radical prostatectomy. *J Clin Oncol* 2004; 22:439–445.

250. Giovannucci E, Rimm EB, Liu Y *et al.* Body mass index and risk of prostate cancer in US health professionals. *J Natl Cancer Inst* 2003; 95:1240–1244.

251. Eyre H, Kahn R, Robertson RM. Preventing cancer, cardiovascular disease, and diabetes: a common agenda for the American Cancer Society, the American Diabetes Association, and the American Heart Association. *CA Cancer J Clin* 2004; 54:190–207.

2

The current state of biomarkers for prostate cancer

Eddy S. Leman, Robert H. Getzenberg

INTRODUCTION

Prostate cancer is perhaps the only cancer type in which biomarkers have changed the clinical course of the disease. As recently as 20 years ago, more than half of the men presenting with prostate cancer did so with metastatic disease. Today, this is a rarity. Despite this apparent success, we still are developing better markers for the disease. Prostate cancer is the second leading cause of cancer death in men in the USA. In 2007, the American Cancer Society estimates that there will be 218 890 new cases and 27 050 related deaths [1]. A study by Sakr *et al.* revealed that by the age of 30–39 years, about 29% of men will have microscopic evidence of prostate cancer, which increases to about 65% by the age of 70 [2]. Prostate cancer arises as a multistep process that includes chromosomal and gene expression modifications. This can lead to overgrowth of cells surrounding the prostate gland, inhibition of apoptosis of these cells, invasion and angiogenesis.

The specific cause of prostate cancer is still unidentified. Factors such as age, genetics, race, diet and lifestyle may contribute to a man's risk of developing prostate cancer [3]. The main risk factor for the disease is age. Prostate cancer is diagnosed typically after the age of 50 and the average age at diagnosis is 70 years [3]. There is, however, a trend towards increasing diagnosis in younger men [3]. Prostate cancer in its early stages presents without symptoms, usually through screening, but the diagnosis may also be made in men presenting with pain, difficulty in urinating, haematuria, painful urination and erectile dysfunction. It is often diagnosed incidentally following a routine medical assessment that identifies elevated serum prostate-specific antigen (PSA) and/or an abnormality on digital rectal examination (DRE). The patient presenting with an elevated PSA or abnormal DRE usually requires further investigation with a biopsy of the prostate to establish a histological diagnosis of cancer where malignancy is present.

Despite the widespread use of PSA testing, PSA is not considered an ideal tumour marker. It is estimated that about 25–35 million PSA tests will be performed in the USA every year [4]. Approximately 1.6–1.8 million men proceed to prostate biopsy. Only about one in seven or one in eight of these men is diagnosed with prostate cancer. As a result, the number of men with elevated PSA levels and at least one set of negative biopsies is growing, with more than 25 million men now in this situation in the USA. The availability of PSA has certainly not adequately served all those men tested throughout the world.

Eddy S. Leman, PhD, The Brady Urological Institute, Johns Hopkins Hospital, Baltimore, Maryland, USA
Robert H. Getzenberg, PhD, Director of Urology Research, Professor, Urology and Oncology, The Brady Urological Institute, Johns Hopkins Hospital, Baltimore, Maryland, USA

Initially, a cut-off point of 4.0 ng/ml was established as the upper limit of normal for serum PSA [5]. Using this cut-off, PSA testing was combined with DRE for prostate cancer detection. Nevertheless, over the last 20 years, the choice of 4.0 ng/ml as the optimal PSA threshold for prostate cancer biopsy has been called into question. Recently, a PSA level of 2.5 ng/ml was proposed as the upper limit for the normal range [6–8], although as discussed in the next section, even this cut-off may not be ideal.

Considerable amounts of both clinical and basic science research efforts continue to be devoted to defining the precise factors that will maximize the sensitivity and specificity of PSA for prostate cancer detection. Parallel with ongoing research to optimize the utilization of PSA, there have been increasing efforts to identify novel biomarkers for prostate cancer. Advancements in both genomic and proteomic technologies have resulted in biomarker discovery as a focus in prostate cancer research. Many potential biomarkers are currently being tested for either detection or as prognostic markers for prostate cancer. The primary goal of biomarker research is the development of highly specific markers that can reduce the rate of false positive tests and unnecessary biopsies for prostate cancer, while providing additional information about clinical and pathological characteristics of the disease.

In this chapter, the utilization of PSA as a serum marker in prostate cancer screening, ways to improve the outcome of PSA tests, and the discovery of other blood- and urine-based markers for prostate cancer will be highlighted.

PROSTATE-SPECIFIC ANTIGEN

Prostate-specific antigen (PSA), a member of the kallikrein family of proteases, is an androgen-regulated serine protease produced by the columnar epithelium of the prostate gland [9]. PSA is located on chromosome 19q13.4 and has a molecular weight of 34 kDa [10]. PSA is secreted directly into the lumen of prostatic acini and has a crucial role in the physiology of prostatic fluid. The main function of PSA is to cleave semenogelin I and II in the seminal coagulum; thus, it is responsible for the rapid clotting of seminal fluid, resulting in a gelatinous fluid for secretion [9]. Liquefication of the seminal fluid by PSA contributes to successful sperm motility. PSA is synthesized from an inactive propeptide called preproPSA, which is converted by human kallikrein 2 (hk2) to another precursor called proPSA. ProPSA is then cleaved by proteases such as hk2 and hk4 into active PSA [9].

Active PSA is secreted into the lumen of prostatic gland and can be further cleaved into various inactive forms of PSA [9]. The PSA level in the prostatic fluid is significantly higher than that in the bloodstream, and typically only a small amount of PSA enters the circulation. The small amount of PSA that enters the blood is principally (70–90%) bound to the protease inhibitor α_1-antichymotrypsin [11, 12], whereas the remaining 10–30% circulates as unbound/free PSA [9]. Circulating PSA is also bound to other proteins such as α_2-macroglobulin and α_1-antitrypsin [9]. Total PSA comprises bound and free PSA fractions in the bloodstream, both of which are recognized by antibodies used in a standard PSA test.

One of the characteristics of prostate cancer is the loss of basal epithelium and basement membrane. Disruption of this architecture has been proposed to increase 'direct access' of PSA into the bloodstream [9]. As PSA is almost exclusively produced by the prostate, it is perhaps better classified as an organ-marker rather than a tumour-marker. That is why it was named 'prostate-specific antigen' and not 'prostate *cancer*-specific antigen'. The use of tumour markers in prostate cancer began with the identification of prostate acid phosphatase. However, owing to false-negative results it was replaced by PSA. PSA was first introduced and purified in 1979 by Wang *et al.* as a protein with different properties to prostate acid phosphatase [13]. In 1986, PSA testing was introduced after a reported increase in the incidence of prostate cancer in the USA [14]. The PSA test was originally approved by the US Food and Drug Administration (FDA) to aid in the care of patients who had already been diagnosed with prostate cancer. Since then, the PSA test has also been used for prostate cancer detection, and in 1994 the FDA approved the use of PSA as the first blood test for prostate cancer screening [4]. It is estimated that over 25 million PSA tests are performed in the USA every year [4].

In 1990, an upper threshold of normal PSA level was established at 4.0 ng/ml [5]. Utilizing this cut-off along with DRE increased the reliability of prostate cancer detection. Nevertheless, this cut-off point has continuously been re-evaluated. There is a growing concern that a number of men with prostate cancer actually have PSA values lower than 4.0 ng/ml. Similarly, a PSA level above 4.0 ng/ml does not always indicate the presence of prostate cancer but can be associated with other prostate conditions such as benign prostatic hyperplasia (BPH), inflammation and prostatitis. With no available means other than by prostate biopsy to discriminate which men with 'elevated' PSA levels have prostate cancer, a large number of apparently unnecessary biopsies have been performed. A study by Potter and Partin reported that, in 1998, 15% of the 15 million men screened by the PSA test had PSA levels higher than the established cut-off and therefore underwent biopsies [15].

An important study performed by Thompson *et al.* on 2950 men enrolled in the Prostate Cancer Prevention Trial (PCPT) revealed that 26.9% of men with PSA levels between 3.1 and 4.0 ng/ml had prostate cancer [16]. Furthermore, 17% of men with PSA levels between 1.1 and 2.0 ng/ml also had the disease. This trial has raised further questions regarding any cut-offs that might be used. Most contemporary studies have suggested that a PSA level of 2.5 ng/ml should be the upper threshold for the normal range [6–8, 16]. Table 2.1 summarizes the probability of prostate cancer detection by DRE at different PSA cut-offs.

In over two decades since the introduction of PSA testing, the major limitation of PSA has been its specificity in detecting men without prostate cancer. More than 75% of men who undergo biopsies as a result of PSA levels in the 4.0–10.0 ng/ml range turn out to be cancer free [17]. Another challenge for PSA is its inability to distinguish prostate cancer from other prostatic diseases such as BPH and prostatitis. Several concepts have been proposed to improve the use of PSA as a tumour marker. Age-adjusted PSA, analyses of PSA isoforms (free and bound/complex PSA), PSA kinetics (doubling time and velocity) and PSA density have been recommended to improve the performance of PSA as both a diagnostic and prognostic marker.

Oesterling *et al.* first reported age-specific reference ranges for PSA with the expectation that the use of this concept would increase PSA sensitivity in younger men and improve its specificity in older men [18]. The concept of age-adjusted cut-offs remains controversial and unfavourable because it is likely to lead to a higher number of unnecessary biopsies in younger men and may miss some cancers in older men [19]. Age, however, is certainly a determinant of BPH as well as PSA level.

As stated earlier, PSA in the bloodstream exists as both free and bound PSA isoforms. Another approach utilized to discriminate BPH from cancer is the free/total PSA ratio. A study by Stenman *et al.* demonstrated that circulating bound PSA was higher in men with prostate cancer than in men with BPH [12]. Furthermore, measurement of free PSA or bound PSA can stratify the risk of prostate cancer for men with total PSA ranging from 4.0 or 2.5 to

Table 2.1 Anticipated probability of prostate cancer detection by PSA and DRE[1]

PSA level (ng/ml)	Prostate cancer probability (%)
1.1–2.0	17
2.5–4.0	10–25
4.1–10.00	25
Above 10.00	50 and above

[1]Adapted from refs 16, 17 and 19.

10.0 ng/ml [12]. In an extensively referenced multicentre trial, prostate cancer was detected in 56% of men with free/total PSA ratio of 0.1, whereas 8% of men with free/total PSA ratio greater than 0.25 were found to have the disease [20]. A separate study using banked plasma samples from the Physicians' Health study of 430 men with prostate cancer and 1642 control patients showed that when the free/total PSA ratio cut-off was lowered from 0.25 to 0.20, unnecessary biopsies were decreased by 12.5%, while cancer detection was increased by 10–11% [21]. The authors from this study suggest that free PSA can maintain prostate cancer detection as well as decrease negative biopsies. Used together, the combination of free/total PSA ratio with total PSA level appears to provide a more reliable indication of clinically pertinent prostate cancer.

Another refinement of PSA that has been used is PSA density. PSA density takes into account the ratio of the total PSA level to the size/volume of the prostate gland as measured by transrectal ultrasonography (TRUS) [22–24]. Prostate cancer cells may secrete higher levels of PSA per volume of the prostate gland into the serum. Theoretically, PSA density should correct for higher PSA levels associated with larger volume (i.e. BPH). However, PSA density may not be ideal since determination of prostate volume by TRUS can often be subjective and variable. In addition, PSA density can be influenced by enlargement of the prostate by BPH or prostatitis.

PSA kinetics, including PSA velocity and PSA doubling time, have also been evaluated as a means of improving PSA specificity. A number of studies suggest that PSA kinetics may offer additional information about cancer progression. PSA velocity is defined as an absolute change in PSA level annually (ng/ml/year) [19]. A study by D'Amico et al. showed that men who have an increase in PSA level greater than 2.0 ng/ml/year prior to diagnosis of the disease are more likely to die regardless of undergoing prostatectomy [25]. This study shows that there is an association between the PSA velocity and time to death from prostate cancer after surgery. Thus, PSA velocity may serve as an indicator of mortality after radical prostatectomy.

PSA doubling time is defined as the exponential change in PSA level over time, and therefore it represents a relative change. Pound et al. demonstrated that there was a significantly higher rate of distant metastases in men with short intervals to PSA failure and quick PSA doubling time after surgery [26]. Another study by Zagars and Pollack demonstrated that men with PSA doubling times of less than 8 months had a 54% incidence of subsequent distant metastasis in comparison with 7% of the same incidence in men with PSA doubling time greater than 8 months [27]. In addition, men whose rapid PSA doubling time and escalating PSA levels occurred within the first year after radiation therapy had a 50% chance of developing metastases by 3 years [27]. A recent study at the Brady Urological Institute of the Johns Hopkins Hospital showed that PSA doubling time (less than 3 months vs. 3.0–8.9 months vs. 9.0–14.9 months vs. greater than or equal to 15 months), pathological Gleason scores (less than or equal to 7 vs. 8–10) and time from surgery to biochemical recurrence (less than or equal to 3 years vs. greater than 3 years) were all significant risk factors that can help risk-stratify men for prostate-specific mortality following biochemical recurrence after radical prostatectomy [28]. These findings may serve as a useful guide to patients and their physicians to identify patients at high risk for prostate cancer-specific mortality following biochemical recurrence after surgery to enrol them in early aggressive treatment trials [28]. The concepts of both PSA velocity and PSA doubling time seem to be promising in terms of improving the standard PSA test and are in the process of being applied clinically.

The discovery of PSA more than 25 years ago represented a key development in the early detection of prostate cancer. Widespread use of PSA screening has resulted in stage migration, early intervention with effective treatments and decreased morbidity. However, its advantage for men's health continues to be disputed. Basic science and clinical research efforts are ongoing to improve PSA specificity (Table 2.2) for prostate cancer detection. Of the various refinements that improve the specificity of PSA testing, free/total PSA ratio and

Table 2.2   Refinements for PSA testing

Theory	Purpose	Current state/usefulness
Age-adjusted PSA	To directly correlate PSA levels and age	Still debated
Free/total PSA ratio	To discriminate BPH from cancer and to stratify risk of prostate cancer for men with PSA levels 2.5–10.00 ng/ml	Reduce unnecessary biopsies
PSA density	To adjust PSA level to prostate volume	Prostate volume can be influenced by BPH and prostatitis
PSA velocity	To measure absolute change in PSA levels annually (ng/ml/year)	Being applied clinically (prognostic)
PSA doubling time	To measure exponential change in PSA levels over time (relative change)	Being applied clinically (prognostic)

PSA doubling time seem to be the most promising. Today, the use of PSA as an early marker for prostate cancer detection is still unfortunately a subject of debate.

BIOMARKERS FOR PROSTATE CANCER DETECTION

Although the utilization of PSA as a serum marker in clinical practice has improved the management of men with prostate cancer, the most documented limitation of PSA is its lack of specificity. Clearly, there is a need to identify and characterize additional biomarkers for prostate cancer detection and prognosis. Advances in biotechnology have allowed many researchers to identify additional prostate cancer biomarkers to improve the diagnosis and treatment of this disease. These markers can then be categorized, according to their applications, as either diagnostic or prognostic markers. Emerging technologies such as genomics and proteomics have been used extensively to characterize novel biomarkers for prostate cancer.

Genomics, broadly stated here as the study of nucleic-acid based technologies, represents a new methodological avenue for investigating disease biology. Since prostate cancer behaves according to complex/multiple genetic pathways and networks, genomic analysis has provided a valuable insight into this disease. Molecular signatures of prostate cancer and other prostatic diseases have been explored and defined by genomic analysis. Genomic approaches are leading to identification of gene regulations or 'fingerprints' that can differentiate normal prostate from BPH and prostate cancer. The use of these nucleic acid signatures has resulted in disease-specific fingerprints. These methods need to be validated in multicentre studies and, although promising, they may be difficult to standardize and expensive to run.

Since proteins typically represent the state of biological activity responsible for most cellular function, analysis of protein expression is another complementary approach to define cellular dysfunction underlying development of the disease. Advances in proteomics can detect protein modifications with cellular trafficking, including altered expression through translational as well as post-translational mechanisms. Today, a majority of the diagnostic tests approved by the US FDA are protein based [29]; therefore, proteomics has been utilized extensively in identifying novel markers for prostate cancer. Collectively, both genomic and proteomic techniques have resulted in discovery of several prostate cancer biomarkers that may have potential clinical application (Table 2.3).

Table 2.3 Other potential markers for prostate cancer

Marker(s)	Application(s)	Diagnostic or prognostic	Current state
AMACR	Tissue-based	Prognostic	Being used clinically for identifying aggressive disease
EZH2	Tissue-based	Prognostic	Being used clinically to identify metastatic and aggressive prostate cancer
Hepsin	Tissue-based	Diagnostic	Needs to be validated for its potential usefulness in differentiating prostate cancer from normal and BPH
Proteomics serum profiling	Serum-based	Diagnostic	Needs further validation to differentiate cancer from benign disease
EPCA-1 and EPCA-2	Tissue- and plasma-based (EPCA-1); serum-based (EPCA-2)	Diagnostic	EPCA-2 serum assay is highly specific for prostate cancer. EPCA-2 also separates organ-confined from non-organ-confined disease. Multi-centre study is under way
Autoantibody profile	Serum-based	Diagnostic	Needs further validation and larger sample sets
DD3^{PCA3}	Urine-based	Diagnostic	Needs further validation and larger sample sets

ALPHA-METHYLACYL COENZYME A RACEMACE (AMACR)

A number of genes that appear to be involved in prostate cancer have been reported using genomic analyses. Alpha-methylacyl coenzyme A racemace (*AMACR*) is one of the genes identified via subtractive hybridization and microarray studies [30]. This protein is an enzyme that is involved in peroximal beta-oxidation of branched fatty acids [30]. *AMACR* has been shown to be up-regulated in prostate cancer tissues by approximately ninefold in comparison with normal tissues [31]. A study by Rubin *et al.* using tissue microarrays containing 342 samples with different stages of prostate cancer demonstrated that tissue AMACR protein expression is 97% sensitive and 100% specific in detecting prostate cancer [32]. Using serum samples from 109 patients, the same group further demonstrated that AMACR is more sensitive and specific than PSA (sensitivity and specificity of 78% and 81% versus 46% and 50% respectively) in differentiating prostate cancer from the control subjects [33]. Additional studies have also shown that *AMACR* mRNAs were detected in urine samples following prostatic massage or biopsies. When this transcript was normalized to PSA mRNA, this combination resulted in differentiation of low from high risk prostate cancer patients [34]. Immunohistochemical analysis using samples from 204 men treated by radical prostatectomy and 188 men followed expectantly showed that AMACR tissue expression was lower in patients with poorer outcome, independent of the clinical variables [35]. Among those with low AMACR expression and high Gleason score, the risk of prostate cancer death was 18-fold higher. This study suggests that AMACR can be used as a marker to identify aggressive prostate cancer, and is currently being used clinically.

ENHANCER OF ZESTE HOMOLOG 2 (EZH2)

Another gene that was identified from microarray analysis was the polycomb group protein enhancer of zeste homolog (*EZH2*). *EZH2* has been reported to function as a histone methyltransferase for gene silencing and it is regulated by the pRB/E2F pathway, which is critical for cell proliferation [30]. Varambally *et al.* showed that *EZH2* was overexpressed in hormone-refractory metastatic prostate cancer at the mRNA and protein levels [36]. In addition, clinically localized prostate cancer that expresses higher levels of EZH2 is associated with a poorer prognosis. Other profiling studies have shown that *EZH2* is overexpressed in metastatic prostate cancer in comparison with localized disease [37, 38]. When EZH2 is used in conjunction with the cell adhesion marker E-cadherin, the combination (high EZH2 and low E-cadherin) was found to be associated with PSA recurrence in localized prostate cancer [39]. In addition, this combination remains significant even after adjusting for clinical parameters, such as tumour stage, Gleason score, and PSA level. Taken together, these results suggest that EZH2 may be utilized as a candidate biomarker to identify metastatic and aggressive prostate cancer.

HEPSIN

Hepsin is a transmembrane serine protease that is found to be overexpressed in prostate cancer when compared with normal and benign hyperplastic prostate tissues [30]. An analysis of tissue microarrays from over 700 clinically stratified prostate cancer specimens demonstrated correlation between hepsin expression and measures of clinical outcome [40]. Other studies using 90 matched prostate tissue samples from the tumour and non-tumour sections of the same tissue samples show that hepsin was overexpressed in 90% of the samples [41]. In addition, 53% of the samples show 10-fold higher expression of hepsin in the tumour section.

PROTEOMICS SERUM PROFILING

Using the surface-enhanced laser desorption/ionization time-of-flight (SELDI TOF) mass spectrometry and a genetic algorithm with cluster analysis, Petricoin *et al.* analysed the serum proteomic patterns from a training set of 56 samples and a validation set of 266 samples that consisted of men with cancer and benign diseases [42]. They demonstrated that the proteomic pattern correctly predicted 36 of 38 men (95%) with prostate cancer, whereas 177 of 288 men (78%) were correctly classified as having benign conditions. In addition, their analysis also showed that those with benign conditions (PSA levels ranging from 4 to 10 ng/ml) were correctly classified in 97 of 137 men (71%). A separate serum proteomic pattern analysis was performed by Wright *et al.* using a training set of 326 samples (167 prostate cancer, 77 BPH and 82 normal prostate tissue) and a validation set of 60 samples (30 prostate cancer, 15 BPH and 15 normal prostate tissue) [43]. The results from this study showed that the proteomic pattern correctly identified 96% of the men in the training cohorts and also demonstrated 83% sensitivity and 97% specificity from the validation set. Despite the apparent success of these approaches, the SELDI-based techniques have not held up in further validation studies. Novel mass spectrometry approaches are being utilized now to develop more robust assays that may need to be performed in reference laboratories.

EARLY PROSTATE CANCER ANTIGEN (EPCA) AND EPCA-2

Utilizing a focused proteomics approach, our laboratory has identified novel prostate cancer biomarkers. Our proteomics efforts have concentrated on determining a molecular correlation with histopathological findings. Alterations in nuclear structure and architecture are defining characteristics of cancer. During neoplastic transformation, modifications in nuclear protein compositions arise in concordance with changes in the nuclear structure. Assessment of the protein components that comprise nuclear structure/architecture have resulted in the discovery of biomarkers that are specifically altered in cancer. Alterations in the protein structure of the nucleus are associated with various neoplasms such as breast, prostate, colon, bladder, lung, ovarian, renal and squamous cell carcinoma of the head and neck (reviewed in ref. 44). Our laboratory has identified several biomarkers that are specific for different prostatic diseases. Differences in the protein components of the nuclear structure have been demonstrated in cancer and normal rat prostate [45], a transgenic mouse model for prostate cancer [46], and in BPH and prostate cancer [47–49]. Our group recently identified two prostate cancer biomarkers that are associated with the nuclear structure: early prostate cancer antigen (EPCA) and early prostate cancer antigen 2 (EPCA-2). Both EPCA and EPCA-2 are the human counterparts of proteins that were originally identified from the Dunning rat prostate tumour and are prostate cancer specific [50].

Our previous work demonstrated that EPCA is a plasma-based marker for prostate cancer with sensitivity and specificity of 92% and 94% respectively [51]. EPCA was also demonstrated to be expressed in prostate cancer tissues. Immunohistochemical analyses reveal that EPCA is expressed throughout the prostate and represents a 'field effect' associated with prostate cancer [52, 53]. Using tissues from negative biopsies, subsequent biopsies and prostatectomy specimens, sensitivity of the EPCA immunohistochemical analysis is 84%, with a specificity of 85% [52]. The expression of EPCA in the 'negative biopsies' of men can help reveal if prostate cancer is localized or a non-confined disease. This study was further validated by a separate group [53]. In this study, EPCA staining was positive in 94% of prostate cancer tissues and it was negative in bladder cancer tissues. There was no correlation of EPCA staining intensity with Gleason scores or stage [53]. In non-cancerous tissues adjacent to major cancer foci, EPCA staining was positive in 86% of prostate cancer [53]. These studies suggest that EPCA may reflect alterations in the nuclear structure that occur in the earlier stage of prostate cancer.

Another biomarker, EPCA-2, is not associated with a field effect and appears only in the prostate cancer tissue. We are currently studying EPCA-2 for its potential to serve as a highly specific and sensitive serum-based marker for prostate cancer. Using over 300 serum samples from normal men, men with BPH or prostate cancer, and men with other benign diseases and cancers, our preliminary studies show that EPCA-2 has a sensitivity and specificity of 97% and 94%, respectively, in separating men with prostate cancer from normal men, men with BPH, and those with other types of benign disease and cancer [54]. In addition, EPCA-2 is also able to differentiate men with organ-confined prostate cancer from those with non-organ-confined disease [54]. Despite the fact that EPCA-2 is a nuclear protein, we speculate that it is released into the blood by cellular breakdown or apoptosis and is quite stable once it gets there [55]. Taken together, our current findings demonstrate that EPCA-2, a prostate cancer-associated nuclear protein, can be utilized as a potential serum-based biomarker for prostate cancer. Further validations using larger sample sizes in multicentre studies are clearly warranted, but it appears that EPCA-2 may indeed serve as a desperately needed highly specific marker of prostate cancer.

AUTOANTIBODY PROFILES

A number of studies have demonstrated that cancer patients develop immune responses to cancer-related antigens. These responses can be detected by the immune system in the forms of detectable autoantibodies or 'molecular fingerprints' that may be used as both diagnostic and prognostic markers. A recent study by Chinnaiyan's group demonstrated that autoantibody signature biomarkers may be used to improve prostate cancer detection [56]. Using a technique that combines phage-display technology with protein microarrays, they were able to identify and characterize new autoantibody-binding peptides derived from prostate cancer tissues. A panel of 22 peptides was used to analyse sera from 119 patients with prostate cancer and 138 control subjects. This panel had 88.2% specificity and 81.6% sensitivity in differentiating men with prostate cancer from the control group. In addition, this panel of peptides also showed better performance than PSA in separating the two groups, in particular among men with PSA between 4 and 10 ng/ml. Although this study shows promising results, the roles of autoantibody profiles still have to be validated in much larger multicentre studies.

URINE-BASED MARKERS

In an effort to develop biomarkers that are more specific than PSA, considerable research has been geared towards development of urine-based tests for prostate cancer. The urine-based test is an alternative non-invasive and easily performed assay. The purpose of these tests is to detect modified forms of proteins or nucleic acids that may be shed into the urine by cancer cells. DD3^{PCA3} is a non-coding RNA-based urine marker currently being studied extensively [57, 58]. DD3^{PCA3} is a prostate cancer-specific gene that is overexpressed in more than 95% of primary prostate cancer specimens and prostate cancer metastasis [58]. In addition, DD3^{PCA3} expression appears to be prostate specific. Schalken's laboratory has extensively analysed DD3^{PCA3} transcripts in three separate studies using 238 urine specimens collected after prostate massage. DD3^{PCA3} had specificity that ranged from 76% to 89%, and sensitivity that ranged from 66% to 82% [58]. It is important to note that in these studies, only specimens that expressed PSA greater than 3 ng/ml were included. Therefore, it was possible that only men with higher risk of prostate cancer were evaluated. At this point, DD3^{PCA3} shows great potential as a tool for molecular urine test, nevertheless, a large multicentre clinical trial needs to be performed in order to validate the performance of this marker.

A molecular test to evaluate DD3^{PCA3} (uPM3) was developed by Fradet *et al.* to detect prostate cancer cells in urine [59]. The uPM3 test is based on the amplification of specific target

RNA using nucleic acid sequence-based amplification (NASBA) technology. This test utilizes the ratio of the relative expression of PSA mRNA and DD3^{PCA3} mRNA. Using urine samples from 517 men, the overall uPM3 sensitivity was 66% and the specificity was 89%. The positive predictive values for the uPM3 test were 75% compared with 38% for serum PSA at 4.0 ng/ml. The negative predictive value for uPM3 was 84% compared with 89% and 80% for PSA at cut-offs of 2.5 and 4.0 ng/ml respectively [59]. However, owing to the higher positive predictive values for uPM3, the accuracy of uPM3 was almost twofold higher than that of PSA (81% for uPM3 versus 43% and 47% for PSA cut-offs of 2.5 and 4.0 ng/ml respectively). These results suggest that the uPM3 molecular urine test may be an important supplement to current methods for the detection of early prostate cancer. Although uPM3 bears great promise as a novel diagnostic tool, the results of this study will need to be validated in other clinical trials that should aim at elucidating the relationship of the test results with the extent of cancer, as well as the possible causes of false-positive and false-negative results.

Telomerase activity is often associated with the ability of cells to escape senescence and subsequently proliferate. A study by Crocitto *et al.* using urine specimens from 14 men with prostate cancer and 35 men with negative biopsies for the disease showed that telomerase reverse transcriptase activity had a specificity of 66% and sensitivity of 36% [60]. Studies utilizing telomeric repeat amplification protocol (TRAP) assay to measure telomerase activity in urine specimens have reported specificity that ranged from 87% to 100%, and sensitivity that ranged from 58% to 90% [61, 62]. In addition, a significant association between Gleason scores and telomerase activities was observed.

Other proteins that have been used as urine-based markers for prostate cancer include prostatic inhibin-like peptide and minichromosome maintenance 5 (MCM-5). Prostatic inhibin-like peptide has been reported in the suppression of follicle-stimulating hormone. In two separate studies, Teni *et al.* used urines that were collected for 24 h and stored at 4 °C prior to testing [63, 64]. They reported that this protein had a specificity of 100% and sensitivity greater than 80% [63, 64]. MCM-5 is one of the minichromosome maintenance proteins that are involved in DNA replication and thus may have a critical regulatory role in cancer cell growth. In a study with urine specimens collected from 213 men, Stoeber *et al.* reported that MCM-5 had a specificity of 82% and sensitivity of 92% [65]. Although the specificity of this protein was obtained from over 200 specimens (BPH and non-BPH), the sensitivity was obtained from a small number of specimens (12 men with prostate cancer). Therefore, this marker still needs to be evaluated on a larger number of samples.

Advances in cellular and molecular biology have provided opportunities for both clinical and basic science researchers to identify and characterize urinary markers with high specificity and sensitivity (Table 2.3). However, development of urinary biomarkers for prostate cancer is still in an early phase. A number of markers outlined above appear to show promising results and bear potential usefulness for detection of the disease. One pitfall of the urine-based markers that are currently being tested is the number of specimens analysed. All of these urine-based markers need to be validated using larger samples in multicentre clinical trials. In addition, many of the urine specimens used for these tests are often handled and stored differently, and do not take into account differences in urine protein or nucleic acid content, thus creating another potential pitfall for reproducibility. Future studies for these markers should address these issues in order to potentially apply these urine-based tests on a mass screening basis.

BIOMARKERS FOR PROSTATE CANCER PROGNOSIS

Prostate cancer development and progression involve a series of molecular changes within the prostate cell and its environment. These molecular changes can be influenced by alterations of genetic and epigenetic pathways that will determine the outcome of the disease. Alterations in genetic and epigenetic pathways may involve diverse processes such as cell cycle regulation, androgen receptor signalling, cellular adhesion and angiogenesis. Variations of DNA, RNA or protein levels of molecules involved in these processes may be used as potential candidate markers of prognosis or therapeutic response. These prognostic markers are typically used to provide additional or independent information to the conventional predictors of prostate cancer recurrence and death (Gleason scores, PSA levels at the time of diagnosis, surgical margin involvement and clinical/pathological disease stage). One of the major questions that still exists in prostate cancer is an ability to differentiate the bad ones (aggressive) from the good ones (non-aggressive). We clearly need better tools to allow us to understand which men may die from their disease and who will die with it.

P53 AND BCL-2 AS KEY PLAYERS IN CELL CYCLE REGULATION

Apoptosis is one of the cellular events involved in cell cycle regulation. The predominant apoptotic regulators such as p53 and Bcl-2 have been demonstrated to have abnormal function and expression as prostate cancer progresses. Both p53 and Bcl-2 have also been shown to be mechanistically involved in hormone resistance. p53 functions by regulating transcription of genes involved in G1 phase growth arrest of cells in response to DNA damage, as well as regulating spindle checkpoint, centrosome homeostasis and G2–M phase transition. Nuclear accumulation of p53 as a prognostic indicator has been reported in several types of cancer including prostate, breast, lung and colorectal [66]. The importance of nuclear accumulation of p53 in localized cancer has been debated. Immunohistochemical analysis showing p53 nuclear accumulation is prognostic at different dichotomizing cut-off points based on the number of p53-positive nuclei. These studies either describe a poor prognosis group of men with greater than 20% p53-positive nuclei [67–70] or a group of men with lower percentages of positive cells in a heterogeneous focal staining pattern where either the presence of any nuclear accumulation or the presence of cluster of cells showing nuclear staining is negatively prognostic [71–73]. Other studies have demonstrated that p53 nuclear accumulation expression is higher in metastatic, recurrent and androgen-insensitive prostate cancer in comparison with localized prostate cancer [66]. Borre et al. showed that p53 nuclear accumulation appeared to be predictive of prostate cancer-related death on a population of men who did not receive treatment after diagnosis of the disease [74]. Quinn et al. showed the negative prognostic effect of an increased percentage of cells with p53 nuclear accumulation that was independent of PSA, Gleason score and pathological grade [75]. There are over 100 studies reporting increased p53 nuclear accumulation with increasing grade and stage [66]. This indicates that p53 expression may serve as a prognostic marker that may or may not be independent of tumour grade and/or stage. Clearly, the clinical usefulness of p53 as a prognostic marker needs further evaluation.

Bcl-2 is a member of the apoptosis regulatory proteins that act as death antagonists. Studies have shown that increased Bcl-2 expression contributes to androgen resistance in advanced prostate cancer and that it can facilitate progression to androgen independence. A study by Stattin et al. showed that Bcl-2 expression was increased regardless of castration therapy in men with localized prostate cancer [76]. However, Bcl-2 expression was higher in men who responded to castration therapy [76]. Bcl-2 overexpression was also proposed to play a role in resistance to radiotherapy in prostate cancer [77]. A number of studies reveal that Bcl-2 expression is a poor prognostic market for localized prostate cancer that requires radical prostatectomy [66]. However, Bcl-2 increases with tumour grade and stage, which suggests that Bcl-2 overexpression may be used as a prognostic factor in more advanced cancer that requires either hormonal therapy or radiotherapy [66].

ANDROGEN RECEPTOR

Many prostate cancers become androgen-independent and refractory to hormone therapy as the disease progresses. Transition of prostate cancer from androgen-dependent to androgen-independent represents a significant problem in the treatment of the disease. It remains unclear how prostate cancer cells acquire the ability to become androgen independent. The expression of androgen receptor (AR) can often be used as an indicator for hormonal responsiveness in the disease. Nevertheless, numerous studies on AR expression in prostate cancer have provided conflicting results. Many studies have shown that heterogeneity of AR expression increases significantly with progression through prostatic intraepithelial neoplasia (PIN) and localized prostate cancer to metastatic disease [78–82]. Other studies have demonstrated that AR overexpression is a characteristic of progression, recurrence, lymph node metastases and antiandrogen resistance in prostate cancer [83–88]. However, others showed no association between AR expression and primary prostate cancer, but revealed that AR overexpression in over 70% of lymph node metastases predicted a poorer cancer-specific survival in a subset of patients with lymph node involvement [88, 89].

Several studies have suggested that AR overexpression may correlate with mutation and/or amplification and with androgen resistance. AR gene amplification has been demonstrated in over 30% of prostate cancer recurring after androgen ablation therapy [90, 91]. The clinical significance of AR mutations remains to be elucidated. Frequency of AR mutation in prostate cancer varies from 6% to 44%, before and after hormonal therapy [92]. AR mutation has been shown to be associated with stimulation by different hormones (progesterone, adrenal androgens, oestrogen) or by antiandrogen such as hydroxyl-flutamide [66]. A series of AR point mutations have been identified in 44% of 25 hormonally naive men with the incidence of mutation increasing with tumour stage [66]. These AR mutants have differential binding affinity for different hormones and different downstream effects. Taken together, selected prostate cancer cells may have amplified and/or overexpressed AR that arises to mutations of these receptors. Consequently, this allows for stimulation by different types of hormones and antiandrogens. It is therefore particularly important to examine which mechanisms are active at various stages of prostate cancer progression in order to achieve successful outcome for prostate cancer treatment.

CELLULAR ADHESION AND ANGIOGENESIS

Cellular adhesion plays an important role in cancer cell metastasis. Detachment from the primary tumour and attachment to the endothelium lining are regulated by cell–cell adhesion molecules. E-cadherin is one of the adhesion molecules involved in the regulation of homotypic cell adhesion and cell morphology. E-cadherin has been reported to be down-regulated in localized prostate cancer, but it is up-regulated in metastases [66]. It is suggested that E-cadherin expression is transiently turned off during invasion into the blood vessels and reactivated again at the sites of metastasis [66]. Overall, studies evaluating E-cadherin and prostate cancer outcome suggest a significant prognostic effect. Since clinical application of E-cadherin is limited by heterogeneous expression in prostate cancer, biopsy results may not be predictive. Further studies in large cohorts are necessary to evaluate the potential usefulness of E-cadherin as an independent prognostic marker or whether it could be associated with other predictors such as Gleason scores or PSA.

Tumour angiogenesis is regulated in part by adhesion molecules and vascular endothelial growth factor (VEGF). VEGF is overexpressed in most prostate cancers [93–95]. Higher VEGF tissue expression has been shown to predict biochemical PSA relapse after prostatectomy and death from prostate cancer in a group that underwent observation for clinically localized disease and two other groups of men with hormone-refractory prostate cancer [96–98]. In men undergoing radical prostatectomy, elevated VEGF levels in serum or urine are predictive of earlier disease progression, whereas serum VEGF drops after prostatectomy [99–101]. Recent studies showed that VEGF and one of its receptors, VEGFR2, may have a role in the development of osteoblastic bone metastasis, which is indicative of advanced prostate cancer [102]. Overall, VEGF expression and its receptors (in particular VEGFR2) seem to bear great promise as prognostic markers in prostate cancer and metastasis respectively.

CONCLUDING REMARKS

The discovery of PSA more than 25 years ago represents an important development in the early detection of prostate cancer. Serum PSA measurement along with DRE continues to be the most performed test recommended by most physicians for prostate cancer detection. The cut-off value for PSA has been lowered from 4.0 ng/ml to 2.5 ng/ml in many major healthcare practices. Various concepts have been implemented in order to improve PSA specificity. Of these concepts, the PSA doubling time and free/total PSA ratio seem to be the most promising. The free/total PSA ratio appears to be able to be applied in conjunction with total PSA level to provide an additional indication of the existence of prostate cancer. In addition, PSA doubling time may serve as an indicator of mortality after radical prostatectomy. Both concepts seem to be promising in terms of improving the standard PSA test and are in the process of being applied clinically.

In recent years, biomarker discovery has become a major focus in prostate cancer research. New technologies in both genomics and proteomics play significant parts in the field of biomarker discovery. Ongoing innovative efforts defining new prostate cancer biomarkers will without doubt contribute to future diagnosis, prognosis and prediction of the disease. Those markers that best detect cancer, predict the outcome of disease and influence therapy options will have a most influential role in determining the future of prostate cancer oncology. With PSA being the only 'reliable' prostate cancer marker at the present time, new biomarkers will more than likely be combined with serum PSA to refine both the molecular and clinical evaluation of prostate cancer.

While individual technologies and biomarkers have been presented in this review, their clinical applications will most likely utilize combinations of markers with other clinical data. Current algorithms with large clinical utility are the Partin tables and the Kattan nomograms. The Partin tables, using a combination of serum PSA, biopsy Gleason score and clinical stage, were initially constructed in 1993 to assist urologists in the preoperative prediction of final pathological stage for patients with clinically localized prostate cancer [103]. Since then, the Partin tables have been validated in a multi-institutional study [104], as well as by other investigators [105]. Similarly, the Kattan nomogram was developed in 1998 using a combination of serum PSA, clinical stage and biopsy Gleason score [106]. The Kattan nomogram calculates the 5-year freedom from PSA-defined progression after radical prostatectomy [106]. This nomogram has also been validated in diverse patient populations [107, 108], and it has been widely used as a disease-specific prediction tool in oncology [109]. Both the Partin tables and Kattan nomograms are continuously being updated. As mentioned previously, all of the other biomarkers discussed in this review also need further validation. By incorporating these updated algorithms with new validated biomarkers, management of localized prostate cancer as well as predictions of disease recurrence will be significantly improved.

REFERENCES

1. Jemal A, Siegel R, Ward E *et al.* Cancer statistics, 2007. *CA Cancer J Clin* 2007; 57:43-66.
2. Sakr WA GD, Crissman JD, Heilbrun LK, Cassin BJ, Pontes JJ, Haas GP. High grade prostatic intraepithelial neoplasia (HGPIN) and prostatic adenocarcinoma between the ages of 20–69: an autopsy study of 249 cases. *In Vivo* 1994; 8:439–443.
3. Walsh PC, Worthington JF. *Dr. Patrick Walsh's Guide to Surviving Prostate cancer*, 2nd edn. Warner Books Inc., New York, 2007.

4. Constantinou J, Feneley MR PSA testing: an evolving relationship with prostate cancer screening. *Prostate Cancer Prostatic Dis* 2006; 9:6–13.
5. Cooner WH, Mosley BR, Rutherford CL, Jr. *et al.* Prostate cancer detection in a clinical urological practice by ultrasonography, digital rectal examination and prostate specific antigen. *J Urol* 1990; 143:1146–52; discussion 1152–1154.
6. Catalona WJ, Smith DS, Ornstein DK. Prostate cancer detection in men with serum PSA concentrations of 2.6 to 4.0 ng/ml and benign prostate examination. Enhancement of specificity with free PSA measurements. *JAMA* 1997; 277:1452–1455.
7. Punglia RS, D'Amico AV, Catalona WJ, Roehl KA, Kuntz KM. Effect of verification bias on screening for prostate cancer by measurement of prostate-specific antigen. *N Engl J Med* 2003; 349:335–342.
8. Thompson IM, Ankerst DP, Chi C *et al.* Operating characteristics of prostate-specific antigen in men with an initial PSA level of 3.0 ng/ml or lower. *JAMA* 2005; 294:66–70.
9. Balk SP, Ko YJ, Bubley GJ. Biology of prostate-specific antigen. *J Clin Oncol* 2003; 21:383–391.
10. Yousef GM, Diamandis EP. The new human tissue kallikrein gene family: structure, function, and association to disease. *Endocr Rev* 2001; 22:184–204.
11. Lilja H, Christensson A, Dahlen U *et al.* Prostate-specific antigen in serum occurs predominantly in complex with alpha 1-antichymotrypsin. *Clin Chem* 1991; 37:1618–25.
12. Stenman UH, Leinonen J, Alfthan H, Rannikko S, Tuhkanen K, Alfthan O. A complex between prostate-specific antigen and alpha 1-antichymotrypsin is the major form of prostate-specific antigen in serum of patients with prostatic cancer: assay of the complex improves clinical sensitivity for cancer. *Cancer Res* 1991; 51:222–226.
13. Wang MC, Valenzuela LA, Murphy GP, Chu TM. Purification of a human prostate specific antigen. *Invest Urol* 1979; 17:159–163.
14. Ferro MA, Barnes I, Roberts JB, Smith PJ. Tumour markers in prostatic carcinoma. A comparison of prostate-specific antigen with acid phosphatase. *Br J Urol* 1987; 60:69–73.
15. Potter SR, Partin AW. Prostate cancer: detection, staging, and treatment of localized disease. *Semin Roentgenol* 1999; 34:269–283.
16. Thompson IM, Pauler DK, Goodman PJ *et al.* Prevalence of prostate cancer among men with a prostate-specific antigen level < or =4.0 ng per milliliter. *N Engl J Med* 2004; 350:2239–2246.
17. Barry MJ. Clinical practice. Prostate-specific-antigen testing for early diagnosis of prostate cancer. *N Engl J Med* 2001; 344:1373–1377.
18. Oesterling JE, Jacobsen SJ, Chute CG *et al.* Serum prostate-specific antigen in a community-based population of healthy men. Establishment of age-specific reference ranges. *JAMA* 1993; 270:860–864.
19. Schmid HP, Riesen W, Prikler L. Update on screening for prostate cancer with prostate-specific antigen. *Crit Rev Oncol Hematol* 2004; 50:71–78.
20. Catalona WJ, Partin AW, Slawin KM *et al.* Use of the percentage of free prostate-specific antigen to enhance differentiation of prostate cancer from benign prostatic disease: a prospective multicenter clinical trial. *JAMA* 1998; 279:1542–1547.
21. Gann PH, Ma J, Catalona WJ, Stampfer MJ. Strategies combining total and percent free prostate specific antigen for detecting prostate cancer: a prospective evaluation. *J Urol* 2002; 167:2427–2434.
22. Babaian RJ, Fritsche HA, Evans RB. Prostate-specific antigen and prostate gland volume: correlation and clinical application. *J Clin Lab Anal* 1990; 4:135–137.
23. Benson MC, Whang IS, Olsson CA, McMahon DJ, Cooner WH. The use of prostate specific antigen density to enhance the predictive value of intermediate levels of serum prostate specific antigen. *J Urol* 1992; 147:817–821.
24. Veneziano S, Pavlica P, Querze R, Nanni G, Lalanne MG, Vecchi F. Correlation between prostate-specific antigen and prostate volume, evaluated by transrectal ultrasonography: usefulness in diagnosis of prostate cancer. *Eur Urol* 1990; 18:112–116.
25. D'Amico AV, Chen MH, Roehl KA, Catalona WJ. Preoperative PSA velocity and the risk of death from prostate cancer after radical prostatectomy. *N Engl J Med* 2004; 351:125–135.
26. Pound CR, Partin AW, Eisenberger MA, Chan DW, Pearson JD, Walsh PC. Natural history of progression after PSA elevation following radical prostatectomy. *JAMA* 1999; 281:1591–1597.
27. Zagars GK, Pollack A. Kinetics of serum prostate-specific antigen after external beam radiation for clinically localized prostate cancer. *Radiother Oncol* 1997; 44:213–221.
28. Freedland SJ, Humphreys EB, Mangold LA *et al.* Risk of prostate cancer-specific mortality following biochemical recurrence after radical prostatectomy. *JAMA* 2005; 294:433–439.

29. Ornstein DK, Tyson DR. Proteomics for the identification of new prostate cancer biomarkers. *Urol Oncol* 2006; 24:231–236.
30. Getzenberg RH, Abrahamsson, PA, Canto, EI *et al.* Advances in Biomarkers for Prostate Diseases. In: McConnell J, Denis L, Akaza H, Khoury S, Schalken J eds. *Prostate Cancer*. Editions 21, Paris, 2006, p. 85–146.
31. Luo J, Zha S, Gage WR *et al.* Alpha-methylacyl-CoA racemase: a new molecular marker for prostate cancer. *Cancer Res* 2002; 62:2220–2226.
32. Rubin MA, Zhou M, Dhanasekaran SM *et al.* alpha-Methylacyl coenzyme A racemase as a tissue biomarker for prostate cancer. *JAMA* 2002; 287:1662–1670.
33. Sreekumar A, Laxman B, Rhodes DR *et al.* Humoral immune response to alpha-methylacyl-CoA racemase and prostate cancer. *J Natl Cancer Inst* 2004; 96:834–843.
34. Zielie PJ, Mobley JA, Ebb RG, Jiang Z, Blute RD, Ho SM. A novel diagnostic test for prostate cancer emerges from the determination of alpha-methylacyl-coenzyme a racemase in prostatic secretions. *J Urol* 2004; 172:1130–1133.
35. Rubin MA, Bismar TA, Andren O *et al.* Decreased alpha-methylacyl CoA racemase expression in localized prostate cancer is associated with an increased rate of biochemical recurrence and cancer-specific death. *Cancer Epidemiol Biomarkers Prev* 2005; 14:1424–1432.
36. Varambally S, Dhanasekaran SM, Zhou M *et al.* The polycomb group protein EZH2 is involved in progression of prostate cancer. *Nature* 2002; 419:624–629.
37. Lapointe J, Li C, Higgins JP *et al.* Gene expression profiling identifies clinically relevant subtypes of prostate cancer. *Proc Natl Acad Sci USA* 2004; 101:811–816.
38. LaTulippe E, Satagopan J, Smith A *et al.* Comprehensive gene expression analysis of prostate cancer reveals distinct transcriptional programmes associated with metastatic disease. *Cancer Res* 2002; 62:4499–4506.
39. Rhodes DR, Sanda MG, Otte AP, Chinnaiyan AM, Rubin MA. Multiplex biomarker approach for determining risk of prostate-specific antigen-defined recurrence of prostate cancer. *J Natl Cancer Inst* 2003; 95:661–668.
40. Dhanasekaran SM, Barrette TR, Ghosh D *et al.* Delineation of prognostic biomarkers in prostate cancer. *Nature* 2001; 412:822–826.
41. Stephan C, Yousef GM, Scorilas A *et al.* Hepsin is highly over expressed in and a new candidate for a prognostic indicator in prostate cancer. *J Urol* 2004; 171:187–191.
42. Petricoin EF, III, Ornstein DK, Paweletz CP *et al.* Serum proteomic patterns for detection of prostate cancer. *J Natl Cancer Inst* 2002; 94:1576–1578.
43. Adam BL, Qu Y, Davis JW *et al.* Serum protein fingerprinting coupled with a pattern-matching algorithm distinguishes prostate cancer from benign prostate hyperplasia and healthy men. *Cancer Res* 2002; 62:3609–3614.
44. Konety BR, Getzenberg RH. Nuclear structural proteins as biomarkers of cancer. *J Cell Biochem* 1999; Suppl 32–33:183–191.
45. Getzenberg RH. Nuclear matrix and the regulation of gene expression: tissue specificity. *J Cell Biochem* 1994; 55:22–31.
46. Leman ES, Arlotti JA, Dhir R, Greenberg N, Getzenberg RH. Characterization of the nuclear matrix proteins in a transgenic mouse model for prostate cancer. *J Cell Biochem* 2002; 86:203–212.
47. Lakshmanan Y, Subong EN, Partin AW. Differential nuclear matrix protein expression in prostate cancers: correlation with pathologic stage. *J Urol* 1998; 159:1354–1358.
48. Partin AW, Getzenberg RH, CarMichael MJ *et al.* Nuclear matrix protein patterns in human benign prostatic hyperplasia and prostate cancer. *Cancer Res* 1993; 53:744–746.
49. Pienta KJ, Lehr JE. A common set of nuclear matrix proteins in prostate cancer cells. *Prostate* 1993; 23:61–67.
50. Getzenberg RH, Pienta KJ, Huang EY, Coffey DS. Identification of nuclear matrix proteins in the cancer and normal rat prostate. *Cancer Res* 1991; 51:6514–6520.
51. Paul B, Dhir R, Landsittel D, Hitchens MR, Getzenberg RH. Detection of prostate cancer with a blood-based assay for early prostate cancer antigen. *Cancer Res* 2005; 65:4097–4100.
52. Dhir R, Vietmeier B, Arlotti J *et al.* Early identification of individuals with prostate cancer in negative biopsies. *J Urol* 2004; 171:1419–1423.
53. Uetsuki H, Tsunemori H, Taoka R, Haba R, Ishikawa M, Kakehi Y. Expression of a novel biomarker, EPCA, in adenocarcinomas and precancerous lesions in the prostate. *J Urol* 2005; 174:514–518.

54. Lemon ES, Cannon GW, Trock BJ, *et al.* EPCA-2: a highly specific serum marker for prostate cancer. *Urology* 2007; 69:714–720.
55. Miller TE, Beausang LA, Winchell LF, Lidgard GP. Detection of nuclear matrix proteins in serum from cancer patients. *Cancer Res* 1992; 52:422–427.
56. Wang X, Yu J, Sreekumar A *et al.* Autoantibody signatures in prostate cancer. *N Engl J Med* 2005; 353:1224–1235.
57. Bussemakers MJ, van Bokhoven A, Verhaegh GW *et al.* DD3: a new prostate-specific gene, highly overexpressed in prostate cancer. *Cancer Res* 1999; 59:5975–5979.
58. Hessels D, Klein Gunnewiek JM, van Oort I *et al.* DD3(PCA3)-based molecular urine analysis for the diagnosis of prostate cancer. *Eur Urol* 2003; 44:8–15; discussion 15–16.
59. Fradet Y, Saad F, Aprikian A *et al.* uPM3, a new molecular urine test for the detection of prostate cancer. *Urology* 2004; 64:311–315; discussion 315–316.
60. Crocitto LE, Korns D, Kretzner L *et al.* Prostate cancer molecular markers GSTP1 and hTERT in expressed prostatic secretions as predictors of biopsy results. *Urology* 2004; 64:821–825.
61. Meid FH, Gygi CM, Leisinger HJ, Bosman FT, Benhattar J. The use of telomerase activity for the detection of prostatic cancer cells after prostatic massage. *J Urol* 2001; 165:1802–1805.
62. Vicentini C, Gravina GL, Angelucci A *et al.* Detection of telomerase activity in prostate massage samples improves differentiating prostate cancer from benign prostatic hyperplasia. *J Cancer Res Clin Oncol* 2004; 130:217–221.
63. Teni TR, Bandivdekar AH, Sheth AR, Sheth NA. Prostatic inhibin-like peptide quantified in urine of prostatic cancer patients by enzyme-linked immunosorbent assay. *Clin Chem* 1989; 35:1376–1379.
64. Teni TR, Sheth AR, Kamath MR, Sheth NA. Serum and urinary prostatic inhibin-like peptide in benign prostatic hyperplasia and carcinoma of prostate. *Cancer Lett* 1988; 43:9–14.
65. Stoeber K, Swinn R, Prevost AT *et al.* Diagnosis of genito-urinary tract cancer by detection of minichromosome maintenance 5 protein in urine sediments. *J Natl Cancer Inst* 2002; 94:1071–1079.
66. Quinn DI, Henshall SM, Sutherland RL. Molecular markers of prostate cancer outcome. *Eur J Cancer* 2005; 41:858–887.
67. Grignon DJ, Caplan R, Sarkar FH *et al.* p53 status and prognosis of locally advanced prostatic adenocarcinoma: a study based on RTOG 8610. *J Natl Cancer Inst* 1997; 89:158–165.
68. Kuczyk MA, Serth J, Bokemeyer C *et al.* The prognostic value of p53 for long-term and recurrence-free survival following radical prostatectomy. *Eur J Cancer* 1998; 34:679–686.
69. Osman I, Drobnjak M, Fazzari M, Ferrara J, Scher HI, Cordon-Cardo C. Inactivation of the p53 pathway in prostate cancer: impact on tumor progression. *Clin Cancer Res* 1999; 5:2082–2088.
70. Visakorpi T, Kallioniemi OP, Heikkinen A, Koivula T, Isola J. Small subgroup of aggressive, highly proliferative prostatic carcinomas defined by p53 accumulation. *J Natl Cancer Inst* 1992; 84:883–887.
71. Bauer JJ, Sesterhenn IA, Mostofi FK, McLeod DG, Srivastava S, Moul JW. Elevated levels of apoptosis regulator proteins p53 and bcl-2 are independent prognostic biomarkers in surgically treated clinically localized prostate cancer. *J Urol* 1996; 156:1511–1516.
72. Bauer JJ, Sesterhenn IA, Mostofi KF, McLeod DG, Srivastava S, Moul JW. p53 nuclear protein expression is an independent prognostic marker in clinically localized prostate cancer patients undergoing radical prostatectomy. *Clin Cancer Res* 1995; 1:1295–1300.
73. Yang G, Stapleton AM, Wheeler TM *et al.* Clustered p53 immunostaining: a novel pattern associated with prostate cancer progression. *Clin Cancer Res* 1996; 2:399–401.
74. Borre M, Stausbol-Gron B, Overgaard J. p53 accumulation associated with bcl-2, the proliferation marker MIB-1 and survival in patients with prostate cancer subjected to watchful waiting. *J Urol* 2000; 164:716–721.
75. Quinn DI, Henshall SM, Head DR *et al.* Prognostic significance of p53 nuclear accumulation in localized prostate cancer treated with radical prostatectomy. *Cancer Res* 2000; 60:1585–1594.
76. Stattin P, Westin P, Damber JE, Bergh A. Short-term cellular effects induced by castration therapy in relation to clinical outcome in prostate cancer. *Br J Cancer* 1998; 77:670–675.
77. Rosser CJ, Reyes AO, Vakar-Lopez F *et al.* Bcl-2 is significantly overexpressed in localized radio-recurrent prostate carcinoma, compared with localized radio-naïve prostate carcinoma. *Int J Radiat Oncol Biol Phys* 2003; 56:1–6.
78. Chodak GW, Kranc DM, Puy LA, Takeda H, Johnson K, Chang C. Nuclear localization of androgen receptor in heterogeneous samples of normal, hyperplastic and neoplastic human prostate. *J Urol* 1992; 147:798–803.

79. Miyamoto KK, McSherry SA, Dent GA *et al*. Immunohistochemistry of the androgen receptor in human benign and malignant prostate tissue. *J Urol* 1993; 149:1015–1019.
80. Ruizeveld de Winter JA, Janssen PJ, Sleddens HM *et al*. Androgen receptor status in localized and locally progressive hormone refractory human prostate cancer. *Am J Pathol* 1994; 144:735–746.
81. Sadi MV, Barrack ER. Androgen receptors and growth fraction in metastatic prostate cancer as predictors of time to tumour progression after hormonal therapy. *Cancer Surv* 1991; 11:195–215.
82. van der Kwast TH, Schalken J, Ruizeveld de Winter JA *et al*. Androgen receptors in endocrine-therapy-resistant human prostate cancer. *Int J Cancer* 1991; 48:189–193.
83. Hobisch A, Culig Z, Radmayr C, Bartsch G, Klocker H, Hittmair A. Distant metastases from prostatic carcinoma express androgen receptor protein. *Cancer Res* 1995; 55:3068–3072.
84. Koivisto P, Kolmer M, Visakorpi T, Kallioniemi OP. Androgen receptor gene and hormonal therapy failure of prostate cancer. *Am J Pathol* 1998; 152:1–9.
85. Koivisto P, Kononen J, Palmberg C *et al*. Androgen receptor gene amplification: a possible molecular mechanism for androgen deprivation therapy failure in prostate cancer. *Cancer Res* 1997; 57:314–319.
86. Olapade-Olaopa EO, MacKay EH, Taub NA, Sandhu DP, Terry TR, Habib FK. Malignant transformation of human prostatic epithelium is associated with the loss of androgen receptor immunoreactivity in the surrounding stroma. *Clin Cancer Res* 1999; 5:569–576.
87. Prins GS, Sklarew RJ, Pertschuk LP. Image analysis of androgen receptor immunostaining in prostate cancer accurately predicts response to hormonal therapy. *J Urol* 1998; 159:641–649.
88. Sweat SD, Pacelli A, Bergstralh EJ, Slezak JM, Cheng L, Bostwick DG. Androgen receptor expression in prostate cancer lymph node metastases is predictive of outcome after surgery. *J Urol* 1999; 161:1233–1237.
89. Sweat SD, Pacelli A, Bergstralh EJ, Slezak JM, Bostwick DG. Androgen receptor expression in prostatic intraepithelial neoplasia and cancer. *J Urol* 1999; 161:1229–1232.
90. Koivisto P, Hyytinen E, Palmberg C *et al*. Analysis of genetic changes underlying local recurrence of prostate carcinoma during androgen deprivation therapy. *Am J Pathol* 1995; 147:1608–1614.
91. Visakorpi T, Hyytinen E, Koivisto P *et al*. In vivo amplification of the androgen receptor gene and progression of human prostate cancer. *Nat Genet* 1995; 9:401–406.
92. Foley R, Hollywood D, Lawler M. Molecular pathology of prostate cancer: the key to identifying new biomarkers of disease. *Endocr Relat Cancer* 2004; 11:477–488.
93. Borre M, Nerstrom B, Overgaard J. Association between immunohistochemical expression of vascular endothelial growth factor (VEGF), VEGF-expressing neuroendocrine-differentiated tumor cells, and outcome in prostate cancer patients subjected to watchful waiting. *Clin Cancer Res* 2000; 6:1882–1890.
94. Ferrer FA, Miller LJ, Andrawis RI *et al*. Vascular endothelial growth factor (VEGF) expression in human prostate cancer: in situ and in vitro expression of VEGF by human prostate cancer cells. *J Urol* 1997; 157:2329–2333.
95. Jackson MW, Bentel JM, Tilley WD. Vascular endothelial growth factor (VEGF) expression in prostate cancer and benign prostatic hyperplasia. *J Urol* 1997; 157:2323–2328.
96. George DJ, Halabi S, Shepard TF *et al*. Prognostic significance of plasma vascular endothelial growth factor levels in patients with hormone-refractory prostate cancer treated on Cancer and Leukemia Group B 9480. *Clin Cancer Res* 2001; 7:1932–1936.
97. Small EJ, Meyer M, Marshall ME *et al*. Suramin therapy for patients with symptomatic hormone-refractory prostate cancer: results of a randomized phase III trial comparing suramin plus hydrocortisone to placebo plus hydrocortisone. *J Clin Oncol* 2000; 18:1440–1450.
98. Strohmeyer D, Rossing C, Bauerfeind A *et al*. Vascular endothelial growth factor and its correlation with angiogenesis and p53 expression in prostate cancer. *Prostate* 2000; 45:216–224.
99. Chan LW, Moses MA, Goley E *et al*. Urinary VEGF and MMP levels as predictive markers of 1-year progression-free survival in cancer patients treated with radiation therapy: a longitudinal study of protein kinetics throughout tumor progression and therapy. *J Clin Oncol* 2004; 22:499–506.
100. George DJ, Regan MM, Oh WK *et al*. Radical prostatectomy lowers plasma vascular endothelial growth factor levels in patients with prostate cancer. *Urology* 2004; 63:327–332.
101. Shariat SF, Anwuri VA, Lamb DJ, Shah NV, Wheeler TM, Slawin KM. Association of preoperative plasma levels of vascular endothelial growth factor and soluble vascular cell adhesion molecule-1 with lymph node status and biochemical progression after radical prostatectomy. *J Clin Oncol* 2004; 22:1655–1663.

102. Dai J, Kitagawa Y, Zhang J *et al*. Vascular endothelial growth factor contributes to the prostate cancer-induced osteoblast differentiation mediated by bone morphogenetic protein. *Cancer Res* 2004; 64:994–999.

103. Partin AW, Yoo J, Carter HB *et al*. The use of prostate specific antigen, clinical stage and Gleason score to predict pathological stage in men with localized prostate cancer. *J Urol* 1993; 150:110–114.

104. Partin AW, Kattan MW, Subong EN *et al*. Combination of prostate-specific antigen, clinical stage, and Gleason score to predict pathological stage of localized prostate cancer. A multi-institutional update. *JAMA* 1997; 277:1445–1451.

105. Blute ML, Bergstralh EJ, Partin AW *et al*. Validation of Partin tables for predicting pathological stage of clinically localized prostate cancer. *J Urol* 2000; 164:1591–1595.

106. Kattan MW, Eastham JA, Stapleton AM, Wheeler TM, Scardino PT. A preoperative nomogram for disease recurrence following radical prostatectomy for prostate cancer. *J Natl Cancer Inst* 1998; 90:766–771.

107. Bianco FJ, Jr., Kattan MW, Scardino PT, Powell IJ, Pontes JE, Wood DP, Jr. Radical prostatectomy nomograms in black American men: accuracy and applicability. *J Urol* 2003; 170:73–76; discussion 76–77.

108. Graefen M, Karakiewicz PI, Cagiannos I *et al*. International validation of a preoperative nomogram for prostate cancer recurrence after radical prostatectomy. *J Clin Oncol* 2002; 20:3206–3212.

109. Stephenson AJ, Scardino PT, Eastham JA *et al*. Preoperative nomogram predicting the 10-year probability of prostate cancer recurrence after radical prostatectomy. *J Natl Cancer Inst* 2006; 98:715–717.

3

Histopathological markers and precursor lesions

Isabelle Meiers, David G. Bostwick

PRECURSOR LESIONS IN PROSTATE CANCER

High-grade prostatic intraepithelial neoplasia (PIN) is known to have a high predictive value for prostate cancer. In addition, about 2% of contemporary needle biopsies contain collections of small acini that are suspicious for cancer but which fall below the diagnostic threshold and are reported as atypical small acinar proliferation suspicious for but not diagnostic of malignancy (ASAP). Identification of PIN, ASAP or both in a needle biopsy warrants repeat biopsy for concurrent or subsequent cancer. Prostate cancer has been identified in about 50% of subsequent biopsies for PIN and up to 60% for ASAP, but most early reports were based on quadrant or sextant biopsies. Recent studies with octant or more biopsies have shown that the predictive accuracy for cancer is lower for PIN and ASAP, particularly in highly screened patient populations when compared with previously reported unscreened populations. However, both PIN and ASAP are still significant predictors of cancer compared with historic controls, and their identification warrants repeat biopsy for concurrent or subsequent invasive carcinoma.

PIN and ASAP can occur together in the same biopsy set without concomitant cancer. We refer to the coexistence of the two lesions in the same high-power microscopic field as 'PIN + ASAP'. Androgen deprivation therapy decreases the prevalence and extent of PIN, suggesting that this form of treatment may play a role in chemoprevention.

HIGH-GRADE PIN

High-grade PIN is the earliest accepted stage in carcinogenesis, possessing most of the phenotypic, biochemical and genetic changes of cancer without invasion into the fibromuscular stroma [1–6]. PIN is defined as an abnormal epithelial proliferation within pre-existing ducts and ductules, with nucleolomegaly involving at least 10% of the cells [7–9]. The term 'PIN' is usually used today as a synonym for high-grade PIN (formerly PIN 2 and 3 on a 1–3 scale). The high level of interobserver variability and apparent lack of predictive value with low-grade PIN limits its clinical utility [10], and most pathologists do not routinely report this finding except in research studies. Thus, PIN is now used interchangeably with high-grade PIN by most investigators. Interobserver agreement for high-grade PIN is 'good to excellent' [10–12]. Terms such as dysplasia, malignant transformation, carcinoma *in situ* and intraductal carcinoma are discouraged [13].

Isabelle Meiers, MD, Bostwick Laboratories, Regents Park, London, UK
David G. Bostwick, MD MBA FCAP, CEO, President, Medical Director, Bostwick Laboratories, Glen Allen, Virginia, USA

EPIDEMIOLOGY OF PIN

In the USA, an estimated 1 300 000 prostate biopsies are performed annually. Annually, around 27 350 Americans die of prostate cancer and 234 460 new cases are diagnosed [14]. The mean incidence of isolated high-grade PIN is 9% (range 4–16%) of prostate biopsies [15, 16]. This is similar to our personal experience in Richmond, Virginia, where, in 2005, 115 000 new cases of high-grade PIN without cancer were diagnosed.

The incidence and extent of PIN increases with patient age [17–20]. An autopsy study of step-sectioned whole mount prostates from older men showed that the prevalence of PIN in prostates with cancer increased with age, predating the onset of carcinoma by more than 5 years [19]. A similar study of young men revealed that PIN is first seen in men in their twenties and thirties (9% and 22% frequency respectively), and preceded the onset of carcinoma by more than 10 years [19, 21]. Most foci of PIN in young men were low-grade, with increasing frequency of high-grade PIN with advancing age. The volume of high-grade PIN also increased with patient age [17].

Race and geographic location also appear to influence the incidence of high-grade PIN [3]. When specific age groups were compared between races, there were notable differences in the frequency of high-grade PIN. For example, African-American men had a greater prevalence of high-grade PIN than Caucasians in the 50- to 60-year-old age group, the decade preceding the manifestation of most clinically detected prostate cancers. African-American men also had the highest incidence of prostate cancer (about 50% more than Caucasians) [22, 23]. In contrast, Japanese men living in Osaka, Japan, had a significantly lower incidence of high-grade PIN than men residing in the USA, and Asians have the lowest clinically detected rate of prostate cancer [24]. Interestingly, Japanese men diagnosed with high-grade PIN also had an increased likelihood of developing prostate cancer, indicating that high-grade PIN is also a precursor of clinical prostate cancer in Asian men [25]. The differences in the frequency of high-grade PIN in the 50–60 years age group across races essentially mirror the rates of clinical prostate cancer observed in the 60- to 70-year-old age group [24].

The likely causal association of high-grade PIN with prostatic adenocarcinoma is supported by the observation that the prevalence of both high-grade PIN and cancer increases with patient age and that high-grade PIN precedes the onset of prostate cancer by less than one decade [19, 26]. The severity and frequency of high-grade PIN in prostates with cancer is greatly increased (73% of 731 specimens) when compared to prostates without cancer (32% of 876 specimens) [17, 27–29]. When high-grade PIN is found on sextant needle biopsy, there is a 50% risk of finding carcinoma on subsequent biopsies within 3 years [30], although this risk is lower when more than six cores are obtained [31–33]. This decline in predictive value is expected given the increased sampling for cancer with a greater number of core biopsies.

INCIDENCE OF PIN

The incidence of PIN varies according to the population of men under study (Table 3.1). The lowest likelihood is in men participating in prostate-specific antigen (PSA) screening and early detection studies, with an incidence of PIN in biopsies ranging from 0.7% to 20%.

Men seen by urologists in practice have PIN in 4.4–25% of contemporary needle biopsies. In those undergoing transurethral resection, the rate of PIN may be higher, varying from 2.8% to 33% [34–36]. In such cases, all tissue should be examined, but serial sections of suspicious foci are usually not necessary. Unfortunately, needle biopsy specimens fail to show the suspicious focus on deeper levels in about half of cases, often precluding assessment by immunohistochemistry and compounding the diagnostic dilemma.

Table 3.1 Incidence of isolated high-grade PIN in prostatic needle biopsies

Reference	Patient population	No. of men	Incidence of PIN (%)
Screening programmes			
Mettlin *et al.*, 1991 [161]	American Cancer Society National Prostate Cancer Detection Project	327	5.2
Feneley *et al.*, 1997 [162]	Screening population in Gwent, UK, 1991–1993	212	19.8
Hoedemaeker *et al.*, 1999 [43]	PSA screening study in Rotterdam, Netherlands	1824	0.7
Postma *et al.*, 2004 [103]	Screening population in Rotterdam, Netherlands (primary round)	4117	0.8
Postma *et al.*, 2004 [103]	Screening population in Rotterdam, Netherlands (secondary round, performed at a 4-year interval from the primary round)	1840	2.5
Urology practice			
Lee *et al.*, 1989 [18]	Consecutive biopsies of hypoechoic lesions at St Joseph Mercy Hospital	256	11
Bostwick *et al.*, 1995 [163]	Consecutive biopsies at Mayo Clinic	200	16.5
Bostwick *et al.*, 1995 [163]	Consecutive biopsies at Glendale Hospital (CA)	200	10.5
Langer *et al.*, 1996 [44]	Consecutive biopsies at University of Pennsylvania Medical Center	1275	4.4
Wills *et al.*, 1997 [45]	Consecutive biopsies at Johns Hopkins Hospital	439	2.7
Feneley *et al.*, 1997 [162]	Consecutive biopsies at University College London Hospitals, 1988–1994	1205	10.9
Feneley *et al.*, 1997 [162]	Consecutive biopsies of symptomatic men at St Bartholomew's Hospital, London, 1993–1994	118	24.6
Skjorten *et al.*, 1997 [34]	Consecutive biopsies from 1974–1975 at Ullevaal and Lovisenberg Hospitals, Oslo, Norway	79	7.6
Perachino *et al.*, 1997 [46]	Consecutive biopsies	148	14.1
O'Dowd *et al.*, 2000 [47]	Consecutive biopsies at UroCor Inc., Oklahoma City, 1994–1998	132426	3.7
Borboroglu *et al.*, 2001 [97]	Consecutive biopsies	1391	5.5
Lefkowitz *et al.*, 2001 [101]	Consecutive biopsies at the Manhattan Veterans Administration Medical Center	619	16.6
San Francisco *et al.*, 2003 [96]	Consecutive biopsies 1996–1997	387	12.6
Roscigno *et al.*, 2004 [95]	Consecutive biopsies at San Raffaele Hospital, Milan, Italy	2314	3.9
Abdel-Khalek *et al.*, 2004 [110]	Consecutive biopsies at Urology and Nephrology Center, Mansoura University, Mansoura, Egypt, 1997–2002	3081	2.7
Alsikafi *et al.*, 2001 [108]	Consecutive biopsies at Section of Urology, University of Chicago, 1998–1999	485	4.3
Gupta *et al.*, 2004 [164]	Consecutive biopsies at St John Hospital and Medical Center, Detroit, 2001–2002	933	12.3

Continued overleaf

Reference	Patient population	No. of men	Incidence of PIN (%)
Gupta et al., 2004 [164]	Consecutive biopsies at St. John Hospital and Medical Center, Detroit, 1998–2000	515	13.5
Kobayashi et al., 2004 [165]	Consecutive biopsies at Hamamatsu Rosai Hospital, Hamamatsu, Japan	104	20.2
Naya et al., 2004 [98]	Consecutive biopsies at University of Texas M. D. Anderson Cancer Center, Houston, 1997–2003	1086	8.7
Moore et al., 2005 [102]	Consecutive biopsies at Albany Medical College and Stratton Veterans Administration Med. Center 1998–2003	1188	2.5
Tunc et al., 2005 [166]	Consecutive biopsies at University of Istanbul, Turkey	505	12.8
Girasole et al., 2006 [106]	Consecutive biopsies at OUR Lab™ 1998–2004	40 966	3

DIAGNOSTIC CRITERIA OF PIN

There are four main patterns of high-grade PIN: tufting, micropapillary, cribriform and flat [37]. The tufting pattern is the most common and is present in 97% of cases (Figure 3.1), although most cases have multiple patterns. There are no known clinically important differences between the architectural patterns, and their recognition appears to be only of diagnostic utility. Sporadic retrospective reports have suggested that the cribriform or micro-

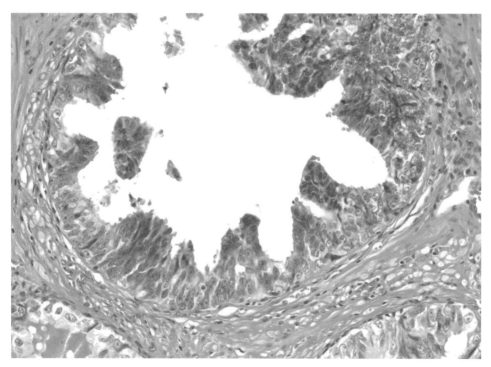

Figure 3.1 High-grade PIN, tufting pattern (H&E, 200×).

papillary patterns may indicate higher risk of coexistent cancer, but this has been repeatedly refuted. Other unusual patterns of PIN include the signet ring-cell pattern, small cell neuroendocrine (oat cell) pattern, mucinous pattern, microvacuolated (foamy gland) pattern and inverted (hobnail) pattern [38]. The presence of extensive PIN appears to be more predictive of cancer than the more common isolated single acinus with PIN.

There is inversion of the normal orientation of epithelial proliferation with PIN; proliferation in the benign epithelium normally occurs in the basal cell compartment, whereas in PIN the greatest proliferation occurs on the luminal surface, similar to preinvasive lesions in the colon (tubular adenoma) and other sites.

PIN spreads through prostatic ducts in multiple different patterns, similar to prostatic carcinoma. In the first pattern, neoplastic cells replace the normal luminal secretory epithelium, with preservation of the basal cell layer and basement membrane. This pattern often has a cribriform or near-solid appearance. Foci of high-grade PIN are usually indistinguishable from intraductal/intra-acinar spread of carcinoma by routine light microscopy [39]. In the second pattern, there is direct invasion through the ductal or acinar wall, with disruption of the basement membrane and basal cell layer. In the third pattern, neoplastic cells invaginate between the basal cell layer and columnar secretory cell layer ('pagetoid spread'), a very rare finding.

Early stromal invasion, the earliest evidence of carcinoma, occurs at sites of acinar outpouching and basal cell disruption in acini with high-grade PIN. Such microinvasion is present in about 2% of high-power microscopic fields of PIN, and is seen with equal frequency in all architectural patterns [37].

The mean volume of PIN in prostates with cancer is $1.2–1.32\,cm^3$, and the volume increases with increasing pathological stage, Gleason grade, positive surgical margins and perineural invasion [17, 40]. These findings emphasize the close spatial and biological relationship of PIN and cancer, and may result from an increase in PIN with increasing cancer volume.

PIN and cancer are usually multicentric [6, 17, 37]. PIN is multicentric in 72% of radical prostatectomy specimens with cancer, including 63% of those involving the non-transition zone and 7% of those involving the transition zone. In addition 2% of cases have concomitant single foci in all zones [17]. The peripheral zone of the prostate, the area in which the majority (70% or more) of prostatic carcinomas occur is also the most common location for PIN [17, 19, 22–29, 34–37, 41–47]. Cancer and PIN are frequently multicentric in the peripheral zone, indicating a 'field effect' similar to the multicentricity of urothelial carcinoma of the bladder.

High-grade PIN and prostate cancer are morphometrically and phenotypically similar. High-grade PIN occurs primarily in the peripheral zone and is seen in areas that are in continuity with prostate cancer [4, 17, 29, 48]. High-grade PIN and prostate cancer are multifocal and heterogeneous [17, 49, 50]. Increasing rates of aneuploidy and angiogenesis as the grade of PIN progresses are further evidence that high-grade PIN is a precancerous [1, 51, 52]. Prostate cancer and high-grade PIN also have similar proliferative and apoptotic indices [1, 24, 53–55].

It is often difficult with small foci in needle biopsies to separate cancer from suspicious foci [atypical small acinar proliferation suspicious for but not diagnostic of malignancy (ASAP)] when there is coexistent high-grade PIN. This difficulty is based on the inability to separate tangential cutting of the larger preexisting acini of PIN (that may appear as small separate adjacent acini) from the smaller discrete acini of cancer. In such cases, we prefer the term 'PIN + ASAP' (referring to the coexistence of the two lesions, high-grade PIN and ASAP in the same high-power microscopic field) to avoid overdiagnosis of tangential cutting of PIN and cancer.

Recent renewed efforts to introduce the term 'intraductal carcinoma' rely on the abandoned concept that dysplasia (defined here as malignancy arising at that specific site within the epithelium) can be separated reliably from intraductal/intra-acinar spread of cancer (defined here as extension of malignant cells through the pre-existing lumens of the prostate). However, this concept has been rejected by consensus on multiple occasions owing to lack of reproducible criteria for making this distinction. The non-committal term 'intraepithelial neoplasia' was internationally adopted and repeatedly reconfirmed since it begs the question of site of origin of the process. Those who persist with the belief that 'intraductal carcinoma' can be diagnosed, rely on proximity of the epithelial abnormality to invasive cancer, but this criterion is arbitrary and not based on valid objective confirmatory data. More importantly, there is no clinical utility at present that requires separation of dysplasia and intraductal/intra-acinar spread of cancer as the clinical response is the same. It is conceivable that future studies may allow diagnostic separation of dysplasia and intraductal/intra-acinar spread of cancer. If this is so, it may be shown that these steps in the biologic progression of prostate cancer may have differential predictive value for prostate cancer. We agree that identification of subsets of high-grade PIN that indicate greater risk of cancer is a clinically important area of investigation, but attempts at separation to date have been fruitless.

USEFUL IMMUNOHISTOCHEMICAL MARKERS FOR THE DIAGNOSIS OF PIN

Select antibodies such as antikeratin 34βE12 (high-molecular-weight keratin) or p63 may be used to stain tissue sections for the presence of basal cells [56], recognizing that PIN retains an intact or fragmented basal cell layer whereas cancer does not.

Monoclonal basal cell-specific antikeratin 34βE12 stains virtually all the normal basal cells of the prostate, with continuous intact circumferential staining in many instances. There is no staining in the secretory and stromal cells. This marker is the most commonly used immunostain for prostatic basal cells [57, 58], and methods of use with paraffin-embedded sections have been optimized [59].

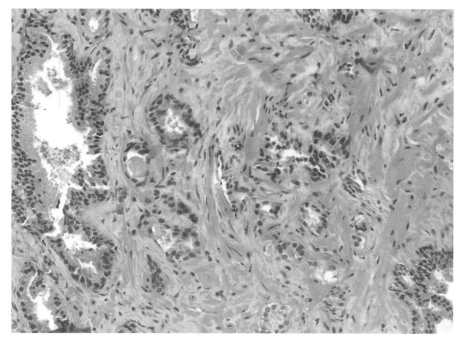

Figure 3.2 High-grade PIN, micropapillary pattern. Immunostain for 34βE12 reveals basal cell layer disruption in high-grade PIN (stained slide, 400×).

Increasing grades of PIN are associated with progressive disruption of the basal cell layer, according to studies utilizing antikeratin 34βE12. Basal cell layer disruption is present in 56% of cases of high-grade PIN, and is more frequent in acini adjacent to invasive carcinoma than in distant acini (Figure 3.2). The amount of disruption increases with increasing grades of PIN. Early invasive carcinoma occurs at sites of glandular outpouching and basal cell discontinuity in association with PIN [9]. The cribriform pattern of PIN may be mistaken for the cribriform pattern of adenocarcinoma, and the use of antikeratin staining is often useful in making this distinction [60]. Cancer cells consistently fail to react with this antibody, although admixed benign acini may be misinterpreted as cancerous staining. Thus, immunohistochemical stains for antikeratin 34βE12 may show the presence or absence of basal cells in a small focus of atypical glands, helping to establish a benign or malignant diagnosis respectively. We believe that this antibody can be employed successfully if one judiciously interprets the results in combination with the light microscopic findings. Relying solely on the absence of immunoreactivity (absence of basal cell staining) to render the diagnosis of cancer is without precedent in diagnostic immunohistochemistry and is discouraged [61]. Nonetheless, some studies have noted that the rate of equivocal cases can be reduced considerably [62], by 68% [57] or from 5.1% to 1.0% [63], by addition of this immunohistochemical marker. Evaluation of prostate biopsies following therapy such as radiation therapy may be one of the most useful roles for antikeratin 34βE12 (see below) [64].

In addition to PIN and cancer, basal cell layer disruption or loss also occurs in inflamed acini, atypical adenomatous hyperplasia and postatrophic hyperplasia, and may be misinterpreted as cancer if one relies exclusively on the immunohistochemical profile of a suspicious focus. Furthermore, basal cells of Cowper's glands may not express keratin 34βE12 [65], although this has been disputed [66]. Rare (0.2%) cases of adenocarcinoma have been reported that express keratin 34βE12, including foci of metastatic high-grade adenocarcinoma. These cases did not appear phenotypically to be basal cell/adenoid cystic carcinoma [67].

Basal cell hyperplasia is a histological mimic of cancer, and use of antikeratin 34βE12 is recommended in any equivocal cases that include this lesion in the differential considerations as it is invariably positive in that lesion [68, 69].

We routinely generate unstained intervening sections of all prostate biopsies for possible future immunohistochemical staining, recognizing that small foci of concern are often lost when the tissue block is re-cut. One study reported loss of the suspicious focus in 31 of 52 cases [70].

Other markers of basal cells include proliferation markers, differentiation markers and genetic markers. The preferential localization of many of these markers in basal cells but not in secretory cells suggests that they play a role in growth regulation. P63 is a recently introduced nuclear marker that may be useful for separating PIN and cancer from a benign mimic. Basal cells display immunoreactivity at least focally for keratins 5, 10, 11, 13, 14, 16 and 19 and, of these, only keratin 19 is also found in secretory cells [71–73]. Keratins found exclusively in the secretory cells include 7, 8 and 18. Basal cells usually do not display immunoreactivity for PSA, prostate acid phosphatase (PAP) and S-100 protein, and only rare single cells stain with chromogranin and neuron-specific enolase. Conversely, the normal secretory luminal cells invariably stain with PSA and PAP. Prostatic basal cells do not usually display myoepithelial differentiation [72, 74], in contrast to basal cells in the breast, salivary glands, pancreas and other sites.

A new molecular marker, racemase (alpha-methylacyl-CoA racemase, P504S), was introduced for separating benign and neoplastic acini [75]. This marker has proven useful for evaluation of ASAP and separation of cancer from hormonally treated benign acini. Its advantage over antikeratin 34βE12 is its positive granular cytoplasmic staining in cancer cells, with little or no staining in benign acini. In PIN, monoclonal and polyclonal antibodies to alpha-methylacyl-CoA racemase, P504S, were positive in 77% and 91%, respectively [76], consistent with previously published studies [77–81]. Helpap suggested that moderate to strong racemase expression in PIN of biopsy specimens is indicative of an associated adeno-carcinoma and may be helpful in the choice of therapy [82]. Since racemase is not specific for prostate cancer and is present in high-grade PIN (> 90%), this staining must be interpreted with caution and the diagnosis of PIN or prostate cancer should be rendered only with convincing histological evidence [83].

DIFFERENTIAL DIAGNOSIS OF PIN

The histological differential diagnosis of PIN includes lobular atrophy, post-atrophic hyper-plasia, atypical basal cell hyperplasia, cribriform hyperplasia and metaplastic changes asso-ciated with radiation, infarction and prostatitis. Many of these display architectural and cytologic atypia, including enlarged nucleoli, and consist of small specimens, and cauterized or distorted specimens. Cribriform adenocarcinoma, ductal (endometrioid) carcinoma, and urothelial carcinoma involving prostatic ducts and acini may also be confused with PIN. Biopsies submitted with incomplete patient history should be interpreted with caution. In one study, the authors reported that the proliferative activity, defined as Ki-67 labelling index, was higher in ductal carcinoma than in PIN (33% vs. 6%) [84]. Stratified epithelium in non-cribriform glands of prostate cancer can also resemble high-grade PIN. Recognition of this fact and immunohistochemical evaluation of stratified glands may be indicated to cor-rectly diagnose those glands as prostate cancer [85].

PIN may be overdiagnosed as adenocarcinoma. Our retrospective review of transurethral resections from the Mayo Clinic files between 1960 and 1970 revealed that PIN was often diagnosed as adenocarcinoma [86]. Similarly, fine needle aspiration of the prostate may yield cell clusters of PIN that are overdiagnosed as cancer; this issue is critically important to consider in evaluating studies from Sweden and other countries that have, perhaps errone-ously, relied on fine-needle aspiration diagnoses for patients treated with watchful waiting (expectant management).

CLINICAL SIGNIFICANCE OF PIN

PIN Does Not Elevate PSA
Biopsy remains the definitive method for detecting PIN and early invasive cancer. Serum PSA concentration may be elevated in patients with PIN [87], although these results have been refuted [88, 89]. There is also a poor correlation between PIN and PSA density accord-ing to studies of radical prostatectomy specimens and preoperative serum [89]. Mean PSA increased from 8.4 to 11.6 ng/ml in patients with PIN who developed cancer within 2 years. Those patients with PIN who did not develop cancer during this interval had an increase in PSA from 4.8 to 5.9 ng/ml or decrease from 5.1 to 4.6 ng/ml. These findings have not been confirmed.

The ratio of free to total PSA is the same for patients with high-grade PIN and cancer, distinct from low-grade PIN and hyperplasia, although this has also been refuted. Many patients in these studies were later found to have cancer, so the elevation in serum PSA concentration and its derivatives may have resulted from the undetected cancer.

Transrectal Ultrasound Cannot Detect PIN
The appearance of PIN at transrectal ultrasound may be hypoechoic like carcinoma, although these findings have not been confirmed [18, 90]. Today, most urologists and radiologists do not believe that PIN is detectable by transrectal ultrasound because PIN is a microscopic finding that is below the detection threshold for this form of imaging.

Men with PIN Develop Prostate Cancer

As a risk factor, the presence of isolated PIN in a set of sextant needle biopsies connotes a risk ratio of 14.9. PIN is a far stronger predictor for subsequent cancer than the independent predictors of patient age (> 65 years old vs. ≤65 years old) and serum PSA (> 4 ng/ml vs. ≤4 ng/ml); for these, the respective risk ratios are 3.5 and 3.64 [91]. PIN coexists with cancer in more than 85% of cases, according to studies employing whole-mounted totally embedded prostates. In one report, the likelihood of finding cancer increased with the biopsy time interval. The investigators reported a 32% incidence of cancer if repeat biopsy was performed within 1 year, compared with a 38% incidence in biopsies obtained after 1 year [91]. Other series have also found a high predictive value of PIN for cancer, although recent reports based on obtaining a greater number of cores shows a lower predictive value (Table 3.2) [32, 44, 47, 91–115]. These data emphasize the strong association of PIN and adenocarcinoma and indicate that vigorous diagnostic follow-up is needed.

Multiple factors account for the decline in the predictive accuracy of high-grade PIN for cancer. The main factor is use of extended biopsy techniques that result in more thorough

Table 3.2　Cancer detection in patients with high-grade PIN

Publication date	Study dates	Cores	Reference	No. of subjects with repeat biopsy(ies)	PIN cases with PCa at follow-up (%)
1995	1987–1993	1–8	Davidson [91]	100	35
1996	1990–1994	NS	Raviv [93]	48	48
1996	1991–1993	F	Langer [44]	53	27
1996	Not stated	4	Shepherd [94]	66	47
2000	1995–1998	Mixed	Kamoi [107]	45	22
2000	1994–1998	Mixed	O'Dowd [47]	1306	23
2001	1991–1998	NS	Kronz [92]	245	32
2001	1998–1999	NS	Alsikafi [108]	21	14
2001	Not stated	6	Maatman [109]	86	16
2001	1995–2000	6	Borboroglu [97]	45	44
2001	1999–2001	12	Lefkowitz [101]	43	2
2002	1995–2002	10–12	Roscigno [95]	47	45
2003	1996–1997	EXT	San Francisco [96]	47	24
2003	2001–2003	6	Goeman [99]	63	27
2004	1997–2003	EXT	Naya [98]	47	11
2004	1999–2002	4–15	Bishara [100]	132	29
2004	Not stated	20	Rabets [115]	38	18
2004	1997–2002	11	Abdel-Khalek [110]	83	36
2004	2000–2003	6	Postma [103]	101	13
2005	1998–2003	EXT	Moore [102]	22	5
2005	2000–2002	6–18	Schlesinger [104]	204	23
2005	1996–2000	6	Gokden [105]	190	30
2005	1998–2003	6 or EXT	El-Fakharany [111]	585	25
2005	2001–2003	NS	Leite [112]	142	13
2006	1997–2001	Mixed	Herawi [32]	332	21
2006	1997–2001	Mixed	Herawi [32]	323	13
2006	1998–2004	2–4	Girasole [106]	358	22
2006	1999–2004	6	Hussein [113]	17	41
2006	1999–2005	12	Keith [114]	48	31

EXT, extended in all cases (≥8); F, fewer than sextant; NS, not specified; PCa, prostate cancer.

prostate sampling and in higher cancer detection rates. As a result, there is a smaller group of patients with an isolated diagnosis of PIN. Another factor is the lower detection rate for, and difficulty in the detection of, the remaining small cancers. Larger significant tumours may also escape detection. These factors lead to a higher frequency of negative repeat biopsies. These results may reflect a new steady state and a newly reached low plateau in the predictive accuracy of these markers. In a recent report, the investigators demonstrated that with six core biopsies for both the initial and re-biopsy, the risk of cancer was 14.1%, compared with 31.9% in a group that had eight or more core biopsies on follow-up. They also observed that the risk of cancer on biopsy within 1 year following a diagnosis of PIN (13.3%) is relatively low if good sampling (eight or more cores) is initially performed [32].

Another plausible explanation for these observations may relate to the fact that backward probability is usually based on retrospective evidence, whereas forward probability is usually based on prospective evidence. Consequently, backward probability is often easier to determine. Many researchers do not distinguish between these two probabilities, falsely concluding that the probability of a risk factor in patients with the disease is the probability of the disease occurring in people with the risk factor. The use of backward probability as a substitute for forward probability is a common fallacy in medical practice and may result in false attribution of causation [116].

High-grade PIN in transurethral resection specimens is also an important predictive factor for prostate cancer [35, 117, 118]. Among 14 patients with PIN and benign prostatic hyperplasia (BPH) followed for up to 7 years (mean 5.9 years), three (21.4%) developed prostatic cancer [118]. Mean serum PSA concentration was higher than in those who did not develop cancer (8.1 vs. 4.6 ng/ml respectively). All subsequent cancers apparently arose in the peripheral zone and were detected by needle biopsy. Thus, all tissue should be submitted by the pathologist for examination when high-grade PIN is found in transurethral resection of the prostate (TURP) specimens. The high predictive value of PIN for the development of subsequent cancer warrants reporting the presence of PIN in TURP specimens, according to the Cancer Committee of the College of American Pathologists. Conversely, a study showed that PIN in the transition zone and central zone from Norwegian men is not predictive of subsequent cancer development [117].

The significance of PIN in initial biopsies as a marker of prostate cancer in repeat biopsies has been extensively investigated (see Table 3.2) but little is known of the actual rate of cancer in the whole prostate in this setting because repeat biopsies may miss the area of cancer. Some investigators aimed to define a more precise, positive predictive value of isolated PIN in initial biopsies in predicting cancer in the prostate gland and found that clinically significant prostate cancer was associated with 4 out of 11 biopsies positive for PIN compared with 3 out of 21 biopsies negative for PIN. The positive predictive value of PIN was 64%, with a sensitivity of 28% and a specificity of 81% [119].

Androgen Deprivation Therapy Eliminates PIN

There is a marked decrease in the prevalence and extent of high-grade PIN in cases after androgen deprivation therapy when compared with untreated cases [120–122]. This decrease is accompanied by epithelial hyperplasia, cytoplasmic clearing and prominent glandular atrophy, with decreased ratio of glands to stroma. These findings indicate that the dysplastic prostatic epithelium is hormone-dependent. In the normal prostatic epithelium, luminal secretory cells are more sensitive to the absence of androgen than basal cells, and these results indicate that the cells of high-grade PIN share this androgen sensitivity. The loss of some normal, hyperplastic and dysplastic epithelial cells with androgen deprivation is probably due to acceleration of programmed single-cell death. One report suggested that PIN is not substantially decreased after hormonal therapy, but those authors failed to use current criteria for PIN, so the results are not comparable [123].

Neoadjuvant hormone deprivation with monthly leuprolide and flutamide 250 mg p.o. t.i.d. for 3 months resulted in a 50% reduction in high-grade PIN. Longer therapy with 6 months of neoadjuvant androgen deprivation therapy prior to radical prostatectomy in the European Randomized Study of Screening for Prostate Cancer (ERSPC) study reduced high-grade PIN even more [30]. Flutamide has been shown to decrease the prevalence and extent of high-grade PIN and to induce epithelial atrophy [124]. There is also evidence that cessation of flutamide results in return of high-grade PIN [125, 126].

The effects of a 5α-reductase inhibitor for treatment of high-grade PIN are controversial and the cumulative number of cases that have been studied is probably too small for any firm conclusions [127]. Two reports found no apparent effect on the histological appearance or extent of high-grade PIN [128, 129], whereas a third study of three cases described atrophy and involution with decreased prevalence [130].

Radiation Therapy Eliminates PIN

The prevalence and extent of PIN are decreased after radiation therapy [131–133]. However, one study paradoxically noted a higher than expected incidence (70%) of PIN after radiation therapy [132]. The authors failed to employ accepted diagnostic criteria for PIN, so their results are not comparable with others. A report from Memorial Sloan-Kettering found PIN in 8.8% of biopsies following a course of three-dimensional (3-D) external beam conformal radiation therapy [133].

Following radiation therapy, PIN retains the features characteristic of untreated PIN, and is readily recognized in tissue specimens. The key pathological features include nuclear crowding, nuclear overlapping and stratification, nuclear hyperchromasia and prominent nucleoli. The basal cell layer is present, but often fragmented; racemase shows strong apical to diffuse cytoplasmic staining [134]. The most common patterns of PIN are tufting and micropapillary, similar to those reported in untreated PIN.

The long-term efficacy of radiation treatment may depend on eradication of cancer as well as precancerous lesions that may otherwise lead to evolution of secondary metachronous invasive cancers. Identification of residual or recurrent cancer portends a worse prognosis. The questions remain whether recurrent cancer after irradiation is due to regrowth of incompletely eradicated tumour or progression from incompletely eradicated PIN. Further studies of salvage prostatectomy specimens and post-radiation needle biopsies are justified in an attempt to establish the significance of high-grade PIN as a source of long-term treatment failure among these patients. If PIN is associated with treatment failure, adjuvant chemoprevention strategies that ablate this lesion may reduce the risk of late cancer recurrence.

Should Men with High-Grade PIN Be Treated?

The clinical importance of recognizing PIN is based on its strong association with prostatic carcinoma. PIN has a high predictive value as a marker for adenocarcinoma, so its identification in biopsy specimens warrants further search for concurrent invasive carcinoma. If all procedures fail to identify coexistent carcinoma, close surveillance and follow-up are indicated. As high-grade PIN progresses, the likelihood of basal cell layer disruption increases, in a similar way to that observed for carcinoma in situ (CIS) of the urinary bladder. CIS of the urinary bladder, like PIN, may become invasive and is treated aggressively. The standard of care for management of CIS of the bladder is intravesical instillation of chemotherapy or BCG, and, in some cases, radical cystectomy.

Follow-up biopsy is suggested for patients with PIN at 3- to 6-month intervals for 2 years, and thereafter at 12-month intervals for life [91, 135]. Some urologists perform 'saturation' biopsies, consisting of more than 12–15 biopsies in one session, often with brief general anaesthesia in the operating theatre, in an effort to definitively exclude cancer. Most authors agree that the identification of PIN in the prostate should not influence or dictate therapeutic decisions [135]. We are aware of 21 radical prostatectomies that were purposely (three cases) or inadvertently performed (18 cases) in patients whose biopsies contained only high-grade PIN; all but two of the cases contained adenocarcinoma in the surgical specimen (DG Bostwick, personal communication, 2003).

Currently, routine treatment is not available for patients who have high-grade PIN. Prophylactic radical prostatectomy or radiation is not an acceptable treatment for patients who have high-grade PIN only [136]. The development and identification of acceptable agents to treat high-grade PIN would fill a therapeutic void. As noted above, androgen deprivation therapy and radiation therapy induce acinar atrophy and apoptosis that result in regression of high-grade PIN [120–122, 130, 136–139].

Chronic therapy, however, would most probably be required to prevent new high-grade PIN lesions from invading and becoming clinical prostate cancer. Although more toxicity may be acceptable for patients wishing to have treatment for PIN, compared with cancer preventatives in healthy men, androgen deprivation therapy would have too many adverse effects to be appropriate in this setting. New agents with a low side effect profile are greatly needed if they are to be taken until the age of 70 years or greater [136]. Toremifene (Acapodene™) is a selective oestrogen receptor modulator that eliminates high-grade PIN and reduces the incidence of prostate cancer. After 4 months of toremifene (60 mg/day orally for 4 months), 72% of men treated (vs. 17.9% of controls) had no high-grade PIN on subsequent prostate biopsies [140]. In another study, cumulative risk of prostate cancer was reduced in patients taking toremifene 20 mg compared with placebo (24.4% vs. 31.2%) with an annualized rate of prevention of 6.8 cancers per 100 men treated [141]. Among patients with no biopsy evidence of cancer at baseline and 6 months, the 12-month incidence of prostate cancer was reduced by 48.2% with toremifene 20 mg compared with placebo (9.1% vs. 17.4%). The 20-mg dose was most effective, but the cumulative and 12-month incidence of prostate cancer was reduced at each toremifene dose compared with placebo (cumulative risk: 29.2% for 40 mg, 28.1% for 60 mg; 12-month incidence: 14.3% for 40 mg, 13.0% for 60 mg) [141].

Green tea catechins (GTCs) may also reduce the incidence of prostate cancer. Catechins are antioxidants in the class of polyphenols called flavonols. After 6 months of GTCs (600 mg/day orally), 3.3% of the men with PIN had cancer compared with 30% of those who took placebo. Selenium and vitamin E are also under investigation as putative chemopreventive agents.

PIN offers promise as an intermediate endpoint in studies of chemoprevention of prostatic carcinoma. Recognizing the slow growth rate of prostate cancer and the considerable amount of time needed in animal and human studies for adequate follow-up, the non-invasive precursor lesion PIN is a suitable intermediate histological marker to indicate subsequent likelihood of cancer.

PIN Does Not Predict Cancer Recurrence after Radical Prostatectomy

PIN was not predictive of PSA (biochemical) failure at 32 months in patients undergoing radical prostatectomy and androgen deprivation therapy [120].

ATYPICAL SMALL ACINAR PROLIFERATION SUSPICIOUS FOR BUT NOT DIAGNOSTIC OF MALIGNANCY (ASAP)

WHAT ARE THE DIAGNOSTIC CRITERIA FOR ASAP?

ASAP represents our inability to render an incontrovertible diagnosis of cancer in a needle biopsy. The focus of concern is invariably no larger than two dozen acini, less than the size of the head of a pin, and so the major concern is overdiagnosis of cancer based on insufficient evidence. The quandary in cases in which ASAP is diagnosed usually results from one or a combination of the reasons listed in Table 3.3 [142]. All of these may hinder a definitive diag-

Table 3.3   Reasons for the diagnosis of ASAP

Small size of focus
Small number of acini in the focus of concern (invariably less than two dozen acini)
Small focus size, average 0.4 mm in diameter
Focus present at core tip or biopsy edge, indicating that the focus is incompletely sampled
Loss of focus of concern in deeper levels

Conflicting morphological findings
Distortion of acini raising concern for atrophy
Lack of convincing features of cancer (insufficient nucleomegaly or nucleolomegaly)
Clustered growth pattern mimicking a benign process such as atypical adenomatous hyperplasia
Foamy cytoplasm raising concern for foamy gland carcinoma

Conflicting immunohistochemical findings
Focally positive high-molecular-weight cytokeratin
Focally positive p63 staining
Negative racemase immunostain

Confounding findings
Histological artefacts such as thick sections or overstained nuclei
Tangential cutting of adjacent high-grade PIN
Architectural or cytological changes (nucleomegaly and nucleolomegaly) owing to inflammation or other lesions

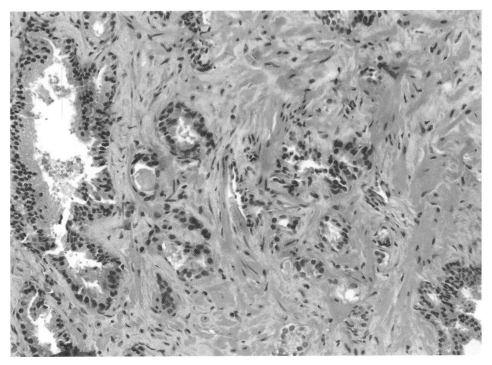

Figure 3.3   Atypical small acinar proliferation suspicious for but not diagnostic of malignancy (ASAP). Small focus has acini with microvacuolated cytoplasm and prominent nucleoli (H&E, 200×).

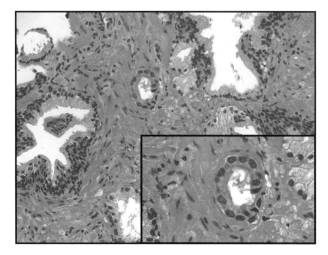

Figure 3.4 Atypical small acinar proliferation highly suspicious for but not diagnostic of malignancy (ASAP). Small focus has one single acinus (inset) with nuclear enlargement, prominent and double nucleoli, and luminal eosinophilic secretions. Small size of focus precludes a definite diagnosis of cancer (H&E, 200×; inset 400×).

nosis of carcinoma but, in such cases, the possibility cannot be definitively excluded (Figures 3.3 and 3.4). The need for this category is based on our 'absolute uncertainty' regarding the diagnosis. That this need exists is manifested by the variety of terms or synonyms currently in use that include the word 'atypical' to describe this diagnosis, although ASAP is now the preferred term that is most widely used clinically around the world. The diagnosis of ASAP indicates to the clinician that the biopsy in question exhibits histological features that are neither clearly malignant nor clearly benign and that follow-up of the patient is warranted.

For pathologists, three questions need to be answered prior to the diagnosis of ASAP or cancer in a small lesion: 'Would you be absolutely confident of this biopsy diagnosis if it were followed by a negative radical prostatectomy?'; 'Would another colleague pathologist agree with the diagnosis of cancer?'; and, finally, 'Can you confidently support the diagnosis of adenocarcinoma based solely on this biopsy?'. If the answer to any of these questions is 'No', then we recommend use of the more conservative diagnosis of ASAP. In this setting, we believe that ASAP is a valid diagnostic category as long as it is employed judiciously and maximum information has been obtained from the available tissue. Other evidence useful in supporting a cancer diagnosis, including patient age, serum PSA concentration and keratin 34βE12, p63, and racemase expression, cannot substitute for convincing haematoxylin and eosin (H&E) microscopic findings. To avoid bias, the above information should be considered only in combination with routine microscopic examination.

Iczkowski and colleagues found that the histological features that most often preclude a definitive diagnosis of malignancy are the small size of the focus (70% of cases), disappearance on step levels (61%), lack of significant cytological atypia such as nucleolomegaly (55%) and associated inflammation (9%), raising the possibility of one of many mimics of adenocarcinoma [143]. Other causes include negative high-molecular-weight cytokeratin or p63 immunostain in the focus, atrophic or inflamed glands lacking a basal cell layer and the presence of associated PIN.

DO SUBSETS OF ASAP EXIST?

Stratification of ASAP is not differentially predictive of cancer on repeat biopsy despite multiple attempts. We stratified suspicion in each ASAP case into three levels: ASAPB (atypical small acinar proliferation suspicious for but not diagnostic of malignancy, favour benign); ASAPS (atypical small acinar proliferation suspicious for but not diagnostic of malignancy); and ASAPH (atypical small acinar proliferation *highly* suspicious for but not diagnostic of malignancy). ASAPB was employed for cases in which we deemed the focus of concern unlikely to be cancer but could not with absolute certainty exclude the possibility. Conversely, ASAPH was employed for cases in which the focus was almost certainly carcinoma, but a confident diagnosis of cancer could not be rendered. ASAPS was employed for cases with intermediate suspicion.

Multiple studies [143, 144] revealed non-significant trends for increasing risk of subsequent cancer with increasing suspicion. Stratification of ASAP also did not predict the normalized per cent of involvement by cancer on positive repeat biopsy [145]. Thus, at present, the level of suspicion should not alter follow-up recommendations.

DOES ASAP PREDICT CANCER ON REPEAT BIOPSY?

In studies published between 1997 and 2001, the reported incidence of prostate cancer in repeat biopsies following a diagnosis of ASAP ranged from 34% to 60% (Table 3.4) [97, 102, 104, 143–150]. We recently reported the results of needle biopsies in patients with long-term follow-up who were biopsied after 2000 in order to accurately reflect the current state of clinical practice. Subsequent cancer was detected at a rate comparable to earlier reported cohorts of patients, in whom longitudinal repetitive PSA screening had been more recently introduced (37% vs. 34–60%; see Table 3.4) [104].

WHAT IS THE CLINICAL SIGNIFICANCE OF ASAP?

Similar to high-grade PIN, ASAP holds a significant predictive value for cancer on repeat biopsy [143–145]. ASAP represents undersampled cancer in at least 40% of cases [145, 149, 151]. Iczkowski et al. observed that some men with ASAP in the first set of biopsies and benign findings or high-grade PIN in the second biopsy may still have cancer that was not detected [145, 149].

False-negative results on repeat sextant biopsy in untreated men with documented adenocarcinoma occurred in 23% of repeat sextant biopsies [152]. These results suggest that the

Table 3.4 Cancer detection in patients with ASAP

Date of publication	Study dates	References	No.of subjects with repeat biopsy(ies)	Frequency of diagnosis (%)	ASAP CA (%)
1997	1993–1995	Cheville et al. [144]	25	4.8	60
1997	1993–1996	Iczkowski et al. [143]	33	100	45
1998	1991–1995	Iczkowski et al. [145]	295	100	42
1998	1989–1996	Renshaw et al. [147]	59	18	34
1999	1992–1993	Chan et al. [146]	92	100	49
2001	1991–1998	Park et al. [148]	45	100	51
2001	1995–2000	Borboroglu et al. [97]	48	3.8	48
2002	1990–2001	Iczkowski et al. [149]	129	3.2	45
2004	2001–2003	Fadare et al. [150]	24	2.8	38
2005	1998–2003	Moore et al. [102]	53	100	36
2005	2000–2002	Schlesinger et al. [104]	78	23	37

current practice of performing 6–12 biopsies per prostate does not lower the frequency of ASAP. A declining volume of cancer at prostatectomy was noted 5 years ago [153], and is probably reflective of increased screening and multiple sampling. Thus, as smaller volume cancers are detected through increased sampling, many will be undersampled and their diagnosis will not be resolvable by immunostaining: an irreducible rate of ASAP diagnosis may therefore be anticipated.

What prostatic sites should be sampled at repeat biopsy? In one report, the investigators found that that sampling only the side or sextant site initially diagnosed as ASAP missed cancer in 39% of patients whose cancer was later detected exclusively at other sites, suggesting that the entire prostate should be rebiopsied [145].

In a recent provocative report, the investigators recommended immediate radical prostatectomy in patients with a biopsy diagnosis of ASAP. They suggested that the risk of subsequent cancer is 100% in radical prostatectomy specimens [154]. We urge caution in recommending expansion of the indications for prostatectomy to include patients with ASAP. ASAP is best considered as a diagnostic risk category and not a true entity.

The recent development of immunohistochemical stains for alpha-methylacyl coenzyme A racemase (P504S) has greatly facilitated the diagnostic support provided by basal cell specific antikeratin and p63, particularly in equivocal biopsies such as ASAP. We routinely use these important techniques in the diagnostic work-up of atypical prostate lesions on needle biopsies, thereby decreasing the incidence of ASAP and reducing the risk of false-negatives and the need for additional biopsies, similar to other reports [155–158]; a technical limitation is preservation of the focus of concern on the levels used for immunostaining [159].

WHAT IS THE SIGNIFICANCE OF ASAP IN COMBINATION WITH PIN?

We recently reported that the combination of high-grade PIN and ASAP lesions (Figures 3.5 and 3.6), found in up to 16% of biopsy sets, had an intermediate predictive value of 33% for cancer [104]. Thus, it is slightly lower than isolated ASAP (37%), but higher than isolated PIN (23%), and the predictive value of the diagnosis of PIN/ASAP combined is similar to that of ASAP alone. In previous reports, associated PIN occurred in 23% ($n = 56$) [142] and 31% ($n = 54$) [144] of cases. We found that the frequency of associated PIN was higher, occurring in 41% of total cases with ASAP ($n = 132$) [104] but most foci were not adjacent or contiguous.

In a similar investigation, a lesion containing both PIN and ASAP ($n = 51$) was reported to have cancer in 46% of follow-up biopsies. This lesion was carefully defined, and corresponded to our definition of contiguous PIN + ASAP lesions [92]. Three reasons might account for the difference in predictive values, 33% vs. 46%, seen in our recent report and this study. First, the latter study was restricted to contiguous cases; this type of lesion might have an intrinsically higher predictive value for cancer than in our series, in which the frequency of contiguous lesions was about half. The selection bias present in cases referred for consultation also may have influenced the study results compared with unselected primary cases in another study cohort. Finally, only a modest number of patients were reported in each study so that skewing of data may have occurred. The best available evidence today indicates that the presence of either or both lesions in needle biopsies is still a predictor for concurrent/subsequent cancer compared with patients lacking these lesions.

A novel finding was that high-grade PIN was more than twice as frequent in association with minimal cancer (57%) as ASAP (23%). High-grade PIN accompanied 14% [143] to 31% [144] of ASAP foci, but only 13% of cancers in biopsies [160]. About half of cases of ASAP are probably undersampled cancer [143–145], and the smaller mean size of the foci in contemporary specimens decreases the likelihood of sampling accompanying high-grade PIN.

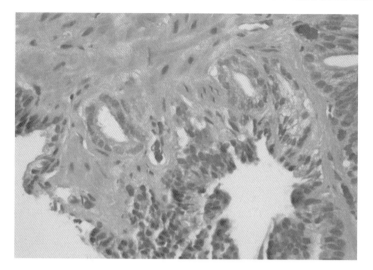

Figure 3.5 PIN+ASAP. Small acini with architectural distortion and prominent nuclei and nucleoli in association with high-grade prostatic intraepithelial neoplasia (PIN). An unequivocal diagnosis cannot be rendered due to the small size of this focus and full complement of architectural and cytological abnormalities (H&E, 400×).

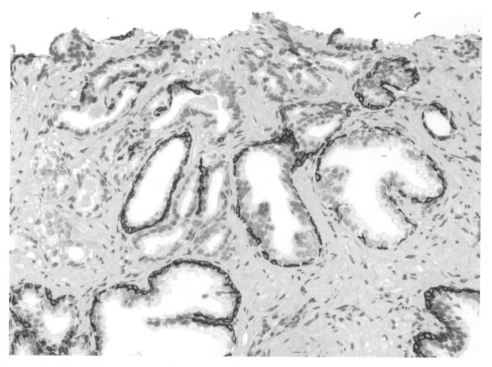

Figure 3.6 PIN+ASAP. Immunostain for keratin 34βE12 reveals lack of basal cell staining in the small acini suspicious but not diagnostic of malignancy (stained slide, 200×).

CONCLUSION

High-grade PIN is the most likely precursor of prostatic adenocarcinoma, according to virtually all available evidence. The clinical importance of recognizing PIN is based on its strong association with prostatic carcinoma. PIN has a high predictive value as a marker for adenocarcinoma, and its identification in biopsy specimens of the prostate warrants further search for concurrent invasive carcinoma. Studies to date have not determined whether PIN remains stable, regresses or progresses, although the implication is that it can progress.

The predictive accuracy for cancer is lower for both PIN and for ASAP in a highly screened patient population compared with previously reported populations. However, the presence of either or both histological markers in a biopsy set is still a significant predictor for concurrent/subsequent cancer compared to the cohorts of patients lacking these lesions. Thus, even though the predictive value of these lesions has decreased, they remain significant risk factors for prostate cancer.

REFERENCES

1. Bostwick DG, Pacelli A, Lopez-Beltran A. Molecular biology of prostatic intraepithelial neoplasia. *Prostate* 1996; 29:117–134.
2. Foster CS, Bostwick DG, Bonkhoff H *et al.* Cellular and molecular pathology of prostate cancer precursors. *Scand J Urol Nephrol Suppl* 2000:19–43.
3. Bostwick DG, Norlen BJ, Denis L. Prostatic intraepithelial neoplasia: the preinvasive stage of prostate cancer. Overview of the prostate committee report. *Scand J Urol Nephrol Suppl* 2000:1–2.
4. Bostwick DG, Montironi R, Sesterhenn IA. Diagnosis of prostatic intraepithelial neoplasia: Prostate Working Group/consensus report. *Scand J Urol Nephrol Suppl* 2000:3–10.
5. Bostwick DG. Prostatic intraepithelial neoplasia is a risk factor for cancer. *Semin Urol Oncol* 1999; 17:187–198.
6. Bostwick DG, Shan A, Qian J *et al.* Independent origin of multiple foci of prostatic intraepithelial neoplasia: comparison with matched foci of prostate carcinoma. *Cancer* 1998; 83:1995–2002.
7. McNeal JE, Bostwick DG. Intraductal dysplasia: a premalignant lesion of the prostate. *Hum Pathol* 1986; 17(1):64–71.
8. McNeal JE, Yemoto CE. Spread of adenocarcinoma within prostatic ducts and acini. Morphologic and clinical correlations. *Am J Surg Pathol* 1996; 20:802–814.
9. Bostwick DG, Brawer MK. Prostatic intra-epithelial neoplasia and early invasion in prostate cancer. *Cancer* 1987; 59:788–794.
10. Egevad L, Allsbrook WC, Epstein JI. Current practice of diagnosis and reporting of prostatic intraepithelial neoplasia and glandular atypia among genitourinary pathologists. *Mod Pathol* 2006; 19:180–185.
11. Allam CK, Bostwick DG, Hayes JA *et al.* Interobserver variability in the diagnosis of high-grade prostatic intraepithelial neoplasia and adenocarcinoma. *Mod Pathol* 1996; 9:742–751.
12. Epstein JI, Grignon DJ, Humphrey PA *et al.* Interobserver reproducibility in the diagnosis of prostatic intraepithelial neoplasia. *Am J Surg Pathol* 1995; 19:873–886.
13. Montironi R, Bostwick DG, Bonkhoff H *et al.* Origins of prostate cancer. *Cancer* 1996; 78:362–365.
14. Jemal A, Siegel R, Ward E *et al.* Cancer statistics, 2006. *CA Cancer J Clin* 2006; 56:106–130.
15. Greenlee R H-HM, Murray T *et al.* Cancer statistics, 2001. *CA Cancer J Clin* 2001; 51:15–36.
16. Steiner MS, Raghow S, Neubauer BL. Selective estrogen receptor modulators for the chemoprevention of prostate cancer. *Urology* 2001; 57(4 Suppl 1):68–72.
17. Qian J, Wollan P, Bostwick DG. The extent and multicentricity of high-grade prostatic intraepithelial neoplasia in clinically localized prostatic adenocarcinoma. *Hum Pathol* 1997; 28:143–148.
18. Lee F, Torp-Pedersen ST, Carroll JT, Siders DB, Christensen-Day C, Mitchell AE. Use of transrectal ultrasound and prostate-specific antigen in diagnosis of prostatic intraepithelial neoplasia. *Urology* 1989; 34(6 Suppl):4–8.
19. Sakr WA, Haas GP, Cassin BF, Pontes JE, Crissman JD. The frequency of carcinoma and intraepithelial neoplasia of the prostate in young male patients. *J Urol* 1993; 150(2 Pt 1):379–385.
20. Yin M, Becich MJ, Delo A, Dhir R. Prevalence of incidental prostate cancer in the general population. [Abstract]. *Lab Invest* 2006; 86:169A.

21. Sakr WA, Sarkar FH, Sreepathi P, Drozdowicz S, Crissman JD. Measurement of cellular proliferation in human prostate by AgNOR, PCNA, and SPF. *Prostate* 1993; 22:147–154.
22. Fowler JE, Jr., Bigler SA, Lynch C, Wilson SS, Farabaugh PB. Prospective study of correlations between biopsy-detected high grade prostatic intraepithelial neoplasia, serum prostate specific antigen concentration, and race. *Cancer* 2001; 91:1291–1296.
23. Angwafo FF, III, Zaher A, Befidi-Mengue R *et al*. High-grade intra-epithelial neoplasia and prostate cancer in Dibombari, Cameroon. *Prostate Cancer Prostatic Dis* 2003; 6:34–38.
24. Sakr WA. Prostatic intraepithelial neoplasia: A marker for high-risk groups and a potential target for chemoprevention. *Eur Urol* 1999; 35(5–6):474–478.
25. Fujita MQ, Shin M, Yasunaga Y *et al*. Incidence of prostatic intra-epithelial neoplasia in Osaka, Japan. *Int J Cancer* 1997; 73:808–811.
26. Sakr WA, Grignon DJ, Crissman JD *et al*. High grade prostatic intraepithelial neoplasia (HGPIN) and prostatic adenocarcinoma between the ages of 20–69: an autopsy study of 249 cases. *In Vivo* 1994; 8:439–443.
27. Helpap B, Bonkhoff H, Cockett A *et al*. Relationship between atypical adenomatous hyperplasia (AAH), prostatic intraepithelial neoplasia (PIN) and prostatic adenocarcinoma. *Pathologica* 1997; 89:288–300.
28. Bostwick DG, Aquilina JW. Prostatic intraepithelial neoplasia (PIN) and other prostatic lesions as risk factors and surrogate endpoints for cancer chemoprevention trials. *J Cell Biochem Suppl* 1996; 25:156–164.
29. Qian J, Bostwick DG. The extent and zonal location of prostatic intraepithelial neoplasia and atypical adenomatous hyperplasia: relationship with carcinoma in radical prostatectomy specimens. *Pathol Res Pract* 1995; 191:860–867.
30. Rochester M. International consultation on prostatic intraepithelial neoplasia pathologic staging of prostatic carcinoma, 3–4 November, 1995. *Cancer* 1996; 78:320–381.
31. Epstein JI, Herawi M. Prostate needle biopsies containing prostatic intraepithelial neoplasia or atypical foci suspicious for carcinoma: implications for patient care. *J Urol* 2006; 175(3 Pt 1):820–834.
32. Herawi M, Kahane H, Cavallo C, Epstein JI. Risk of prostate cancer on first re-biopsy within 1 year following a diagnosis of high grade prostatic intraepithelial neoplasia is related to the number of cores sampled. *J Urol* 2006; 175:121–124.
33. Epstein JI. What's new in prostate cancer disease assessment in 2006? *Curr Opin Urol* 2006; 16:146–151.
34. Skjorten FJ, Berner A, Harvei S, Robsahm TE, Tretli S. Prostatic intraepithelial neoplasia in surgical resections: relationship to coexistent adenocarcinoma and atypical adenomatous hyperplasia of the prostate. *Cancer* 1997; 79:1172–1179.
35. Gaudin PB, Sesterhenn IA, Wojno KJ, Mostofi FK, Epstein JI. Incidence and clinical significance of high-grade prostatic intraepithelial neoplasia in TURP specimens. *Urology* 1997; 49:558–563.
36. Brawer MK, Bigler SA, Sohlberg OE, Nagle RB, Lange PH. Significance of prostatic intraepithelial neoplasia on prostate needle biopsy. *Urology* 1991; 38:103–107.
37. Bostwick DG, Amin MB, Dundore P, Marsh W, Schultz DS. Architectural patterns of high-grade prostatic intraepithelial neoplasia. *Hum Pathol* 1993; 24:298–310.
38. Reyes AO, Swanson PE, Carbone JM, Humphrey PA. Unusual histologic types of high-grade prostatic intraepithelial neoplasia. *Am J Surg Pathol* 1997; 21:1215–1222.
39. Bock BJ, Bostwick DG. Does prostatic ductal adenocarcinoma exist? *Am J Surg Pathol* 1999; 23:781–785.
40. de la Torre M, Haggman M, Brandstedt S, Busch C. Prostatic intraepithelial neoplasia and invasive carcinoma in total prostatectomy specimens: distribution, volumes and DNA ploidy. *Br J Urol* 1993; 72:207–213.
41. Richie JP, Kavoussi LR, Ho GT *et al*. Prostate cancer screening: role of the digital rectal examination and prostate-specific antigen. *Ann Surg Oncol* 1994; 1:117–120.
42. Feneley MR, Busch C. Precursor lesions for prostate cancer. *J R Soc Med* 1997; 90:533–539.
43. Hoedemaeker RF, Kranse R, Rietbergen JB, Kruger AE, Schroder FH, van der Kwast TH. Evaluation of prostate needle biopsies in a population-based screening study: the impact of borderline lesions. *Cancer* 1999; 85:145–152.
44. Langer JE, Rovner ES, Coleman BG *et al*. Strategy for repeat biopsy of patients with prostatic intraepithelial neoplasia detected by prostate needle biopsy. *J Urol* 1996; 155:228–231.
45. Wills ML, Hamper UM, Partin AW, Epstein JI. Incidence of high-grade prostatic intraepithelial neoplasia in sextant needle biopsy specimens. *Urology* 1997; 49:367–373.
46. Perachino M, di Ciolo L, Barbetti V *et al*. Results of rebiopsy for suspected prostate cancer in symptomatic men with elevated PSA levels. *Eur Urol* 1997; 32:155–159.

47. O'Dowd GJ, Miller MC, Orozco R, Veltri RW. Analysis of repeated biopsy results within 1 year after a noncancer diagnosis. *Urology* 2000; 55:553–559.

48. Montironi R, Diamanti L, Pomante R, Thompson D, Bartels PH. Subtle changes in benign tissue adjacent to prostate neoplasia detected with a Bayesian belief network. *J Pathol* 1997; 182:442–449.

49. Qian J, Jenkins RB, Bostwick DG. Detection of chromosomal anomalies and c-myc gene amplification in the cribriform pattern of prostatic intraepithelial neoplasia and carcinoma by fluorescence in situ hybridization. *Mod Pathol* 1997; 10:1113–1119.

50. Qian J, Jenkins RB, Bostwick DG. Genetic and chromosomal alterations in prostatic intraepithelial neoplasia and carcinoma detected by fluorescence in situ hybridization. *Eur Urol* 1999; 35(5–6):479–483.

51. Montironi R, Mazzucchelli R, Algaba F, Lopez-Beltran A. Morphological identification of the patterns of prostatic intraepithelial neoplasia and their importance. *J Clin Pathol* 2000; 53:655–665.

52. Qian J, Jenkins RB, Bostwick DG. Determination of gene and chromosome dosage in prostatic intraepithelial neoplasia and carcinoma. *Anal Quant Cytol Histol* 1998; 20:373–380.

53. Sakr WA, Partin AW. Histological markers of risk and the role of high-grade prostatic intraepithelial neoplasia. *Urology* 2001; 57(4 Suppl 1):115–120.

54. Qian J, Jenkins RB, Bostwick DG. Potential markers of aggressiveness in prostatic intraepithelial neoplasia detected by fluorescence in situ hybridization. *Eur Urol* 1996; 30:177–184.

55. Montironi R, Filho AL, Santinelli A *et al.* Nuclear changes in the normal-looking columnar epithelium adjacent to and distant from prostatic intraepithelial neoplasia and prostate cancer. Morphometric analysis in whole-mount sections. *Virchows Arch* 2000; 437:625–634.

56. Zhou M, Shah R, Shen R, Rubin MA. Basal cell cocktail (34betaE12 + p63) improves the detection of prostate basal cells. *Am J Surg Pathol* 2003; 27:365–371.

57. Novis DA, Zarbo RJ, Valenstein PA. Diagnostic uncertainty expressed in prostate needle biopsies. A College of American Pathologists Q-probes Study of 15,753 prostate needle biopsies in 332 institutions. *Arch Pathol Lab Med* 1999; 123:687–692.

58. Wojno KJ, Epstein JI. The utility of basal cell-specific anti-cytokeratin antibody (34 beta E12) in the diagnosis of prostate cancer. A review of 228 cases. *Am J Surg Pathol* 1995; 19:251–260.

59. Varma M, Linden MD, Amin MB. Effect of formalin fixation and epitope retrieval techniques on antibody 34betaE12 immunostaining of prostatic tissues. *Mod Pathol* 1999; 12:472–478.

60. Amin MB, Schultz DS, Zarbo RJ. Analysis of cribriform morphology in prostatic neoplasia using antibody to high-molecular-weight cytokeratins. *Arch Pathol Lab Med* 1994; 118:260–264.

61. Ramnani DM, Bostwick DG. Basal cell-specific anti-keratin antibody 34betaE12: optimizing its use in distinguishing benign prostate and cancer [editorial; comment]. *Mod Pathol* 1999; 12:443–444.

62. Shin M, Fujita MQ, Yasunaga Y, Miki T, Okuyama A, Aozasa K. Utility of immunohistochemical detection of high molecular weight cytokeratin for differential diagnosis of proliferative conditions of the prostate. *Int J Urol* 1998; 5:237–242.

63. Freibauer C. Diagnosis of prostate carcinoma on biopsy specimens improved by basal-cell-specific anti-cytokeratin antibody (34 beta E12). *Wien Klin Wochenschr 18* 1998; 110:608–611.

64. Brawer MK, Nagle RB, Pitts W, Freiha F, Gamble SL. Keratin immunoreactivity as an aid to the diagnosis of persistent adenocarcinoma in irradiated human prostates. *Cancer* 1989; 63:454–460.

65. Saboorian MH, Huffman H, Ashfaq R, Ayala AG, Ro JY. Distinguishing Cowper's glands from neoplastic and pseudoneoplastic lesions of prostate: immunohistochemical and ultrastructural studies. *Am J Surg Pathol* 1997; 21:1069–1074.

66. Cina SJ, Silberman MA, Kahane H, Epstein JI. Diagnosis of Cowper's glands on prostate needle biopsy. *Am J Surg Pathol* 1997; 21:550–555.

67. Yang XJ, Lecksell K, Gaudin P, Epstein JI. Rare expression of high-molecular-weight cytokeratin in adenocarcinoma of the prostate gland: a study of 100 cases of metastatic and locally advanced prostate cancer. *Am J Surg Pathol* 1999; 23:147–152.

68. Devaraj LT, Bostwick DG. Atypical basal cell hyperplasia of the prostate. Immunophenotypic profile and proposed classification of basal cell proliferations. *Am J Surg Pathol* 1993; 17:645–659.

69. Bonkhoff H, Stein U, Remberger K. The proliferative function of basal cells in the normal and hyperplastic human prostate. *Prostate* 1994; 24:114–118.

70. Green R, Epstein JI. Use of intervening unstained slides for immunohistochemical stains for high molecular weight cytokeratin on prostate needles biopsies. *Am J Surg Pathol* 1999; 23:567–570.

71. O'Malley FP, Grignon DJ, Shum DT. Usefulness of immunoperoxidase staining with high-molecular-weight cytokeratin in the differential diagnosis of small-acinar lesions of the prostate gland. *Virchows Arch A Pathol Anat Histopathol* 1990; 417:191–196.

72. Srigley JR, Dardick I, Hartwick RW, Klotz L. Basal epithelial cells of human prostate gland are not myoepithelial cells. A comparative immunohistochemical and ultrastructural study with the human salivary gland. *Am J Pathol* 1990; 136:957–966.

73. Shah IA SM, Stinnett P *et al.* Cytokeratin immunohistochemistry as a diagnostic tool for distinguishing malignant from benign epithelial lesions of the prostate [see comments]. *Mod Pathol* 1991; 4:220–224.

74. Howat AJ, Mills PM, Lyons TJ, Stephenson TJ. Absence of S-100 protein in prostatic glands. *Histopathology* 1988; 13:468–470.

75. Adley BP, Yang XJ. Application of alpha-methylacyl coenzyme A racemase immunohistochemistry in the diagnosis of prostate cancer: a review. *Anal Quant Cytol Histol* 2006; 28:1–13.

76. Kunju LP, Chinnaiyan AM, Shah RB. Comparison of monoclonal antibody (P504S) and polyclonal antibody to alpha methylacyl-CoA racemase (AMACR) in the work-up of prostate cancer. *Histopathology* 2005; 47:587–596.

77. Kunju LP, Rubin MA, Chinnaiyan AM, Shah RB. Diagnostic usefulness of monoclonal antibody P504S in the workup of atypical prostatic glandular proliferations. *Am J Clin Pathol* 2003; 120:737–745.

78. Rubin MA, Zhou M, Dhanasekaran SM *et al.* alpha-Methylacyl coenzyme A racemase as a tissue biomarker for prostate cancer. *JAMA* 2002; 287:1662–1670.

79. Luo J, Zha S, Gage WR *et al.* Alpha-methylacyl-CoA racemase: a new molecular marker for prostate cancer. *Cancer Res* 2002; 62:2220–2226.

80. Beach R, Gown AM, De Peralta-Venturina MN *et al.* P504S immunohistochemical detection in 405 prostatic specimens including 376 18-gauge needle biopsies. *Am J Surg Pathol* 2002; 26:1588–1596.

81. Jiang Z, Woda BA, Rock KL *et al.* P504S: a new molecular marker for the detection of prostate carcinoma. *Am J Surg Pathol* 2001; 25:1397–1404.

82. Helpap B. The significance of the P504S expression pattern of high-grade prostatic intraepithelial neoplasia (HGPIN) with and without adenocarcinoma of the prostate in biopsy and radical prostatectomy specimens. *Virchows Arch* 2006; 448:480–4.

83. Gologan A, Bastacky S, McHale T *et al.* Age-associated changes in alpha-methyl CoA racemase (AMACR) expression in nonneoplastic prostatic tissues. *Am J Surg Pathol* 2005; 29:1435–1441.

84. Rioux-Leclercq N, Leray E, Patard JJ *et al.* The utility of Ki-67 expression in the differential diagnosis of prostatic intraepithelial neoplasia and ductal adenocarcinoma. *Hum Pathol* 2005; 36:531–535.

85. Hameed O, Humphrey PA. Stratified epithelium in prostatic adenocarcinoma: a mimic of high-grade prostatic intraepithelial neoplasia. *Mod Pathol* 2006; 19:899–906.

86. Bostwick DG, Chang L. Overdiagnosis of prostatic adenocarcinoma. *Semin Urol Oncol* 1999; 17:199–205.

87. Kilic S, Kukul E, Danisman A, Guntekin E, Sevuk M. Ratio of free to total prostate-specific antigen in patients with prostatic intraepithelial neoplasia. *Eur Urol* 1998; 34:176–180.

88. Ronnett BM, Carmichael MJ, Carter HB, Epstein JI. Does high grade prostatic intraepithelial neoplasia result in elevated serum prostate specific antigen levels? *J Urol* 1993; 150(2 Pt 1):386–389.

89. Alexander EE, Qian J, Wollan PC, Myers RP, Bostwick DG. Prostatic intraepithelial neoplasia does not appear to raise serum prostate-specific antigen concentration. *Urology* 1996; 47:693–698.

90. Ozden E, Gogus C, Karamursel T, Baltaci S, Kupeli S, Gogus O. Transrectal sonographic features of prostatic intraepithelial neoplasia: correlation with pathologic findings. *J Clin Ultrasound* 2005; 33:5–9.

91. Davidson D, Bostwick DG, Qian J *et al.* Prostatic intraepithelial neoplasia is a risk factor for adenocarcinoma: predictive accuracy in needle biopsies. *J Urol* 1995; 154:1295–1299.

92. Kronz JD, Allan CH, Shaikh AA, Epstein JI. Predicting cancer following a diagnosis of high-grade prostatic intraepithelial neoplasia on needle biopsy: data on men with more than one follow-up biopsy. *Am J Surg Pathol* 2001; 25:1079–1085.

93. Raviv G, Janssen T, Zlotta AR, Descamps F, Verhest A, Schulman CC. Prostatic intraepithelial neoplasia: influence of clinical and pathological data on the detection of prostate cancer. *J Urol* 1996; 156:1050–1055.

94. Shepherd D, Keetch DW, Humphrey PA, Smith DS, Stahl D. Repeat biopsy strategy in men with isolated prostatic intraepithelial neoplasia on prostate needle biopsy. *J Urol* 1996; 156(2 Pt 1):460–463.

95. Roscigno M, Scattoni V, Freschi M *et al.* Monofocal and plurifocal high-grade prostatic intraepithelial neoplasia on extended prostate biopsies: factors predicting cancer detection on extended repeat biopsy. *Urology* 2004; 63:1105–1110.

96. San Francisco IF, Olumi AF, Kao J, Rosen S, DeWolf WC. Clinical management of prostatic intraepithelial neoplasia as diagnosed by extended needle biopsies. *BJU Int* 2003; 91:350–354.

97. Borboroglu PG, Sur RL, Roberts JL, Amling CL. Repeat biopsy strategy in patients with atypical small acinar proliferation or high grade prostatic intraepithelial neoplasia on initial prostate needle biopsy. *J Urol* 2001; 166:866–870.

98. Naya Y, Ayala AG, Tamboli P, Babaian RJ. Can the number of cores with high-grade prostate intraepi-thelial neoplasia predict cancer in men who undergo repeat biopsy? *Urology* 2004; 63:503–508.

99. Goeman L JS, Ponette D, Van der Aa F, Roskams T, Oyen R, Van Poppel H. Is low-grade prostatic intraepithelial neoplasia a risk factor for cancer? *Prostate Cancer Prostatic Dis* 2003; 6:305–310.

100. Bishara T, Ramnani DM, Epstein JI. High-grade prostatic intraepithelial neoplasia on needle biopsy: risk of cancer on repeat biopsy related to number of involved cores and morphologic pattern. *Am J Surg Pathol* 2004; 28:629–633.

101. Lefkowitz GK, Sidhu GS, Torre P, Lepor H, Taneja SS. Is repeat prostate biopsy for high-grade prostatic intraepithelial neoplasia necessary after routine 12-core sampling? *Urology* 2001; 58:999–1003.

102. Moore CK, Karikehalli S, Nazeer T, Fisher HA, Kaufman RP, Jr., Mian BM. Prognostic significance of high grade prostatic intraepithelial neoplasia and atypical small acinar proliferation in the contempo-rary era. *J Urol* 2005; 173:70–72.

103. Postma R RM, Schroder FH, van der Kwast TH. Lesions predictive for prostate cancer in a screened population: first and second screening round findings. *Prostate* 2004; 61:260–6.

104. Schlesinger C, Bostwick DG, Iczkowski KA. High-grade prostatic intraepithelial neoplasia and atypical small acinar proliferation: predictive value for cancer in current practice. *Am J Surg Pathol* 2005; 29:1201–1207.

105. Gokden N, Roehl KA, Catalona WJ, Humphrey PA. High-grade prostatic intraepithelial neoplasia in needle biopsy as risk factor for detection of adenocarcinoma: current level of risk in screening popula-tion. *Urology* 2005; 65:538–542.

106. Girasole CR, Cookson MS, Putzi MJ *et al.* Significance of atypical and suspicious small acinar prolifera-tions, and high grade prostatic intraepithelial neoplasia on prostate biopsy: implications for cancer detection and biopsy strategy. *J Urol* 2006; 175:929–933.

107. Kamoi K, Troncoso P, Babaian RJ. Strategy for repeat biopsy in patients with high grade prostatic intraepithelial neoplasia. *J Urol* 2000; 163:819–823.

108. Alsikafi NF, Brendler CB, Gerber GS, Yang XJ. High-grade prostatic intraepithelial neoplasia with adjacent atypia is associated with a higher incidence of cancer on subsequent needle biopsy than high-grade prostatic intraepithelial neoplasia alone. *Urology* 2001; 57:296–300.

109. Maatman TJ, Papp SR, Carothers GG, Shockley KF. The critical role of patient follow-up after receiving a diagnosis of prostatic intraepithelial neoplasia. *Prostate Cancer Prostatic Dis* 2001; 4:63–66.

110. Abdel-Khalek M, El-Baz M, Ibrahiem el H. Predictors of prostate cancer on extended biopsy in patients with high-grade prostatic intraepithelial neoplasia: a multivariate analysis model. *BJU Int* 2004; 94:528–533.

111. El-Fakharany MM, Wojno KJ. Significance of high-grade prostatic intraepithelial neoplasia in the era of extended prostatic needle biopsies [Abstract]. *Mod Pathol* 2005; 18:152A.

112. Leite KRM, Mittledorf CATS, Camara-Lopes LH. Prostate biopsies following the diagnosis of PIN and ASAP: numbers and findings in the Brazilian population. [Abstract]. *Mod Pathol* 2005; 18:152A.

113. Hussein S, Leung CS, Kapusta L, Srigley JR. Temporal trends and cancer prediction rates for atypi-cal small acinar proliferation (ASAP) with or without associated high grade prostatic intraepithelial neoplasia (PIN). [Abstract]. *Lab Invest* 2006; 86:142A.

114. Keith JD, Akhavan A, McHale T *et al.* Predictive value of high-grade prostatic intraepithelial neoplasia (HGPIN) for prostatic adenocarcinoma (CaP) on 12-core prostate needle biopsy (Bx). [Abstract]. *Lab Invest* 2006; 86:144A.

115. Rabets JC, Jones JS, Patel A, Zippe CD. Prostate cancer detection with office based saturation biopsy in a repeat biopsy population. *J Urol* 2004; 172:94–97.

116. Burke HB, Hoang A, Bostwick DG. Determining a causal relationship between prostatic intraepithelial neoplasia (risk factor) and prostate cancer (disease): the fallacy of substituting backward and forward probabilities. *Submitted.*

117. Harvei S, Skjorten FJ, Robsahm TE, Berner A, Tretli S. Is prostatic intraepithelial neoplasia in the transi-tion/central zone a true precursor of cancer? A long-term retrospective study in Norway. *Br J Cancer* 1998; 78:46–49.

118. Pacelli A, Bostwick DG. Clinical significance of high-grade prostatic intraepithelial neoplasia in transurethral resection specimens. *Urology* 1997; 50:355–359.

119. Roustan Delatour NLD, Mai KT, Park PC, Burns BF. Positive predictive value of an isolated HGPIN in needle biopsy cores for prostatic adenocarcinoma. A study with complete sampling of hemi-prostates with correlating negative biopsies. [Abstract]. *Lab Invest* 2006; 86:158A.

120. Balaji KC, Rabbani F, Tsai H, Bastar A, Fair WR. Effect of neoadjuvant hormonal therapy on prostatic intraepithelial neoplasia and its prognostic significance. *J Urol* 1999; 162(3 Pt 1):753–757.

121. Ferguson J, Zincke H, Ellison E, Bergstrahl E, Bostwick DG. Decrease of prostatic intraepithelial neoplasia following androgen deprivation therapy in patients with stage T3 carcinoma treated by radical prostatectomy. *Urology* 1994; 44:91–95.

122. Vailancourt L, Têtu B, Fradet Y *et al.* Effect of neoadjuvant endocrine therapy (combined androgen blockade) on normal prostate and prostatic carcinoma. A randomized study. *Am J Surg Pathol* 1996; 20:86–93.

123. van der Kwast TH, Labrie F, Tetu B. Persistence of high-grade prostatic intra-epithelial neoplasia under combined androgen blockade therapy. *Hum Pathol* 1999; 30:1503–1507.

124. Alers JC, Krijtenburg PJ, Vissers KJ, Bosman FT, van der Kwast TH, van Dekken H. Interphase cytogenetics of prostatic adenocarcinoma and precursor lesions: analysis of 25 radical prostatectomies and 17 adjacent prostatic intraepithelial neoplasias. *Genes Chromosomes Cancer* 1995; 12:241–250.

125. Prostatic Intraepithelial Neoplasia and the Origins of Prostatic Carcinoma. Proceedings of the first international consultation meeting. Ancona, Italy, September 11–12, 1994. *Pathol Res Pract* 1995; 191:828–959.

126. Steiner MS. High-grade prostatic intraepithelial neoplasia and prostate cancer risk reduction. *World J Urol* 2003; 21:15–20.

127. Andriole G, Bostwick D, Civantos F *et al.* The effects of 5alpha-reductase inhibitors on the natural history, detection and grading of prostate cancer: current state of knowledge. *J Urol* 2005; 174:2098–2104.

128. Civantos F, Watson RB, Pinto JE *et al.* Finasteride effect on benign prostatic hyperplasia and prostate cancer. A comparative clinico-pathologic study of radical prostatectomies. *J Urol Pathol* 1997; 6:1–8.

129. Yang XJ, Lecksell K, Short K *et al.* Does long-term finasteride therapy affect the histologic features of benign prostatic tissue and prostate cancer on needle biopsy? PLESS Study Group. Proscar Long-Term Efficacy and Safety Study. *Urology* 1999; 53:696–700.

130. Montironi R, Pomante R, Diamanti L, Hamilton PW, Thompson D, Bartels PH. Evaluation of prostatic intraepithelial neoplasia after treatment with a 5-alpha-reductase inhibitor (finasteride). A methodologic approach. *Anal Quant Cytol Histol* 1996; 18:461–470.

131. Bostwick DG, Neumann R, Qian J, Cheng L. Reversibility of prostatic intraepithelial neoplasia: implications for chemoprevention. *Eur Urol* 1999; 35(5–6):492–495.

132. Arakawa A, Song S, Scardino PT, Wheeler TM. High grade prostatic intraepithelial neoplasia in prostates removed following irradiation failure in the treatment of prostatic adenocarcinoma. *Pathol Res Pract* 1995; 191:868–872.

133. Gaudin PB, Zelefsky MJ, Leibel SA, Fuks Z, Reuter VE. Histopathologic effects of three-dimensional conformal external beam radiation therapy on benign and malignant prostate tissues. *Am J Surg Pathol* 1999; 23:1021–1031.

134. Martens MB, Keller JH. Routine immunohistochemical staining for high-molecular weight cytokeratin 34-beta and alpha-methylacyl CoA racemase (P504S) in postirradiation prostate biopsies. *Mod Pathol* 2006; 19:287–290.

135. Bostwick DG. Prostatic intraepithelial neoplasia (PIN): current concepts. *J Cell Biochem Suppl* 1992; 16H:10–19.

136. Abbas F, Hochberg D, Civantos F, Soloway M. Incidental prostatic adenocarcinoma in patients undergoing radical cystoprostatectomy for bladder cancer. *Eur Urol* 1996; 30:322–326.

137. Montironi R, Pomante R, Diamanti L, Magi-Galluzzi C. Apoptosis in prostatic adenocarcinoma following complete androgen ablation. *Urol Int* 1998; 60 (Suppl 1):25–30.

138. Bostwick DG, Qian J. Effect of androgen deprivation therapy on prostatic intraepithelial neoplasia. *Urology* 2001; 58(2 Suppl 1):91–93.

139. Montironi R, Magi-Galluzzi C, Muzzonigro G, Prete E, Polito M, Fabris G. Effects of combination endocrine treatment on normal prostate, prostatic intraepithelial neoplasia, and prostatic adenocarcinoma. *J Clin Pathol* 1994; 47:906–913.

140. Steiner MS, Pound CR. Phase IIA clinical trial to test the efficacy and safety of Toremifene in men with high-grade prostatic intraepithelial neoplasia. *Clin Prostate Cancer* 2003; 2:24–31.

141. Price D, Stein B, Sieber P *et al.* Toremifene for the prevention of prostate cancer among men with high-grade prostatic intraepithelial neoplasia: results of a double-blind, placebo-controlled, phase IIB clinical trial. *In press.*

142. Iczkowski KA, Bostwick DG. Criteria for biopsy diagnosis of minimal volume prostatic adenocarcinoma: analytic comparison with nondiagnostic but suspicious atypical small acinar proliferation. *Arch Pathol Lab Med* 2000; 124:98–107.

143. Iczkowski KA, MacLennan GT, Bostwick DG. Atypical small acinar proliferation suspicious for malignancy in prostate needle biopsies: clinical significance in 33 cases. *Am J Surg Pathol* 1997; 21:1489–1495.

144. Cheville JC, Reznicek MJ, Bostwick DG. The focus of 'atypical glands, suspicious for malignancy' in prostatic needle biopsy specimens: incidence, histologic features, and clinical follow-up of cases diagnosed in a community practice. *Am J Clin Pathol* 1997; 108:633–640.

145. Iczkowski KA, Bassler TJ, Schwob VS *et al.* Diagnosis of 'suspicious for malignancy' in prostate biopsies: predictive value for cancer. *Urology* 1998; 51:749–758.

146. Chan TY, Epstein JI. Follow-up of atypical prostate needle biopsies suspicious for cancer. *Urology* 1999; 53:351–355.

147. Renshaw AA, Santis WF, Richie JP. Clinicopathological characteristics of prostatic adenocarcinoma in men with atypical prostate needle biopsies. *J Urol* 1998; 159:2018–2022.

148. Park S, Shinohara K, Grossfeld GD, Carroll PR. Prostate cancer detection in men with prior high grade prostatic intraepithelial neoplasia or atypical prostate biopsy. *J Urol* 2001; 165:1409–1414.

149. Iczkowski KA, Chen HM, Yang XJ, Beach RA. Prostate cancer diagnosed after initial biopsy with atypical small acinar proliferation suspicious for malignancy is similar to cancer found on initial biopsy. *Urology* 2002; 60:851–854.

150. Fadare O, Wang S, Mariappan MR Practice patterns of clinicians following isolated diagnoses of atypical small acinar proliferation on prostate biopsy specimens. *Arch Pathol Lab Med* 2004; 128:557–560.

151. Walsh PC. Prostate cancer diagnosed after initial biopsy with atypical small acinar proliferation suspicious for malignancy is similar to cancer found on initial biopsy. *J Urol* 2003; 170:316.

152. Rabbani F, Stroumbakis N, Kava BR, Cookson MS, Fair WR. Incidence and clinical significance of false-negative sextant prostate biopsies. *J Urol* 1998; 159:1247–1250.

153. DiGiuseppe JA, Sauvageot J, Epstein JI. Increasing incidence of minimal residual cancer in radical prostatectomy specimens. *Am J Surg Pathol* 1997; 21:174–178.

154. Brausi M, Castagnetti G, Dotti A, De Luca G, Olmi R, Cesinaro AM. Immediate radical prostatectomy in patients with atypical small acinar proliferation. Over treatment? *J Urol* 2004; 172:906–909.

155. Shah RB, Zhou M, LeBlanc M, Snyder M, Rubin MA. Comparison of the basal cell-specific markers, 34betaE12 and p63, in the diagnosis of prostate cancer. *Am J Surg Pathol* 2002; 26:1161–1168.

156. Browne TJ, Hirsch MS, Brodsky G, Welch WR, Loda MF, Rubin MA. Prospective evaluation of AMACR (P504S) and basal cell markers in the assessment of routine prostate needle biopsy specimens. *Hum Pathol* 2004; 35:1462–1468.

157. Jiang Z, Woda BA. Diagnostic utility of alpha-methylacyl CoA racemase (P504S) on prostate needle biopsy. *Adv Anat Pathol* 2004; 11:316–321.

158. Molinié V, Fromont G, Sibony M *et al.* Diagnostic utility of a p63/alpha-methyl-CoA-racemase (p504s) cocktail in atypical foci in the prostate. *Mod Pathol* 2004; 17:1180–1190.

159. Iczkowski KA. Current prostate biopsy interpretation: criteria for cancer, atypical small acinar proliferation, high-grade prostatic intraepithelial neoplasia, and use of immunostains. *Arch Pathol Lab Med* 2006; 130:835–843.

160. Epstein JI. Diagnostic criteria of limited adenocarcinoma of the prostate on needle biopsy. *Hum Pathol* 1995; 26:223–229.

161. Mettlin C, Lee F, Drago J, Murphy GP. The American Cancer Society National Prostate Cancer Detection Project. Findings on the detection of early prostate cancer in 2425 men. *Cancer* 1991; 67:2949–2958.

162. Feneley MR, Green JS, Young MP *et al.* Prevalence of prostatic intra-epithelial neoplasia (PIN) in biopsies from hospital practice and pilot screening: clinical implications. *Prostate Cancer Prostatic Dis* 1997; 1:79–83.

163. Bostwick DG, Qian J, Frankel K. The incidence of high grade prostatic intraepithelial neoplasia in needle biopsies. *J Urol* 1995; 154:1791–1794.

164. Gupta C, Ren JZ, Wojno KJ. Individual submission and embedding of prostate biopsies decreases rates of equivocal pathology reports. *Urology* 2004; 63:83–86.

165. Kobayashi T, Nishizawa K, Watanabe J, Ogura K, Mitsumori K, Ide Y. Effects of sextant transrectal prostate biopsy plus additional far lateral cores in improving cancer detection rates in men with large prostate glands. *Int J Urol* 2004; 11:392–396.

166. Tunc M, Sanli O, Kandirali E *et al.* Should high-grade prostatic intraepithelial neoplasia change our approach to infravesical obstruction? *Urol Int* 2005; 74:332–336.

4

Prostate cancer screening

Sarah Marietti, Peter C. Albertsen

When planning a screening programme for any disease, five key questions should be addressed [1]. Is the test screening for a significant, serious disease? Are the tests used to screen for the condition accurate? Is the outcome of the disease changed or improved by the use of the screening test? Does screening cause the patient harm? Does the screening produce more good than harm? This chapter will review each of these questions in an attempt to address the appropriateness of prostate cancer screening in contemporary medical practice.

IS THE TEST SCREENING FOR A SIGNIFICANT, SERIOUS DISEASE?

After lung cancer, prostate cancer is the second leading cause of cancer death in men in both the USA and Canada [2]. By the age of 79, men have a 1 in 8 chance of being diagnosed with prostate cancer, but a much lower chance of dying from the disease. African-American men are at a particularly high risk of developing prostate cancer. Between 1998 and 2002 the estimated prostate cancer incidence among African-American men was 272 per 100 000 men, one of the highest rates in the world [2, 3].

In the USA, prostate cancer incidence rates rose steadily from 1969 through the 1980s and then much more rapidly during the late 1980s and early 1990s, peaking in 1992 (Figure 4.1). Epidemiologists attribute the widespread use of transurethral resection of the prostate during the 1970s and 80s and the subsequent rise in testing for prostate-specific antigen (PSA) as the primary explanation for these trends [4]. Since 1992, US prostate cancer incidence rates have fallen by more than 11%, but now appear to be rising again. Contemporary incidence rates are considerably higher than previously recorded during the 1970s. From 1998 through to 2002, the US prostate cancer incidence rate was estimated to be 164 per 100 000 men, age-adjusted to the 2000 US standard population [3].

In the USA, mortality from prostate cancer has risen slowly for many decades, peaking in 1998 at a rate of 42 per 100 000 men, age adjusted to the 2000 US standard population [2] (Figure 4.2). Since then mortality rates have fallen by more than 25%. In 2006, the prostate cancer mortality rate was estimated to be 30.3 per 100 000 men, age adjusted to the 2000 US standard population [3]. When death rates are age-adjusted to the World Health Organization world standard population, the rates of prostate cancer seen in the USA are similar to rates seen in countries such as France, Germany and the UK, and somewhat lower than rates seen in Scandinavia. In contrast, the mortality rates from prostate cancer are much lower in Asia. Recently, rates have been rising in the more industrialized countries in Asia such as Japan. In 2002 the mortality rate from prostate cancer in Japan was 5.7 per 100 000, age adjusted to the World Health Organization world standard population [5].

Sarah Marietti, MD, Division of Urology, University of Connecticut Health Center, Farmington, Connecticut, USA
Peter C. Albertsen, MD, Division of Urology, University of Connecticut Health Center, Farmington, Connecticut, USA

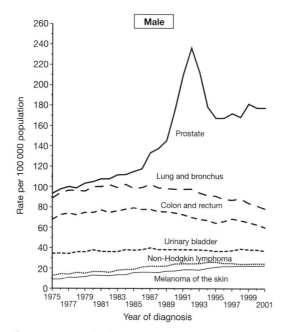

Figure 4.1   Incidence of prostate cancer in the USA 1975–2001 [5].

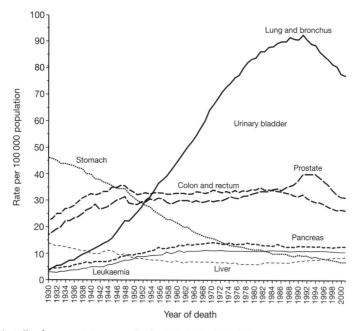

Figure 4.2   Mortality from prostate cancer in the USA 1975–2001 [5].

Prostate cancer poses an epidemiological conundrum. Recent studies have shown that the lifetime risk of prostate cancer diagnosis is about 16%, but the lifetime risk of dying from this disease is only 3.4% [6]. A recent paper by Thompson *et al.* [7] reported an extraordinarily high incidence of prostate cancer among 2950 healthy men participating in a prostate cancer chemoprevention study comparing finasteride and placebo. All of these men had PSA below 4.0 ng/ml at the start of the study, and in most men PSA remained below 4.0 during the 7 years of follow-up. Remarkably, 6.6% of the men with PSA less than 0.5 ng/ml had prostate cancer and 26.9% of the men with PSA between 3.1 and 4.0 ng/ml had prostate cancer. Clearly most of these men are not destined to die from prostate cancer.

These findings highlight a difficult paradox. Many prostate cancers are significant, serious problems resulting in the deaths of many otherwise healthy men. In addition, however, there are a significant number of indolent prostate cancers that are not destined to cause any harm. Does widespread PSA testing identify clinically significant disease or are a high percentage of screen-detected cancers likely to be indolent tumours that do not require diagnosis or treatment?

ARE THE TESTS USED TO SCREEN FOR THE CONDITION ACCURATE?

Screening for prostate cancer in contemporary practice usually consists of a digital rectal examination (DRE) and a serum PSA test. DRE alone has a very low positive predictive value in men with a PSA less than 3.0 ng/ml. However, when the DRE is used in combination with PSA, prostate cancer detection rates almost double [8]. PSA is a glycoprotein that is produced within normal prostate gland epithelium. PSA is not specific for prostate cancer. Serum PSA levels can increase either because of increased production or secondary to disruption of the epithelial barrier separating blood from prostate tissue. Prostate cancer, benign prostate hypertrophy (BPH), inflammation or manipulation can all raise serum PSA levels [9].

In 1991, Catalona et al. [10] first proposed using PSA testing as a screening tool and suggested 4.0 ng/ml as the upper limit of normal. In an effort to improve the sensitivity of PSA testing, many urologists have suggested lowering the cut point to 2.6 ng/ml in all men, but in particular for African-Americans [11]. While additional prostate cancers will be identified, lowering the cut point will also increase the number of false-positive tests and will increase the number of men without cancer who will be advised to undergo prostate ultrasound and biopsy.

To evaluate the accuracy of PSA testing, Gann et al. [12] performed a case–control study using data collected as part of the Physicians' Health Study. During this 10-year study designed to determine the effect of beta-carotene, 366 men developed clinical evidence of prostate cancer and 48 men died of their disease. By comparing PSA levels in stored sera from these men with sera from three matched controls from the study, they found that men with prostate cancer had a much higher probability of having an elevated PSA. Using the cut-off point of 4.0 ng/ml, they estimated that PSA testing had a 46% sensitivity of identifying clinically significant prostate cancer within the following 10 years and a 73% sensitivity of finding prostate cancer within the next 4 years. The overall specificity was 91% and changed little by year of follow-up.

To improve the utility of PSA testing, some researchers have proposed measuring the percentage of PSA that is bound to the enzyme α-chymotrypsin and the percentage that is free. Men with a very low ratio of free to bound PSA have a higher probability of having prostate cancer [13]. Unfortunately, in most instances this ratio is not helpful in distinguishing clinically significant from clinically insignificant prostate cancer.

PSA testing is often confounded by the presence of BPH. As prostates enlarge with age they produce greater quantities of PSA. This increases serum PSA values and leads to a large number of false-positive screening tests. To increase both the sensitivity and specificity of PSA testing, Benson et al. [14] proposed measuring PSA density. This is calculated by dividing the PSA value by the prostate volume as measured by transrectal ultrasonography (TRUS). Oesterling et al. [15] recognized that PSA values rise with age because of the increasing prevalence of BPH. They proposed age-specific reference ranges as a method to decrease the number of false-positive tests. They determined, for example, that the cut point for men aged 70–79 years should be 6.5 ng/ml rather than 4.0 ng/ml. Unfortunately, neither adjustment is widely accepted because many physicians are concerned about potentially missing a clinically significant cancer and are willing to tolerate a high rate of false-positive tests.

IS THE OUTCOME OF THE DISEASE CHANGED OR IMPROVED BY THE USE OF THE SCREENING TEST?

In order to determine whether the outcome of prostate cancer has been improved by PSA testing, it is imperative to know the natural history of screen-detected disease. Several studies have increased our understanding of the natural history of prostate cancer. In a series of four articles published between 1989 and 2004, Johanssen *et al.* [16–19] reported the long-term outcome of a cohort of 648 men diagnosed with prostate cancer between 1977 and 1984 in the Orebro Medical Center in Sweden. Five hundred and forty-two men were diagnosed with prostate cancer following aspiration biopsy and 106 were diagnosed following transurethral resection of the prostate (TRUP). Of the 648 men diagnosed with cancer, 300 had localized disease and of these 223 received no treatment for their disease. Initial reports revealed very low 5 and 10-year mortality rates. However, after a longer follow-up period of 15–20 years, Johanssen *et al.* noted an increase in prostate cancer mortality rates. After 20 years, 90% of the men had died, but only 16% appeared to have died from prostate cancer. They noted that the majority of prostate cancer deaths were among men with poorly differentiated tumours. Based on these studies, Johanssen *et al.* concluded that men with low-grade tumours and a life experience of less than 20 years are unlikely to die from prostate cancer. These findings are based on a cohort of men diagnosed with prostate cancer before the advent of PSA testing. Therefore, contemporary patients may require an even longer follow-up to benefit from aggressive screening and treatment.

Albertsen *et al.* [20] have documented the long-term outcomes of 767 Connecticut men diagnosed with clinically localized prostate cancer between 1971 and 1984, who were managed conservatively (Figure 4.3). All men were aged 55–74 at the time of diagnosis and were followed for over 20 years. Original pathology slides were re-examined to obtain accurate Gleason grading. Cause of death was determined from the death certificates on file with the Connecticut Vital Statistics Bureau. Older men with Gleason 2–4 tumours were much more likely to die of causes other than prostate cancer. Younger men, especially those men with high-grade cancers had a very high probability of dying from prostate cancer. Men with intermediate-grade cancers had an outcome in between. Men with Gleason 6 tumours had a 27% 20-year risk of dying from prostate cancer, while men with Gleason 7 tumours had a 45% 20-year risk of dying from prostate cancer. The age at diagnosis did not impact the prostate cancer-specific mortality rate, but did impact the risk of dying from other causes.

While these studies have advanced our understanding of the natural history of prostate cancer, there is still much we do not know about this disease. PSA testing has identified a large cohort of men with relatively low-grade tumours. Do these tumours progress in the same manner as described by the studies above? Are most low-grade prostate cancers identified by PSA testing truly indolent, or do they progress to clinically significant disease as men age? Do clinically significant tumours metastasize early in their course, or do they remain localized in the prostate for many years? PSA is only valuable as a screening tool if it is able to identify clinically significant disease while it is confined to the prostate.

DOES SCREENING CAUSE THE PATIENT HARM?

Although screening for PSA only involves obtaining a single blood test, several subsequent events must be considered before the test can be deemed innocuous. A positive test result affects the patient not only mentally but also physically, as it often leads to a transrectal

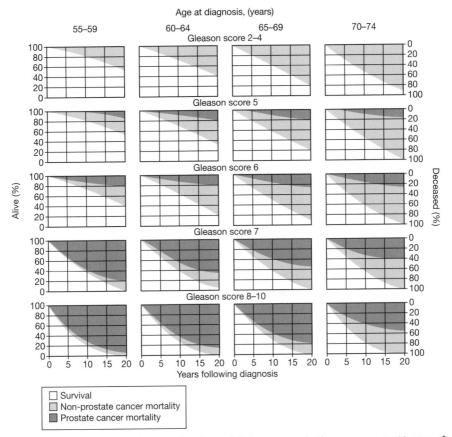

Figure 4.3 Survival and cumulative mortality from prostate cancer and other causes up to 20 years after diagnosis stratified by age at diagnosis and Gleason score ©2007 American Medical Association. All rights reserved [20].

ultrasound and prostate biopsy [21]. Although the procedure is uncomfortable it is well tolerated by most men and usually is performed as an office procedure under local anaesthesia. The risks of a biopsy are small but not insignificant. Haemorrhage and/or infection occurs in 1–4% of cases.

Most of the morbidity associated with PSA testing is related to the treatment procedures that are currently available. In men with clinically significant prostate cancers, complications associated with treatment are considered acceptable if the treatments cure the disease or prolong life. In men who harbour indolent disease, however, any morbidity from treatment lowers overall quality of life.

Options currently available to treat prostate cancer include surgical prostatectomy, external beam radiation, internal radioactive seed placement and cryotherapy. Unfortunately, no data are available that document the relative efficacy of these treatments to cure screendetected prostate cancer. To date, only one large randomized trial has reported a survival advantage among men undergoing surgery to treat localized prostate cancer. In 2005, Bill-Axelson et al. [22] reported the 10-year outcomes of a randomized trial involving 695 men with localized prostate cancer who were randomized to receive radical prostatectomy versus conservative management. After 10 years, the prostate cancer-specific mortality rate was 14% for the group treated conservatively versus 8% for the group undergoing radical prostatectomy. Overall survival between the two groups favoured those men undergoing radical prostatectomy, but the difference was relatively small. Among men undergoing radical prostatectomy 76% were alive after 10 years compared with only 69% of the men undergoing conservative management. Comparable data supporting the efficacy of radiation therapy or cryotherapy are not available. Large case series suggest that results may be similar, but this remains to be determined. Furthermore, it is unclear whether similar results can be achieved in a population of screen-detected men.

The Prostate Cancer Outcomes Study was developed to obtain information concerning the impact of treatment on quality of life. Patients participating in the study were identified by five sites participating in the Surveillance Epidemiology and End Results (SEER) programme sponsored by the National Cancer Institute [23]. The study was a large, prospective population-based study that followed men with localized prostate cancer diagnosed in 1994 and 1995. Men enrolled in the study completed surveys shortly after diagnosis and again 12, 24 and 60 months later. The questions were designed to evaluate sexual, bowel and bladder function over time following treatment for prostate cancer. The questions also evaluated the overall impact on quality of life. Of the 1291 men undergoing radical prostatectomy, 59.9% were impotent and 8.4% were incontinent 18 months after surgery. Forty-one per cent answered that sexual performance was a moderate to large problem after treatment. Of the 497 patients who received external beam radiation, 43% of the previously potent men were impotent within 2 years and 5.4% had significant bowel dysfunction [24]. Similar findings have been noted in the large Swedish randomized trial comparing radical prostatectomy with conservative management. In 2002, Steineck *et al.* [25] reported that 80% of men undergoing surgery had erectile dysfunction compared with only 45% of those managed by observation alone. Incontinence in the surgical group was as high as 49% compared with only 21% in the observation group. Several case series have also reported serious side-effects associated with radioactive seed implants and with cryosurgery.

DOES THE SCREENING PRODUCE MORE GOOD THAN HARM?

The primary purpose of screening for prostate cancer is to decrease the morbidity and mortality associated with this disease. Since 1998, prostate cancer mortality rates in the USA have been falling, but epidemiologists are uncertain what is driving these changes. Some researchers speculate that the decline is a direct result of intensive PSA testing and aggressive treatment of the disease [26]. Others argue that the declines in prostate cancer mortality have occurred much earlier than would be expected from screening and treatment and suggest other hypotheses such as the early widespread use of antiandrogen therapy or other environmental factors [27]. Cooperberg *et al.* [28] have reported an increase in the use of hormonal therapy for the treatment of prostate cancer during the same time period as the decline in mortality rates. These and other data suggest that the early use of hormonal therapy may yield a survival benefit.

Why do some epidemiologists express doubt that PSA testing has produced a decline in prostate cancer mortality? One issue is lead time. Screening identifies disease earlier in its natural course. Patients diagnosed with prostate cancer often appear to survive longer than patients who are diagnosed with prostate cancer when it presents clinically. Once lead time is accounted for, the presumed survival advantage associated with screening may disappear.

The widespread use of PSA testing has caused many men to be diagnosed with prostate cancer much earlier in their lives when compared with the pre-PSA era. Gann *et al.* [12] originally estimated that the lead time associated with PSA testing was 3–5 years. More recently Draisma *et al.* [29] estimated the potential lead time associated with PSA testing as part of the large European Randomized Study of Screening for Prostate Cancer. In 2003, they published a model that suggested that prostate cancer diagnosis was advanced by as much as 10 years among men aged 55 years at the time of diagnosis and 5 years for men aged 75. Since men undergoing conservative management for localized prostate cancer can survive on average at least 10 years, it would take 15–20 years to demonstrate a significant decline in prostate cancer mortality based on a programme of PSA testing and treatment.

Widespread PSA screening appears to have raised another significant concern: the overdetection of indolent disease. Overdetection refers to the ability of a screening test to identify a condition that would have remained silent and caused a patient no morbidity during his lifetime. Epidemiologists have long known that repeated use of a screening test will, over time, more frequently identify relatively asymptomatic, slow-growing tumours compared with aggressive tumours. They often refer to this concept as 'length time bias'. Several studies have clearly shown that there is a high prevalence of indolent prostate cancer. Draisma *et al.* [29] estimated that at age 55, the lead time associated with PSA testing is approximately 12.3 years and results in an overdetection rate of 27%. By age 75, lead time decreases to 6.0 years, while the rate of overdetection increases to 56%. They concluded that while lead time decreases with age, screening all men aged 55–67 years annually would overdetect this disease by as much as 50%. Therefore, widespread testing for PSA could possibly result in identifying indolent cancers in approximately half of all new diagnoses.

Changes in the application of Gleason scoring have also contributed to the prostate cancer screening conundrum. The previously reported studies describing the natural history of prostate cancer stratified patients according to Gleason score, one of the most powerful predictors of prostate cancer mortality. Most researchers and clinicians agree that Gleason 2–5 tumours pose little threat of prostate cancer mortality over 20 years. Unfortunately, these tumours are rarely reported in contemporary practice. In an analysis of changes in the application of Gleason scoring, Albertsen *et al.* [30] analysed 1858 men who were diagnosed between 1990 and 1992 with localized prostate cancer. Original pathology slides were identified and re-read using contemporary Gleason grading criteria. A comparison of the contemporary readings with the historical readings demonstrated a significant shift towards higher grades in the contemporary cohort (Figure 4.4). As a consequence, men with contemporary Gleason 6 and 7 tumours on biopsy have a superior prognosis when compared with historical controls.

Most researchers agree that the patients most likely to benefit from PSA testing are those who are destined to harbour higher grade tumours. Unfortunately, the shift in the applica-

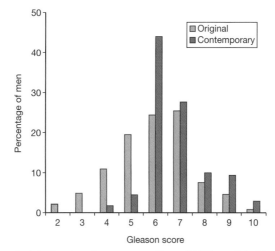

Figure 4.4 Distribution of original and contemporary readings of 1850 prostate biopsies performed between 1990 and 1992 [30].

tion of Gleason scoring has moved many men with indolent disease into higher categories thereby altering our understanding of the risk posed by this disease. From an epidemiological standpoint, this further amplifies length time bias and will make it even more difficult to determine whether PSA testing has yielded a positive net effect in contemporary practice.

Enthusiastic supporters of PSA screening frequently cite improvements in 5- and 10-year survival rates as proof of the effectiveness of PSA screening. Unfortunately, this is an inappropriate metric to evaluate the effectiveness of a screening programme because it is significantly affected by the lead time associated with screening. In 2000, Welch and Black [31] discussed the impact of lead time on cancer mortality rates. They found that both the prevalence of disease and the consequences of its treatment modalities depend on the level of screening for that disease in the population. Improvements in 5- and 10-year survival rates do not always correlate with mortality rate decreases. From 1950 to 1966, the 5-year survival rates for prostate cancer in the USA increased by 50%. During this same time period the prostate cancer mortality rates also increased by 10%. Thus, the increased survival rates did not proportionally affect the mortality rates.

Two large randomized trials are currently in progress to test whether PSA screening reduces prostate cancer mortality rates. They include the European Randomized Study of Prostate Cancer sponsored by the European Organisation for Research and Treatment of Cancer (EORTC) and the Prostate, Lung, Colon and Ovary (PLCO) trial sponsored by the National Cancer Institute. The former study is expected to report findings in 2–3 years and the latter shortly thereafter. Both studies have been in progress for approximately 12 years and have yet to demonstrate a clinically significant survival advantage for those men in the screening arm.

The US Preventative Task Force recently readdressed the issue of PSA testing. Again, the study deemed the evidence supporting PSA screening insufficient to support its use [32]. They did not believe that the benefit of using PSA as a screening test in asymptomatic men was appropriate given the possible treatment complications and false-positive results with negative biopsies. Those who support PSA screening believe that the results of screening have already been demonstrated because disease has been identified at an earlier stage and 5- and 10-year survival rates have improved. PSA screening detractors worry that too many indolent cancers are being identified and treated resulting in unnecessary morbidity to patients. Hopefully, this debate will be resolved during the next several years.

Education and informed consent must play an active role in an individual's decision to undergo screening or not. A thorough discussion between patient and doctor should take place to educate the patient on both the possible risks and benefits of screening, including the possibility of false-positive or false-negative results and the lack of evidence demonstrating that screening actually decreases mortality from prostate cancer. Natural history studies suggest that younger men between the ages of 50 and 70 years with a life expectancy greater than 10 years are most likely to gain from screening. Similarly, men with a family history of prostate cancer and African-American men are at a higher risk of developing prostate cancer. They also may benefit from prostate cancer screening.

SUMMARY

Prostate cancer is a serious disease affecting one in eight men by the age of 79. As recently demonstrated by Thompson *et al.*, subclinical disease is far more prevalent than previously thought. PSA testing is capable of detecting prostate cancer at an early stage, however, it is unclear whether the majority of cancers identified are clinically significant or not.

Studies have clearly shown that high-grade prostate cancers (Gleason scores 7–10) are often lethal if left untreated. Unfortunately, screening with PSA often detects lower grade tumours (Gleason score 2–6). It is unclear how many of these tumours are likely to progress to metastatic disease during a patient's lifetime. Many men are being treated for PSA-detected cancers and a significant percentage will become impotent. Other complications include bowel and bladder dysfunction including incontinence. These outcomes would often be accepted by patients and clinicians if treatment resulted in a significant decline in prostate cancer mortality. This may or may not be the case. The challenge to urologists is no longer whether they can find early prostate cancer, but whether they can differentiate clinically significant cancer from indolent disease. With the increasing prevalence of PSA testing, overdetection has become a more pressing problem.

Some may argue that the benefits of screening have already been proven because mortality rates are falling and there has been a dramatic shift from advanced to early stage disease. Unfortunately, diagnostic lead time may account for these findings. Results from two large randomized trials concerning prostate cancer screening should become available during the next 2–3 years. Until then clinicians and patients should understand that the efficacy of prostate cancer testing remains in doubt. Some men will surely benefit, but when the test is applied to an entire population of patients, the benefits may not balance or exceed the potential harms. Therefore, the decision to undergo PSA testing for prostate cancer remains a personal decision between the patient and his physician.

REFERENCES

1. Hulka BS. Cancer screening. Degrees of proof and practical application. *Cancer* 1988; 62(8 Suppl.):1776–1780.
2. McDavid K, Lee J, Fulton JP *et al.* Prostate cancer incidence and mortality rates and trends in the United States and Canada. *Public Health Rep* 2004; 119:174–186.
3. Jemal A, Murray T, Ward E *et al.* Cancer statistics, 2005. *CA Cancer J Clin* 2005; 55:10–30.
4. Potosky AL, Miller BA, Albertsen PC *et al.* The role of increasing detection in the rising incidence of prostate cancer. *JAMA* 1995; 273:548–552.
5. Jemal A, Siegel R, Ward E *et al.* Cancer statistics, 2006. *CA Cancer J Clin* 2006; 56:106–130.
6. Ries L. SEER Cancer Statistics Review, 1973–1997. National Cancer Institute , Bethesda, MD, 2000.
7. Thompson IM, Pauler DK, Goodman PJ *et al.* Prevalence of prostate cancer among men with a prostate-specific antigen level < or =4.0 ng per milliliter. *N Engl J Med* 2004; 350(22):2239–2246.
8. Schroder FH, van der Maas P, Beemsterboer P *et al.* Evaluation of the digital rectal examination as a screening test for prostate cancer. Rotterdam section of the European Randomized Study of Screening for Prostate Cancer. *J Natl Cancer Inst* 1998; 90:1817–1823.
9. Nadler RB, Humphrey PA, Smith DS *et al.* Effect of inflammation and benign prostatic hyperplasia on elevated serum prostate specific antigen levels. *J Urol* 1995; 154(2 Pt 1):407–413.
10. Catalona WJ, Smith DS, Ratliff TL *et al.* Measurement of prostate-specific antigen in serum as a screening test for prostate cancer. *N Engl J Med* 1991; 324:1156–1161.
11. Catalona WJ, Smith DS, Ornstein DK. Prostate cancer detection in men with serum PSA concentrations of 2.6 to 4.0 ng/ml and benign prostate examination. Enhancement of specificity with free PSA measurements. *JAMA* 1997; 277:1452–1455.
12. Gann PH, Hennekens CH, Stampfer MJ. A prospective evaluation of plasma prostate-specific antigen for detection of prostatic cancer. *JAMA* 1995; 273:289–294.
13. Catalona WJ, Smith DS, Wolfert RL *et al.* Evaluation of percentage of free serum prostate-specific antigen to improve specificity of prostate cancer screening. *JAMA* 1995; 274:1214–1220.
14. Benson MC, Olsson CA. Prostate specific antigen and prostate specific antigen density. Roles in patient evaluation and management. *Cancer* 1994; 74:1667–1673.
15. Oesterling JE, Jacobsen SJ, Chute CG *et al.* Serum prostate-specific antigen in a community-based population of healthy men. Establishment of age-specific reference ranges. *JAMA* 1993; 270:860–864.
16. Johansson JE, Adami HO, Andersson SO *et al.* High 10-year survival rate in patients with early, untreated prostatic cancer. *JAMA* 1992; 267:2191–2196.
17. Johansson JE, Adami HO, Andersson SO *et al.* Natural history of localised prostatic cancer. A population-based study in 223 untreated patients. *Lancet* 1989; 1(8642):799–803.
18. Johansson JE, Andren O, Andersson SO *et al.* Natural history of early, localized prostate cancer. *JAMA* 2004; 291:2713–2719.

19. Johansson JE, Holmberg L, Johansson S *et al.* Fifteen-year survival in prostate cancer. A prospective, population-based study in Sweden. *JAMA* 1997; 277:467–471.
20. Albertsen PC, Hanley JA, Fine J. 20-year outcomes following conservative management of clinically localized prostate cancer. *JAMA* 2005; 293:2095–2101.
21. Fowler FJ Jr, Barry MJ, Walker-Corkery B *et al.* The impact of a suspicious prostate biopsy on patients' psychological, socio-behavioral, and medical care outcomes. *J Gen Intern Med* 2006; 21:715–721.
22. Bill-Axelson A, Holmberg L, Ruutu M *et al.* Radical prostatectomy versus watchful waiting in early prostate cancer. *N Engl J Med* 2005; 352:1977–1984.
23. Stanford JL, Feng Z, Hamilton AS *et al.* Urinary and sexual function after radical prostatectomy for clinically localized prostate cancer: the Prostate Cancer Outcomes Study. *JAMA* 2000; 283:354–360.
24. Hamilton AS, Stanford JL, Gilliland FD *et al.* Health outcomes after external-beam radiation therapy for clinically localized prostate cancer: results from the Prostate Cancer Outcomes Study. *J Clin Oncol* 2001; 19:2517–2526.
25. Steineck G, Helgesen F, Adolfsson J *et al.* Quality of life after radical prostatectomy or watchful waiting. *N Engl J Med* 2002; 347:790–796.
26. Horninger W, Berger A, Pelzer A *et al.* Screening for prostate cancer: updated experience from the Tyrol study. *Curr Urol Rep* 2004; 5:220–225.
27. Lu-Yao G, Albertsen PC, Stanford JL *et al.* Natural experiment examining impact of aggressive screening and treatment on prostate cancer mortality in two fixed cohorts from Seattle area and Connecticut. *BMJ* 2002; 325(7367):740.
28. Cooperberg MR, Grossfeld GD, Lubeck DP *et al.* National practice patterns and time trends in androgen ablation for localized prostate cancer. *J Natl Cancer Inst* 2003; 95:981–989.
29. Draisma G, Boer R, Otto SJ *et al.* Lead times and overdetection due to prostate-specific antigen screening: estimates from the European Randomized Study of Screening for Prostate Cancer. *J Natl Cancer Inst* 2003; 95:868–878.
30. Albertsen PC, Hanley JA, Barrows GH *et al.* Prostate cancer and the Will Rogers phenomenon. *J Natl Cancer Inst* 2005; 97:1248–1253.
31. Welch HG, Schwartz LM, Woloshin S. Are increasing 5-year survival rates evidence of success against cancer? *JAMA* 2000; 283:2975–2978.
32. Screening for prostate cancer: recommendation and rationale. *Ann Intern Med* 2002; 137:915–916.

Section II

Regional prostate cancer – localized and locally advanced cancer

5

Assessment of treatment strategies in prostate cancer using risk stratification and prediction of clinical outcomes

Denise C. Babineau, Michael W. Kattan

Prostate cancer is a slowly progressing disease that has a variety of treatment options. The choice of treatment for a particular patient is influenced by several factors. Each patient must consider his own tolerance level regarding treatment-specific clinical outcomes. One patient may choose a treatment that has a high risk of some adverse side effect if there is a low risk of disease progression. A similar patient may elect to forgo such treatment due to the lower quality of life that they may develop once the treatment is given. Prediction tools that estimate the risk of a clinical outcome are an invaluable resource to the patient in this context.

This chapter reviews statistical methods that are used to develop prediction tools for risk stratification and prediction of clinical outcomes. Using these sophisticated techniques, many prediction tools have been developed that provide patient-specific risk assessment with respect to clinical outcomes that can occur throughout the course of prostate cancer. This chapter will provide a review of some of these models in an attempt to provide both the treating physician and patient the most current prediction models available to decide an optimal strategy for prostate cancer management.

CLINICAL OUTCOMES AND SIDE-EFFECTS

Prior to prostate cancer diagnosis, it is of most interest in determining the likelihood that a patient has prostate cancer and if prostate cancer is present, if it is of an indolent or aggressive nature. The treating physician and patient must then decide which treatment options are available and which will provide the best possible set of health outcomes for the patient. Each treatment must be assessed with regard to its effect on the time to biochemical progression (sometimes used as a surrogate measure for disease progression), the time to metastatic disease or the time to disease-specific death. Due to the indolent nature of some prostate cancers, these health outcomes may take several years to develop and treatment side-effects must also be considered. Side-effects, such as urinary incontinence, bowel dysfunction, erectile dysfunction and irritative bladder symptoms, may significantly lower a patient's quality of life after treatment and his risk of side-effects must also be considered in conjunction with the risk of developing other clinical outcomes. This chapter will review prediction models that have been developed for some of these outcomes.

Denise C. Babineau, PhD, Assistant Staff, Department of Quantitative Health Sciences, Cleveland Clinic Foundation, Cleveland, Ohio, USA
Michael W. Kattan, PhD, Chairman, Department of Quantitative Health Sciences, Cleveland Clinic Foundation, Cleveland, Ohio, USA

RISK FACTORS

Patients are inherently different with regard to their medical history. Predicting a patient's risk of developing some health outcome must take account of patient heterogeneity to obtain reliable estimates of risk. Factors that are strongly associated with the development of an outcome are called 'risk factors'. However, even strong risk factors may not be useful for risk assessment if their prevalence is extremely low [1] or if they are not routinely collected. These limitations must be considered in the development of any prediction tool.

METHODS USED TO DEVELOP TOOLS FOR RISK STRATIFICATION AND PREDICTION

Several methods are used to predict health outcomes for treatment strategies in prostate cancer. The most basic and easily accessible method is clinical judgement. In this case, the treating physician uses personal experience and knowledge to predict a patient's outcome. This method is highly biased because the physician can only offer his/her opinion based on previous experience, which may or may not include all treatment options. In addition, the physician cannot tailor his opinion to a particular patient due to the inability to simultaneously account for the presence or absence of a wide range of risk factors.

An approach that improves upon clinical judgement is risk grouping, where similar patients are placed into a specific risk category. Although this method is commonly used to predict risk, it is based on some strong assumptions. Risk grouping often reduces continuous factors, such as age, into categorical factors thereby decreasing the precision of risk estimates. In addition, patients placed in the same category may differ substantially with regard to other important risk factors. Both assumptions fail to tailor risk according to a patient's specific set of risk factors. For example, Figure 5.1 illustrates the distribution of nomogram predicted probabilities within risk groups using the CaPSURE (Cancer of the Prostate Strategic Urologic Research Endeavor) database.

In an attempt to develop a tool that predicts risk for each patient separately, predictive tools have been developed that are based on the number of risk factors a patient has. Risk factors are chosen that have a significant association with the outcome based on univariable statistical analyses. The total number of risk factors a patient has is the patient's score. The

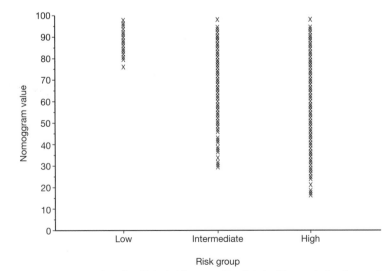

Figure 5.1   Kattan nomogram values by clinical risk group. Reprinted with permission from ref. 48.

higher the score, the higher the patient's risk. Although this method is simple to use, it has several disadvantages. Univariable analyses do not consider the effect that one factor may have on another with regard to risk. Continuous risk factors must still be categorized as well. The strongest assumption that is made, and by far the worst, is that all factors provide the same amount of risk.

To develop tools that can easily account for patient heterogeneity yet still provide easy translation from bench to bedside, sophisticated statistical modelling techniques are required. Three commonly used methods are multivariable models expressed through nomograms, tree-based methods and artificial neural networks (ANNs). These methods do not require categorization of continuous variables and provide a measure of risk that is specifically tailored to each patient based on any set of risk factors. A brief description of each technique follows.

- *Nomograms.* Depending on the outcome of interest, specific statistical methods are needed to predict risk. Typically, continuous outcomes are modelled using regression techniques, categorical outcomes are modelled using logistic regression or proportional odds models, and survival outcomes are modelled using Cox proportional hazards methods. Prediction of risk varies with each of these statistical techniques. A tool that depicts risk, regardless of the method used, is a nomogram. A nomogram provides a graphical depiction of the risk of an outcome based on a multivariable model and can easily be used by physicians and patients alike. Kattan [2] gives a thorough discussion comparing nomograms to staging and risk grouping methods. Figure 5.2 illustrates a nomogram.
- *Tree-based methods.* Tree-based methods are often built using recursive partitioning, an iterative process that splits the data into partitions that are then used to maximize predictive accuracy with regard to risk of an outcome. There are several types of tree-based methods: binary recursive partitioning, tree-structured survival analysis, classification and regression trees (CARTs) and multiple adaptive regression splines (MARS).
- *ANNs.* This method classifies a patient's risk through a learning process. It is based on the assumption of a network made up of computational neurons that are connected

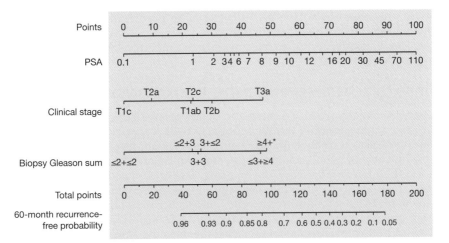

Figure 5.2 Preoperative nomogram based on 983 patients treated at Baylor College of Medicine, Houston, TX, for predicting freedom from recurrence after radical prostatectomy, adapted from Kattan *et al.* [23]. ©1997 Michael W. Kattan and Peter T. Scardino.

to one or more layers of other neurons through weighted signal pathways. Prior to analysis, the weights on all signal pathways are set to small random numbers. The data are then randomly divided into three parts: the training set, the validation (or testing) set and the verification set. The network is then presented with the training set that provides inputs (e.g. one or many factors of interest) and desired outputs (e.g. the outcome of interest) to these inputs. The weights on all signal pathways are adjusted to increase the likelihood that the network will compute the desired output. The validation set is used to decide when to stop training the network and the verification set is used to report the performance of the ANN. A thorough discussion of ANNs is given in Dayhoff and DeLeo [3].

The predictive value of any of these tools must also be assessed objectively. Three areas that are typically evaluated when assessing the accuracy and precision of a predictive model are discrimination, calibration and validation. Discrimination is the ability to separate patients into those that are likely and unlikely to experience the clinical outcome of interest and is measured using the area under the curve (AUC) or concordance index. This index measures the probability that, given two randomly selected patients, the patient who first experiences the outcome was at higher risk of developing the outcome. The concordance index ranges between 0.5 and 1.0, where 0.5 indicates no predictive value and 1.0 indicates a perfect ability to predict outcome. Calibration measures how close the predicted probability is to the actual probability of the outcome and is typically depicted using graphical techniques. Validation refers to consistent performance across different study populations and consists of two types: internal and external. Internal validation uses data drawn from the same population to develop the predictive model. Methods of internal validation include data-splitting, cross-validation, bootstrapping and jackknife techniques. External validation uses data obtained from an external data source.

As will be shown, one or all of these methods may be used to predict risk for a particular outcome. Choosing among them is somewhat difficult and there is some controversy regarding which method of developing prediction models is more accurate. A thorough discussion of this issue is given in Karakiewicz et al. [4] and Kattan [5].

CURRENT PREDICTION MODELS IN PROSTATE CANCER

A variety of prediction tools have been developed to predict the risk of prostate cancer detection and the risk of various health outcomes in response to prostate cancer treatment strategies. The remainder of this chapter reviews recently developed and frequently used predictive models in this area.

PROSTATE CANCER DETECTION PRIOR TO INITIAL PROSTATE BIOPSY

Prostate-specific antigen (PSA) screening and digital rectal examinations (DRE) are used to detect prostate cancer. If either test is abnormal, a patient may receive a recommendation for a prostate biopsy. To reduce the number of unnecessary biopsies, tools that accurately predict the outcome of initial prostate biopsy are useful. Garzotto et al. [6] analysed data on 1433 men with serum PSA levels ≤10 ng/ml using classification and regression tree analysis. Serum PSA, PSA density, ultrasound data, age and prostate volume were used to develop a model with an AUC of 0.74. Alternatively, Karakiewicz et al. [7] developed a nomogram based on a multivariate logistic regression analysis of data obtained from 1762 German men with PSA ≤50 ng/ml. This model predicted the outcome of initial prostate biopsy using patient age, DRE, serum PSA and per cent free PSA, and achieved an AUC of 0.77 on external validation of 514 men from Montreal, Canada. Both models can be easily applied to patients with abnormal PSA or DRE to determine the likelihood of prostate cancer prior to initial prostate biopsy.

PROSTATE CANCER DETECTION AFTER A NEGATIVE RESULT ON INITIAL BIOPSY

If a patient is at high risk of a positive initial prostate biopsy and they are then given a biopsy only to find a negative result, the patient cannot be certain that he is cancer free due to the biopsy's false-negative error rate. In this case, prediction tools that can aid in the decision to perform subsequent prostate biopsies are needed. Several tools are available.

Thompson *et al.* [8] developed a logistic regression model based on data obtained from 5519 men from the Prostate Cancer Prevention Trial to predict the risk of prostate cancer and high-grade disease. Risk factors included in the model were PSA, a family history of prostate cancer, DRE result and a prior negative biopsy result. This model achieved an AUC of 0.70.

Alternatively, it may also be of interest to patients with a previous negative biopsy to determine the time to a positive biopsy. This issue was addressed in Lopez-Corona *et al.* [9] who developed a nomogram based on a Cox regression analysis of data obtained from 343 men with at least one initial negative biopsy. Risk factors included in the model were age, family history of prostate cancer, serum PSA, PSA slope, DRE findings, cumulative number of negatives cores previously obtained and history of high-grade prostatic intraepithelial neoplasia (PIN) or atypical small acinar proliferation. The nomogram had a concordance index of 0.70. This model was externally validated by Yanke *et al.* [10] using data obtained from 230 men from the Brooklyn Veterans Administration Medical Center.

PREDICTING PATHOLOGICAL STAGE USING PREOPERATIVE CLINICAL DATA

Once a patient has been diagnosed with prostate cancer based on biopsy findings, the clinical stage of the tumour, as well as its size and how far it has spread, must be determined to choose an optimal treatment strategy. Clinical stage is mainly determined using the DRE. Other examinations may also be used for clinical staging, such as transrectal ultrasound of the prostate (TRUSP), prostate biopsy and imaging studies.

Alternatively, pathological stage is based on surgical removal and examination of the entire prostate gland and possibly other surrounding tissue. Although pathological stage is more accurate than clinical stage, its assessment involves invasive procedures that may affect the patient's clinical outcomes. To avoid these procedures but still accurately stage a tumour so that the appropriate treatment is chosen, prediction tools have been developed to predict pathological stage based on preoperative clinical data.

Simple models that predict organ-confined disease have been developed. Veltri [11] developed a logistic regression model using data on 386 men with clinical stage T1c disease. Predictors included in the model were quantitative nuclear grade, complexed PSA density and Gleason score, and an AUC of 82.4% was achieved.

Recently, it has been of interest to develop models that predict the presence and side of extracapsular extension. This would be useful information to decide if the patient should undergo nerve-sparing surgery. Ohori *et al.* [12] developed a logistic regression model that predicted side-specific extraprostatic extension based on data from 763 patients with clinical stage T1c–T3 prostate cancer. PSA, clinical T stage on each side and biopsy Gleason sum on each side were independent predictors of extracapsular extension, yielding an accuracy of 0.788. Accuracy was increased to 0.806 if the results of systemic biopsy were incorporated into the model. The resulting nomograms were internally validated and had excellent calibration and discrimination. This same cohort of men was used to develop and internally validate a nomogram to predict seminal vesicle invasion [13]. In this case, the presence and amount of cancer in systematic needle biopsy cores from the base of the prostate strongly predicted the presence of seminal vesicle invasion to within ± 10% in 68% of the cases.

Pathological staging also involves determination of pelvic lymph node invasion (LNI). Several algorithms have been developed to predict LNI using preoperative variables. Briganti *et al.* [14] developed and internally validated a nomogram using data from 602 patients with localized disease undergoing pelvic lymphadenectomy. The logistic regression model predicted LNI based on PSA, clinical stage and biopsy Gleason sums, and achieved a predictive accuracy of 76%. The same level of accuracy was also achieved by a similar nomogram based on data from 5510 patients from six separate institutions treated with radical prostatectomy [15].

Rather than predicting organ-confined disease, extracapsular extension, seminal vesicle invasion or LNI separately, prediction models have also been developed that predict the outcomes simultaneously. Perhaps the most commonly used prediction model of this kind was developed by Partin et al. in 1997 [16] and updated in 2001 [17]. The current model was based on data from 5079 men treated with prostatectomy (without neoadjuvant therapy) between 1994 and 2000 at Johns Hopkins Hospital. A multinomial log-linear regression analysis was used to predict the likelihood of organ-confined disease, extraprostatic extension, seminal vesical or lymph node status based on preoperative PSA, clinical stage and biopsy Gleason score. External validation of this nomogram was done in other academic settings [18], community-based settings [19] and in Europe [20] with comparable accuracy. However, there is some evidence to suggest that this nomogram is less accurate for transition zone cancers compared with peripheral zone cancers [21].

SELECTING A TREATMENT STRATEGY

EXPECTANT MANAGEMENT

Owing to the indolent nature of prostate cancer, watchful waiting is a good alternative to surgical treatment or radiation therapy if a patient has a non-aggressive tumour. However, it is not easy to determine a tumour's aggressiveness based on clinical data alone. Kattan et al. [22] developed three separate nomograms predicting indolent cancer based on logistic regression analyses of data obtained from 409 patients. Risk factors included in the nomograms were clinical stage, Gleason grade, PSA and the amount of cancer in a systematic biopsy specimen (either absent from the nomogram or included as per cent of positive cores, ultrasound prostate volume or millimetres of non-cancerous and cancerous tissue). All models achieved an AUC between 0.64 and 0.79 and had good calibration. These nomograms can be used to select patients who are likely to have indolent disease and are well suited to an expectant management treatment strategy for prostate cancer.

PREDICTION MODELS PRIOR TO PROSTATECTOMY

Owing to the risks and side-effects of prostatectomy, prediction of these clinical outcomes prior to surgery would provide information that could affect a patient's treatment strategy. Several prediction tools have been developed that estimate the likelihood of disease recurrence after prostatectomy. Kattan et al. [23] developed a nomogram based on a Cox proportional hazards model applied to data from 983 men with clinically localized prostate cancer who were treated with radical prostatectomy. Disease recurrence at 5 years after prostatectomy was defined as clinical evidence of recurrence, a rising serum PSA level (two measurements of 0.4 ng/ml or greater and rising) or initiation of adjuvant therapy. Risk factors included in the model were preoperative serum PSA, biopsy Gleason scores and clinical stage. The model achieved an AUC of 0.79 and appeared accurate and discriminating. This nomogram was externally validated in several settings [24, 25]. Improvements to this nomogram have been explored by including information provided by systematic biopsy [26] and adding biological markers of prostate cancer [27] to the existing nomogram. An updated version was subsequently developed in 2006 [28] that predicted the likelihood of disease recurrence 10 years after surgery with a concordance index of 0.79.

Other risk factors have also been explored to examine their predictive ability with respect to biochemical recurrence or disease progression after prostatectomy. Strom et al. [29]

showed that obesity and weight gain were independent predictors of biochemical recurrence. Poulakis *et al.* [30] developed a neural network for predicting biochemical recurrence using results from pelvic magnetic resonance imaging (MRI), PSA and biopsy Gleason score. Percentage of positive scores from the dominant side of the prostate, PSA and biopsy Gleason score were also assessed for the predictive value in estimating the risk of biochemical recurrence after prostatectomy [31]. Note that PSA density has been shown to have very little predictive value for disease progression after prostatectomy [32].

Another clinical outcome of interest that may occur after prostatectomy is death. D'Amico *et al.* [33] developed a Cox proportional hazards model based on PSA velocity 1 year prior to diagnosis, PSA level, Gleason score and clinical stage to predict time to death after prostatectomy. They showed that men whose PSA level increases by more than 2.0 ng/ml during the year before prostate cancer diagnosis have a relatively high risk of death from prostate cancer.

Prediction models have also explored the likelihood of complications after prostatectomy. Preoperative International Index of Erectile Function score, surgical technique and age were found to be independent predictors of postoperative sexual function [34]. An ANN was developed by Poulakis *et al.* [35] to predict positive surgical margins based on MRI results, PSA and Gleason score; this model yielded an AUC of 0.872. Prediction of homologous blood transfusion showed that larger prostate size, use of general anaesthesia, use of neoadjuvant hormonal therapy and annual surgeon case volume were independently associated with an increased likelihood of a blood transfusion after prostatectomy [36].

PREDICTION MODELS AFTER PROSTATECTOMY

If a patient undergoes a prostatectomy, surgical results may improve the predictive value of the previous algorithms that are based solely on preoperative information. This information could be used to decide if patients may benefit from adjuvant treatment. Kattan *et al.* [37] did just this and developed a postoperative nomogram that predicted disease recurrence 5 and 7 years after prostatectomy using data obtained from 996 men with clinical stage T1a–T3c NXM0 prostate cancer. A Cox proportional hazards model that included pretreatment serum PSA, pathological Gleason sum, prostatic capsular invasion, surgical margin status, seminal vesicle invasion and lymph node status yielded an AUC of 0.89. This nomogram has been updated to predict disease recurrence 10 years after prostatectomy by Stephenson *et al.* [38], who have included treatment year as an additional predictor. In this case, the model achieved a concordance index of 0.81 and 0.79 in two external cohorts of patients. Han *et al.* [39] developed a simpler nomogram to predict biochemical recurrence at 3, 5, 7 and 10 years after prostatectomy using pathological Gleason score and organ confinement status as well as PSA. Alternatively, Khan *et al.* [40] used pathological Gleason score, stage and surgical margin status to estimate the probability of biochemical recurrence in 1955 men who were treated with prostatectomy and pelvic lymph node dissection between 1989 and 2001. This model was externally validated in a cohort of 2417 patients [41].

PREDICTION MODELS PRIOR TO RADIATION THERAPY

Preoperative prognostic models have also been developed to examine clinical outcomes after radiation therapy. Using Cox regression and recursive partitioning techniques based on data from 1765 men with stage T1b, T1c and T2 tumours treated between 1988 and 1995 with external beam radiation, Shipley *et al.* [42] developed four prognostic groups to stratify a patient's risk of biochemical recurrence at 5 years after therapy. The groups were based on categorized PSA levels and Gleason scores. Zelefsky *et al.* [43] also developed risk groups based on PSA, clinical stage and Gleason score using clinical data on 772 patients treated with intensity modulated radiation therapy between 1996 and 2001. Both strategies failed to take into consideration patient heterogeneity within individual risk groups. Kattan *et al.* [44] improved upon these earlier attempts at risk stratification by developing a nomogram that predicted the likelihood of biochemical recurrence 5 years after three-dimensional (3-D) conformal radiotherapy using stage, biopsy Gleason score, clinical serum PSA, presence or absence of neoadjuvant androgen deprivation therapy and radiation dose as prognostic factors. The accuracy of this nomogram was superior to that of existing algorithms.

PREDICTION MODELS AFTER RADIATION THERAPY

Once patients have undergone radiation therapy, the previous preoperative prediction models can be improved using data acquired after therapy. Two post-treatment models that focus on PSA nadir levels as a potential prognostic factor of PSA recurrence are given by Ray *et al.* [45] and Kamat *et al.* [46]. Ray *et al.* obtained data on 4839 patients with external beam radiotherapy between 1986 and 1995. The time to PSA failure and the time to clinically apparent distant failure were modelled as separate clinical outcomes. Prognostic factors included in the model were initial PSA, clinical stage, Gleason score, radiation dose, nadir PSA and time to nadir PSA. Alternatively, Kamat *et al.* found that a PSA increase of 1.5 ng/ml or more above the 24-month PSA nadir was an independent predictor of biochemical failure based on data from 745 patients. Both algorithms show that PSA nadir levels are useful when predicting biochemical recurrence after external beam radiotherapy.

PREDICTION MODELS FOR BRACHYTHERAPY

A model that can be used to evaluate brachytherapy as a potential therapy was developed in 2001 by Kattan *et al.* [47]. Data was obtained from 920 patients who received brachytherapy between 1992 and 2000. Prognostic factors included pretreatment serum PSA, clinical stage and biopsy Gleason sum, while recurrence was defined as any post-treatment administration of androgen deprivation, clinical relapse or biochemical failure (defined as three consecutive PSA rises). Using this information, a pretreatment nomogram was developed based on a Cox proportional hazards model. External validation based on data from two other institutions yielded a concordance index between 0.61 and 0.64.

PREDICTION MODELS FOR OTHER TREATMENT STRATEGIES

Other treatment strategies for the management of prostate cancer are hormone therapy, cryosurgery, cryotherapy and chemotherapy. Cryosurgery and cryotherapy are relatively new procedures, and prognostic models have not been developed due to limited data. Chemotherapy is usually used for salvage treatment after other treatments have failed and the patient has advanced prostate cancer. As such, prediction models are of limited use and have not been developed.

This chapter has provided a review of existing prognostic models that can be used to predict clinical outcomes for various treatment strategies of prostate cancer. Application of these models can provide both the treating physician and patient valuable information that can be used to select an optimal treatment strategy.

REFERENCES

1. Grobman WA, Stamilio DM. Methods of clinical prediction. *Am J Obstet Gynecol* 2006; 194:888–894.
2. Kattan MW. Nomograms are superior to staging and risk grouping systems for identifying high-risk patients: preoperative application in prostate cancer. *Curr Opin Urol* 2003; 13:111–116.
3. Dayhoff JE, DeLeo JM. Artificial neural networks: opening the black box. *Cancer* 2001; 91(Suppl. 8): 1615–1635.
4. Karakiewicz PI, Chun FK, Briganti A *et al.* Prostate cancer nomograms are superior to neural networks. *Can J Urol* 2006; 13(Suppl. 2):18–25.

5. Kattan MW. Comparison of Cox regression with other methods for determining prediction models and nomograms. *J Urol* 2003; 170 (6 Pt 2):S6–9.

6. Garzotto M, Beer TM, Hudson RG *et al.* Improved detection of prostate cancer using classification and regression tree analysis. *J Clin Oncol* 2005; 23:4322–4329.

7. Karakiewicz PI, Benayoun S, Kattan MW *et al.* Development and validation of a nomogram predicting the outcome of prostate biopsy based on patient age, digital rectal examination and serum prostate specific antigen. *J Urol* 2005; 173:1930–1934.

8. Thompson IM, Ankerst DP, Chi C *et al.* Assessing prostate cancer risk: Results from the prostate cancer prevention trial. *J Natl Cancer Inst* 2006; 98:529–534.

9. Lopez-Corona E, Ohori M, Scardino PT, Reuter VE, Gonen M, Kattan MW. A nomogram for predicting a positive repeat prostate biopsy in patients with a previous negative biopsy session. *J Urol* 2003; 170(4 Pt 1):1184–1188.

10. Yanke BV, Gonen M, Scardino PT, Kattan MW. Validation of a nomogram for predicting positive repeat biopsy for prostate cancer. *J Urol* 2005; 173:421–424.

11. Veltri RW, Miller MC, Mangold LA, O'Dowd GJ, Epstein JI, Partin AW. Prediction of pathological stage in patients with clinical stage T1c prostate cancer: the new challenge. *J Urol* 2002; 168:100–104.

12. Ohori M, Kattan MW, Koh H *et al.* Predicting the presence and side of extracapsular extension: a nomogram for staging prostate cancer. *J Urol* 2004; 171:1844–1849.

13. Koh H, Kattan MW, Scardino PT *et al.* A nomogram to predict seminal vesicle invasion by the extent and location of cancer in systematic biopsy results. *J Urol* 2003; 170(4 Pt 1):1203–1208.

14. Briganti A, Chun FK, Salonia A *et al.* Validation of a nomogram predicting the probability of lymph node invasion among patients undergoing radical prostatectomy and an extended pelvic lymphadenectomy. *Eur Urol* 2006; 49:1019–1026.

15. Cagiannos I, Karakiewicz P, Eastham HA *et al.* A preoperative nomogram identifying decreased risk of positive pelvic lymph nodes in patients with prostate cancer. *J Urol* 2003; 170:1798–1803.

16. Partin AW, Subong ENP, Walsh PC *et al.* Combination of prostate-specific antigen, clinical stage, and Gleason score to predict pathological stage of localized prostate cancer: A multi-institutional update. *JAMA* 1997; 277:1445–1451.

17. Partin AW, Mangold LA, Lamm DM, Walsh PC, Epstein JI, Pearson JD: Contemporary update of prostate cancer nomograms (Partin tables) for the new millennium. *Urology* 2001; 58:843.

18. Blute ML, Bergstralh EJ, Partin AW *et al.* Validation of Partin tables for predicting pathological stage of clinically localized prostate cancer. *J Urol* 2000; 164:1591–1595.

19. Penson DF, Grossfeld GD, Li YP, Henning JM, Lubeck DP, Carroll PR. How well does the Partin nomogram predict the pathological stage after radical prostatectomy in a community based population? Results of the cancer of the prostate strategic urological research endeavor. *J Urol* 2002; 167:1653–1657.

20. Graefen M, Augustin H, Karakiewicz PI *et al.* Can predictive models for prostate cancer patients derived in the United States of America be utilized in European patients? A validation study of the Partin tables. *Eur Urol* 2003; 43:6–10.

21. Steuber T, Karakiewicz PI, Augustin H *et al.* Transition zone cancers undermine the predictive accuracy of Partin table stage predictions. *J Urol* 2005; 173:737–741.

22. Kattan MW, Eastham JA, Wheeler TM *et al.* Counseling men with prostate cancer: a nomogram for predicting the presence of small, moderately differentiated, confined tumors. *J Urol* 2003; 170:1792–1797.

23. Kattan MW, Eastham JA, Stapleton AMF, Wheeler TM, Scardino PT. A preoperative nomogram for disease recurrence following radical prostatectomy for prostate cancer. *J Natl Cancer Inst* 1998; 90: 766–771.

24. Greene KL, Meng MV, Elkin EP *et al.* Validation of the Kattan preoperative nomogram for prostate cancer recurrence using a community based cohort: results from Cancer of the Prostate Strategic Urological Research Endeavor (CaPSURE). *J Urol* 2004; 171(6 pt 1):2255–2259.

25. Graefen M, Karakiewicz PI, Cagiannos I *et al.* A validation of two preoperative nomograms predicting recurrence following radical prostatectomy. *Urol Oncol* 2002; 7:141–146.

26. Graefen M, Ohori M, Karakiewicz PI *et al.* Assessment of the enhancement in predictive accuracy provided by systematic biopsy in predicting outcome for clinically localized prostate cancer. *J Urol* 2004; 171:200–203.

27. Kattan MW, Shariat SF, Andrews B *et al.* The addition of interleukin-6 soluble receptor and transforming growth factor beta1 improves a preoperative nomogram for predicting biochemical progression in patients with clinically localized prostate cancer. *J Clin Oncol* 2003; 21919:3573–3579.

28. Stephenson AJ, Scardino PT, Eastham JA *et al.* Preoperative nomogram predicting the 10-year probability of prostate cancer recurrence after radical prostatectomy. *J Natl Cancer Inst* 2006; 98:715–717.

29. Strom SS, Wang X, Pettaway CA *et al.* Obesity, weight gain, and risk of biochemical failure among prostate cancer patients following prostatectomy. *Clin Cancer Res* 2005;11(19 Pt 1):6889–6894.

30. Poulakis V, Witzsch U, de Vries R *et al.* Preoperative neural network using combined magnetic resonance imaging variables, prostate-specific antigen and Gleason score for predicting prostate cancer biochemical recurrence after radical prostatectomy. *Urology* 2004; 64:1165–1170.

31. Freedland SJ, Aronson WJ, Terris MK *et al.* The percentage of prostate needle biopsy cores with carcinoma from the more involved side of the biopsy as a predictor of prostate specific antigen recurrence after radical prostatectomy: results from the Shared Equal Access Regional Cancer Hospital (SEARCH) database. *Cancer* 2003; 98:2344–2350.

32. Freedland SJ, Kane CJ, Presti JC Jr. *et al.* Comparison of preoperative prostate specific antigen density and prostate specific antigen for predicting recurrence after radical prostatectomy: results from the search database. *J Urol* 2003; 169:969–973.

33. D'Amico AV, Chen MH, Roehl KA, Catalona WJ. Preoperative PSA velocity and the risk of death from prostate cancer after radical prostatectomy. *N Engl J Med* 2004; 351920:125–135.

34. Michl UH, Friedrich MG, Graefen M, Haese A, Heinzer H, Huland H. Prediction of postoperative sexual function after nerve sparing radical retropubic prostatectomy. *J Urol* 2006; 176:227–231.

35. Poulakis V, Witzsch U, de Vries R *et al.* Preoperative neural network using combined magnetic resonance imaging variables, prostate-specific antigen and Gleason score to predict positive surgical margins. *Urology* 2004; 64:516–521.

36. Dash A, Dunn RL, Resh J, Wei JT, Montie JE, Sanda MG. Patient, surgeon, and treatment characteristics associated with homologous blood transfusion requirements during radical retropubic prostatectomy: multivariate nomogram to assist patient counseling. *Urology* 2004; 64:117–122.

37. Kattan MW, Wheeler TM, Scardino PT. Postoperative nomogram for disease recurrence after radical prostatectomy for prostate cancer. *J Clin Oncol* 1999; 17:1499–1507.

38. Stephenson AJ, Scardino PT, Eastham JA *et al.* Postoperative nomogram predicting the 10 year probability of prostate cancer recurrence after radical prostatectomy. *J Clin Oncol* 2005; 23:7005–7012.

39. Han M, Partin AW, Zahurak M, Piatadose S, Epstein JI, Walsh PD: Biochemical (prostate specific antigen) recurrence probability following radical prostatectomy for clinically localized prostate cancer. *J Urol* 2003; 169:517–523.

40. Khan MA, Partin AW, Mangold LA, Epstein JI, Walsh PC. Probability of biochemical recurrence by analysis of pathologic stage, Gleason score, and margin status for localized prostate cancer. *Urology* 2003; 62:866–871.

41. McAleer SJ, Schultz D, Whittington R *et al.* PSA outcome following radical prostatectomy for patients with localized prostate cancer stratified by prostatectomy findings and the preoperative PSA level. *Urol Oncol* 2005; 23:311–317.

42. Shipley WU, Thames HD, Sandler HM *et al.* Radiation therapy for clinically localized prostate cancer: a multi-institutional pooled analysis. *JAMA* 1999; 281:1598–1604.

43. Zelefsky MJ, Fuks Z, Hunt M *et al.* High-dose intensity-modulated radiation therapy for prostate cancer: early toxicity and biochemical outcome in 772 patients. *Int J Radiat Oncol Biol Phys* 2002; 53:1111–1116.

44. Kattan MW, Zelefsky MJ, Kupelian PA, Scardino PT, Fuks Z, Leibel SA. Pretreatment nomogram for predicting the outcome of three-dimensional conformal radiotherapy in prostate cancer. *J Clin Oncol* 2000; 18:3352–3359.

45. Ray ME, Thames HD, Levy LB *et al.* PSA nadir predicts biochemical and distant failures after external beam radiotherapy for prostate cancer: a multi-institutional analysis. *Int J Radiat Oncol Biol Phys* 2006; 64:1140–1150.

46. Kamat AM, Rosser CH, Levy LB *et al.* Rise in serum PSA of 1.5 ng/ml above 24-month nadir after external beam radiotherapy is predictive of biochemical failure. *Urology* 2004; 63:1132–1137.

47. Kattan MW, Potters L, Blasko JC, Beyer DC, Fearn P, Cavanagh W *et al.* Pretreatment nomogram for predicting freedom from recurrence after permanent prostate brachytherapy in prostate cancer. *Urology* 2001; 58:393–399.

48. Mitchell JA, Cooperberg MR, Elkin EP *et al.* Ability of 2 pretreatment risk assessment methods to predict prostate cancer recurrence after radical prostatectomy: data from CaPSURE. *J Urol* 2005; 173:1126–1131.

6

Conservative treatment strategies for localized favourable-risk prostate cancer

Laurence Klotz

INTRODUCTION

Prostate cancer screening based on prostate biopsy for men with levels of serum prostate-specific antigen (PSA) above an empirical level, or abnormal digital rectal examination (DRE), results in diagnosing many men with prostate cancer for whom the disease does not pose a threat to their life. Welch has recently calculated that there are 2.74 million US men aged 50–70 with a PSA > 2.5. If all American men in this age group had a PSA blood test, and a PSA > 2.5 is used as an indication for biopsy, this means that in the USA alone 775 000 cases will be diagnosed. This is 543 000 more than the 232 000 cases diagnosed in 2005, and 25 times more than the 30 350 men expected to die of prostate cancer per year in the USA [1].

Several autopsy studies of men dying of other causes have documented the high prevalence of histological prostate cancer [2]. A large proportion of this histological, or 'latent', prostate cancer is never destined to progress or affect the lifespan of the patient. Since the introduction of PSA screening, the lifetime risk of being diagnosed with prostate cancer has almost doubled from around 10%, in the pre-PSA era, to 17% [3]. This means that many cases of localized prostate cancer are overtreated, in that some patients not destined to experience prostate cancer death or morbidity are subject to radical therapy [4].

Cancer aggressiveness can be predicted to some degree using existing clinical parameters. The ones mostly widely used are tumour grade, or Gleason score, PSA and tumour stage. Favourable risk prostate cancer is characterized as Gleason 6 or less, PSA 10 or less and T1c–T2a disease [5]. As a result of stage migration due to PSA screening, the proportion of newly diagnosed patients who fall into the 'favourable risk' category has increased, and now constitutes 50–60% of patients. While patients with these characteristics have a much more favourable natural history and progression rate than those with higher Gleason grade or PSA, some of them still progress to advanced, incurable prostate cancer and death.

An update of a large group of patients in Connecticut who were treated with watchful waiting has recently reported 20-year follow-up [6]. These data confirm the powerful predictive value of Gleason score. In that pre-PSA screening cohort, 23% of untreated Gleason 6 patients died of prostate cancer by 20 years. For Gleason 7 prostate cancer, about 65% died of prostate cancer. In addition, the author recently subjected the original slides to r-analysis using contemporary Gleason scoring [7]. This demonstrated clearly that there has been a shift in grade interpretation over the last 20 years. Many Gleason 6 cancers diagnosed 20 years ago would be called Gleason 7 today. Thus, the Connecticut results are likely to

Laurence Klotz, MD FRCSC, Chief, Division of Urology, Sunnybrook and Women's College Health Sciences Centre, Toronto, Ontario, Canada

represent a 'worse case' scenario for the expected mortality from untreated Gleason 6 prostate cancer. This means that the natural prostate cancer mortality of untreated non-screen-detected contemporary Gleason 6 cancer may be as low as 10% at 20 years.

Autopsy studies have demonstrated that prostate cancer typically begins in the third or fourth decade of life [1]. This means that, in most patients, there can be a period of slow subclinical tumour progression that lasts approximately 30 years, followed by a period of clinical progression (potentially to metastatic disease and death) lasting about 15 years. The implication is that most patients have a long window of curability. This is particularly true for patients with favourable-risk, low-volume disease.

One approach to achieving a prediction of tumour aggressiveness is to use this window of curability to identify patients at higher risk for progression based on a rapid prostate-specific antigen doubling time (PSADT) or histological progression over time.

The results of a watchful waiting approach, meaning no treatment until progression to metastatic or locally advanced disease, at which point androgen ablation therapy is implemented, have been described in numerous cohorts [8–17]. These studies consistently describe non-progression in many patients. However, the results are difficult to apply in the current era for two reasons: (a) the cohorts described are from the pre-PSA era, and constitute patients with more extensive disease at the time of diagnosis, and (b) because they do not offer patients the opportunity for selective definitive therapy where required. In the era of PSA monitoring, patients who are treated conservatively are followed with periodic PSA tests. This raises the tantalizing prospect that treatment of favourable prostate cancer could be deferred indefinitely in the majority, while effective delayed therapy was offered to the subset in whom PSA progresses rapidly or the tumour grade increases [18, 19].

The Prostate Cancer Prevention Trial (PCPT) incorporated a strategy of routine systematic biopsies of the prostate, regardless of PSA level. Twenty-four per cent of patients in the placebo arm were diagnosed with prostate cancer over a 7-year period, a surprisingly high proportion [20]. This means, in sharp contrast to accepted wisdom, that routine prostate biopsy, regardless of PSA, results in the detection of latent microfoci of disease in many men. The lifetime risk of dying from prostate cancer remains less than 3% [3]. As the lifetime risk of being diagnosed approaches the known rate of histological (mostly insignificant) prostate cancer, there is a greater risk of overtreatment. At least two studies have attempted to model the rate of diagnosing clinically insignificant disease, suggesting that it ranges from 30% to 84% [4–5]. The current incidence to mortality ratio of about 7:1 suggests that the higher figure is more likely. Factors contributing to this are the increasing use of PSA screening and more extensive biopsy strategies employing 8–13 cores [21]. Additionally, biopsies are often repeated until a cancer diagnosis is made. More biopsies means more prostate cancer diagnosed, and more clinically insignificant disease (as well as more clinically important disease).

A large series of patients from Johns Hopkins treated with radical prostatectomy [22] showed that a median of 16 years elapses from surgery until death in patients who die of prostate cancer following disease recurrence. Many watchful waiting studies, most of which accrued patients from the pre-PSA era, also demonstrate that disease-related mortality in populations of prostate cancer patients only becomes substantial after 10 years. The lead time afforded by PSA screening probably increases this interval to 15–20 years in screened populations. Low-grade prostate cancer in particular is associated with low progression rates and high survival rates in the intermediate to long term. This is also supported by the Albertson data [6].

The estimated lead time between diagnosis based on PSA, and diagnosis based on clinical factors like the Connecticut series has been estimated to be around 10 years by many authors [23, 24]. Thus, many patients currently diagnosed by PSA screening, with favourable prognostic factors, are diagnosed considerably earlier in disease development than the average patient in this unscreened population. They are likely to have prostate cancer with an even longer and more benign natural history. Add to this the opportunity for radical intervention for patients who become reclassified as higher risk over time, and it seems obvious that the expected prostate cancer mortality in this group is likely to be exceptionally low.

IDENTIFYING INSIGNIFICANT DISEASE

Epstein *et al.* [25] utilized the data from Stamey *et al.* [26] with historical radical prostate-ctomy cohorts from Johns Hopkins School of Medicine [25, 27–29] to define insignificant cancers as those having clinical stage T1c, tumour volume < 0.2 ml, no Gleason pattern of 4 or 5, organ-confined disease and no evidence of seminal vesicle or lymph node invasion. Tumours between 0.2 and 0.5 ml were identified as having a minimal risk of progression. Since this classification was developed, other authors have merged these two categories into one, despite the propensity of some of the 0.2–0.5 ml tumours to display capsular invasion (Table 6.1) [30–36]. Clinical parameters predicting for minimal disease include Gleason 6 or less, < 50% of any one core involved, and a maximum of one to three cores involved (see Table 6.1). Crucially, the designation of 'insignificant' disease is based on histological volume, not natural history. The definition of insignificant cancer as < 0.5 cm³ of low-grade disease has never been validated in a trial with a clinical endpoint. Based on substantial data, including the PCPT trial, and the incontrovertible ratio of 7:1 between the current lifetime likelihood of diagnosis (about 1 in 6) and death (1 in 40), it understates the proportion of patients who have prostate cancer that is not destined to pose a threat to their life (about 6 out of 7).

WHO BENEFITS FROM TREATMENT?

A landmark trial from Sweden recently demonstrated, for the first time, that radical prosta-tectomy improves survival [37]. In that study, about 600 patients were randomized between radical prostatectomy and watchful waiting. The study showed a 5% absolute survival ben-efit at 10 years, and a 50% reduction in prostate cancer mortality with surgery.

However, this cohort was a group with many patients who had intermediate to high-risk disease. Only 5% were diagnosed based on PSA screening, and the median PSA was 12.8. The volume of disease in these patients represented a pre-stage migration cohort. (Even in this group, however, the number needed to treat to prevent one prostate cancer death was 19.) The distribution of disease volume and grade is higher than the expected distribution in a contemporary screened population, where a substantial proportion of newly diagnosed patients have small volume low-grade disease. The Swedish study should not be interpreted to mean that all patients with localized prostate cancer should be treated radically. Many studies emphasize that the patients with Gleason 4–5 pattern disease are at the greatest risk

Table 6.1 Clinical parameters to predict 'insignificant' prostate cancer

Author	PSA density	No. of positive cores	Maximum % of cores positive	Grade	% Tissue positive	Extent (mm)
Epstein [27]	<0.10	<3	<50%	≤6		
Epstein [28]	<0.15	1		≤6		<3
Irwin [34]		1		≤6		<3
Cupp [35]		1		≤6		<3
Goto [30]	<0.10	1		≤6		<2
Epstein [29]	F/T>0.15	<3	<50%	≤6		
Noguchi [33]	<0.15	1		≤6		<3
Augustin [32]	<0.10				<1	
Anast [36]			<10%	≤6		

for death from prostate cancer. In the Swedish study, the mortality improvement began to appear at 5 years. It would be most unusual for a patient with low-grade, low-volume disease to die within 5–7 years of diagnosis. (In the Toronto surveillance cohort, this is 1% of patients.) This means that the majority of the benefit seen in the Swedish trial probably represented mortality reduction in the high-risk group.

We have used these data and the Connecticut watchful waiting data to estimate the number of patients with favourable-risk prostate cancer that would have to be treated at the time of diagnosis for each prostate cancer death averted at 20 years. This is summarized in Table 6.2. The number needed to treat for each cancer death avoided at 10 years in the Swedish trial was 20. It is likely that with additional (i.e. 20-year) follow-up, the survival benefit in the Swedish trial, now 10 years, will increase. This is likely to be balanced by the lead time inherent in PSA screening. Thus, in a screened patient with intermediate grade and PSA similar to the Swedish cohort, the number needed to treat (NNT) at 20 years is estimated to also be 20. The Albertsen data [6] indicate that the mortality for intermediate risk disease was about 2.5 times greater at 20 years than for favourable-risk disease. This number may be an underestimate if the shift in contemporary Gleason scoring is factored in. Thus, at least 50 favourable-risk patients need to be treated for each death prevented by surgery compared with no treatment. However, if one offers selective delayed intervention to those patients who progress, it is likely that at least 50% can be salvaged. (This is a very conservative estimate.) The conclusion is that about 100 radical prostatectomies would be required for each prostate cancer death averted in favourable-risk disease. Correcting the Connecticut data for grade migration, as referred to above, would increase this even further. The Pound data suggest that the prostate cancer deaths averted would have occurred on average 16 years after diagnosis, meaning that the number of life years saved in each of these 1 in 100 averted deaths is modest. For the average 60-year-old, life would be prolonged an average of 5 years by having prostate cancer death averted [7]. If each prostate cancer death averted adds 5 years to that individual's life, each radical prostatectomy would add 0.6 months of life (60 months per 100 operations). This is of dubious merit.

IDENTIFYING AGGRESSIVE DISEASE IN FAVOURABLE-RISK PATIENTS

Egawa *et al.* examined PSADT before radical prostatectomy and found that a doubling time of ≤3 years was more common with pT3 disease at radical prostatectomy [38]. McLaren and coauthors also examined PSADT in a watchful waiting cohort and found that a PSADT of < 3 years was associated with clinical progression (defined as palpable enlargement in the tumour nodule or increase in T stage) in over 80% of patients by 18 months from diagnosis [39]. D'Amico and colleagues reported that a rise in PSA of > 2 ng/ml/year prior to surgery identified a group of patients who had a 15% prostate cancer mortality rate at 7 years [40]. No patients with a PSA rise of < 2.0 ng/ml/year prior to surgery died of the disease. Clearly, therefore, a rise in PSA of > 2.0 ng/ml/year, which corresponds to a PSADT of about 3 years or less in a patient with a PSA of 6 ng/ml, identifies a group at risk. The primary concern with using PSADT as a trigger for curative intervention is that it may act as a marker of aggressive disease that has already progressed and is no longer localized. Importantly, 20% of the favourable-risk patients had a PSA velocity > 2.0 ng/ml/year. Seven per cent of these died at 10 years. Thus only 1.4% of the favourable-risk cohort died of prostate cancer. If one assumes that the 50% reduction in prostate cancer mortality in the Swedish trial also applies to this group, this means that had these patients been managed with watchful waiting, instead of surgery, 2.8% would have died of prostate cancer. Thus, the benefit of surgery in favourable-risk patients can be estimated at 2.8 − 1.4 = 1.4%, remarkably close to the NNT analysis above.

Table 6.2 NNT estimate for screen-detected, favourable-risk prostate cancer: radical prostatectomy vs. active surveillance with selective delayed intervention

	Bill-Axelson [37]	Correct for PSA lead time	Adjust for low grade/grade shift	Adjust for salvage in 'high-risk' patients	Benefit per patient
Factor		10 years (factor 1.5–2.0)	1.5–2.5	Assume 50% curable (factor 2)	5–10 year survival benefit for each death averted
NNT at 10 years	20	30–40	45–75	90–150	
NNT at 20 years	9	20 (from study)	27–45	54–90	1–2 months unadjusted for quality of life

ACTIVE SURVEILLANCE

Because the prediction of clinically insignificant disease is problematic and inaccurate, an alternative strategy has been developed that allows patient entry into an expectant management protocol with rigorous monitoring and the option of curative salvage therapy, should signs of progression develop. This is referred to as 'active surveillance' [18, 19].

Choo and Klotz were the first to report on a prospective active surveillance protocol incorporating selective delayed intervention for the subset with rapid PSA progression or grade progression on repeat biopsy [41, 42]. The eligibility criteria for this included patients with T1c or T2a prostate cancer, who had Gleason ≤6 and PSA ≤10. For patients over age 70, the criteria were relaxed to include Gleason ≤7 (3 + 4) and/or PSA ≤15. The current cohort comprises 299 patients. The median age was 70 years with an age range of 49 to 84 years. Eighty per cent of patients had a Gleason score of 6 or less, and the same proportion had a PSA < 10 ng/ml (median 6.5 ng/ml). Patients were followed with PSA every 3 months for 2 years, then every 6 months (assuming PSA was stable), with repeat biopsy at year 1 and then every 4–5 years until age 80. With a median follow-up of 72 months, 101 patients (34%) came off active surveillance, while 198 have remained on surveillance. Of patients discontinuing surveillance, the reason was rapid biochemical progression in 15%, clinical progression in 3%, histological progression in 4% and patient preference in only 12%. With a median follow-up of 7 years (range 2–11 years), overall survival was 85% and disease-specific survival was 99% (Figures 6.1 and 6.2) [43]. Only 3 out of 299 patients had died of prostate cancer at the time of writing this chapter. All of these patients had a PSADT of < 2 years and death occurred 3.0, 5.1 and 5.2 years after diagnosis. All three patients exhibited the same pattern of clinical progression: initial favourable prognostic factors, a rapid rise in PSA which led to treatment at 6, 9 and 11 months after the initial diagnosis and progressive rise in PSA and clinically apparent bone metastases within 1 year of treatment leading to androgen deprivation therapy. Death occurred within 3 years of initiating hormonal therapy in all three patients. This very rapid progression after diagnosis suggests that these patients had occult metastases at the time of initial disease presentation, and their outcome would not have been altered by earlier treatment. Even in the Swedish trial, there were almost no 'saves' before 5 years.

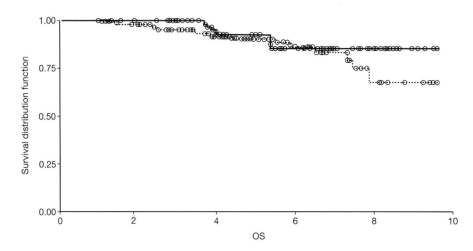

Figure 6.1 Overall survival in 331 patients on active surveillance.

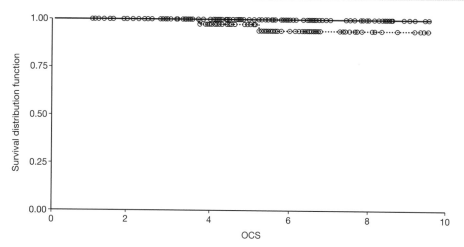

Figure 6.2 Prostate cancer specific survival in 331 patients on active surveillance.

The median PSADT, calculated by logarithmic regression, was 7 years. Twenty-two per cent of patients had a PSADT of < 3 years; 42% had a PSADT of over 10 years, suggesting an indolent course of disease in these patients.

Gleason score remained stable in 92% of patients; 8% demonstrated a significant rise in Gleason score, classed as in increase of ≥2. It is not known whether this represents true grade progression or initial undersampling; however, it is consistent with other similar series, demonstrating a 4% rate of grade progression over 2–3 years [44].

From this group, 29 patients (10% of the cohort) had a radical prostatectomy as a result of a short PSADT or grade progression. Of these patients, all had an initial Gleason score of 5–6, PSA < 10 ng/ml, and tumour stage pT1–2 at study entry. The final pathology was stage pT2 in 18 patients (64%%), pT3a in 11, T3c in 1 and N+ in 1. Amongst the patients with a PSADT < 3 years (18 patients), 7/18 only had positive margins. This suggests that even amongst the worst subset of the cohort, i.e. those reclassified as higher risk over time, the majority remained curable by delayed therapy.

DISCUSSION

The advent of widespread PSA screening has the positive effect of identifying patients with life-threatening prostate cancer at a time when they are more curable, and the negative effect of identifying many patients with non-life-threatening cancer who are susceptible to overtreatment. In a population subjected to regular screening, the latter group is more prevalent. A rational approach to therapy is to offer aggressive treatment to the intermediate and high-risk groups, and little or no treatment to the low-risk group. Since some apparently low-risk patients may reclassify as high risk over time, patients should be followed carefully and treated if they show evidence of rapid PSA progression or grade progression on repeat biopsy.

In young, healthy patients on surveillance, we believe that the optimal PSADT threshold for radical intervention should be around 3 years. In our series patients with a PSADT of 3 years or less constituted 22% of the cohort. This cutpoint for intervention remains empirical and speculative. However, the 20–25% of patients that a 3-year doubling time identifies represent a rough approximation of the proportion of good-risk patients 'at risk' for disease progression. For patients with a PSA in the 6–10 range, this also approximates an annual rise of 2 ng/ml, an adverse predictor of outcome as described by D'Amico.

The psychological effects of living for many years with untreated cancer are a potential concern. Does the cumulative effect, year after year, of knowing one is living with untreated cancer, a time bomb, sword of Damocles, etc., lead to depression or other adverse effects? The best data on this come from a companion study to the Holmberg randomized trial of surgery versus watchful waiting in Sweden. It found absolutely no significant psychological difference after 5 years in any domain. Worry, anxiety and depression were all equal between the two arms [45]. While surveillance is clearly stressful for some men, the reality is that most patients with prostate cancer, whether treated or not, are concerned about the risk of progression. Anxiety about PSA recurrence is common amongst both treated and untreated patients. Patients who are educated to appreciate the very indolent natural history of most good-risk prostate cancers may avoid much of this anxiety.

A follow-up strategy for managing patients with active surveillance and selective delayed intervention is described in Table 6.3.

CONCLUSION

There is good evidence that PSA testing detects prostate cancer at a more curable stage, and that patients with intermediate and high-risk cancer benefit from this earlier detection. However, treating all prostate cancer patients identified with PSA testing will result in hundreds of thousands of patients needlessly subjected to the side-effects of therapy. Conservative management has been adopted with reluctance in many constituencies due to concern about the inaccuracies of clinical staging and grading. This could result in rendering a curable patient incurable because of the delay in intervention.

Some apparently favourable-risk patients harbour more aggressive disease. In these patients there are benefits of curative treatment. A policy of close monitoring with selective intervention for those whose cancers exhibit characteristics of higher risk disease over time is appealing. Intervention is offered for a PSA doubling time < 3 years (depending on patient age, comorbidity, etc.), or grade progression to predominant Gleason 4 pattern. This approach is currently the focus of several clinical trials, and preliminary analysis of these has demonstrated that it is feasible. Most patients who understand the basis for this approach will remain on long-term surveillance. If patients are selected properly (i.e. good-risk and low-volume disease) and followed carefully, with early intervention for evidence of progression, it is likely that the majority of men with indolent disease will not suffer from clinical disease progression or prostate cancer death, and the minority with aggressive disease will

Table 6.3 Active surveillance: suggested algorithm for eligibility and follow-up

Eligibility
Gleason ≤6
T1c–T2a
Depending on age and comorbidity: < 3 cores involved, < 50% of any one core
Follow-up schedule
PSA, DRE every 3 months for 2 years, then every 6 months assuming PSA is stable
10–12 core biopsy at 1 year, and then every 3 years until age 80
Optional: TRUS on alternate visits
Intervention
For PSA doubling time <3 years (in most cases, based on at least eight determinations) (about 20% of patients)
For grade progression to Gleason 7 (4 + 3) or higher (about 5% of patients)

These are guidelines, and should be modified according to patient age and comorbidity

still be amenable to cure. Using two different approaches, we estimate that the NNT, if all such patients were offered radical prostatectomy compared with the strategy described above, is approximately 100 for each patient who avoids a prostate cancer death. Thus, the proportion of patients who die of disease is not likely to be significantly different from the proportion dying in spite of aggressive treatment of all good-risk patients at the time of diagnosis. This approach is currently being evaluated in a large-scale phase III study.

REFERENCES

1. Welch HG, Schwartz LM, Woloshin S. Prostate-specific antigen levels in the United States: implications of various definitions for abnormal. *J Natl Cancer Inst* 2005; 97:1132–1137.
2. Sakr WA, Haas GP, Cassin BF *et al*. The frequency of carcinoma and intraepithelial neoplasia of the prostate in young male patients. *J Urol* 1993; 150:379.
3. Jemal A, Tiwari RC, Murray T *et al*. Cancer Statistics, 2004. *CA Cancer J Clin* 2004; 54:8.
4. Etzioni R, Penson DF, Legler JM *et al*. Overdiagnosis due to prostate-specific antigen screening: lessons from U.S. prostate cancer incidence trends. *J Natl Cancer Inst* 2002; 94:981.
5. D'Amico AV, Whittington R, Malkowicz SB *et al*. Biochemical outcome after radical prostatectomy, external beam radiation therapy, or interstitial radiation therapy for clinically localized prostate cancer. *JAMA* 1998; 280:969–974.
6. Albertsen P, Hanley JA, Fine J. 20-Year Outcomes following conservative management of clinically localized prostate cancer. *JAMA* 2005; 293:2095–2101.
7. Albertsen PC, Hanley JA, Barrows GH *et al*. Prostate cancer and the Will Rogers Phenomenon. *Natl Cancer Inst* 2005; 97:1248–1253.
8. Hanash KA, Utz DC, Cook EN, Taylor WF, Titus JL. Carcinoma of the prostate: a 15-year followup. *J Urol* 1972; 107:450–453.
9. Johansson J-E, Holmberg L, Johansson S *et al*. Fifteen-year survival in prostate cancer. A prospective, population-based study in Sweden. *JAMA* 1997; 277:467.
10. Lerner SP, Seale-Hawkins C, Carlton CE Jr. The risk of dying of prostate cancer in patients with clinically localized disease. *J Urol* 1991; 146:1040–1045.
11. Handley R, Carr TW, Travis D, Powell PH, Hall RR. Deferred treatment for prostate cancer. *Br J Urol* 1988; 62:249–253.
12. Adolfsson J, Carstensen J, Lowhagen T. Deferred treatment in clinically localized prostate carcinoma. *Br J Urol* 1992; 69:183–187.
13. Waaler G, Stenwig AE. Prognosis of localised prostatic cancer managed by 'Watch and Wait' policy. *Br J Urol* 1993; 72:214–219.
14. Whitmore WF Jr, Warner JA, Thompson IM Jr. Expectant management of localized prostatic cancer. *Cancer* 1991; 67:1091–1096.
15. George, N. Natural history of localised prostatic cancer managed by conservative therapy alone. *Lancet* 1988; 1:494.
16. Aus G, Hugosson I, Norlen L. Long-term survival and mortality in prostate cancer treated with noncurative intent. *J Urol* 1995; 154:460.
17. Sandblom G. Long-term survival in a Swedish population-based cohort of men with prostate cancer. *Urology* 2000; 56:442–447.
18. Parker C. Active surveillance: towards a new paradigm in the management of early prostate cancer. *Lancet Oncol* 2004; 5:101.
19. Parker C. Active surveillance: an individualized approach to early prostate cancer. *BJU Int* 2003; 92:2.
20. Thompson IM, Goodman PJ, Tangen CM *et al*. The influence of finasteride on the development of prostate cancer. *N Engl J Med* 2003; 349:215.
21. Presti JC Jr. Prostate biopsy: how many cores are enough? *Urol Oncol* 2003, 21:135.
22. Pound CR, Partin AW, Eisenberger MA, Chan DW, Pearson JD, Walsh PC. Natural history of progression after PSA elevation following radical prostatectomy. *JAMA* 1999; 281:1591–1597.
23. Draisma G, Schroeder FH *et al*. Lead times and overdetection due to PSA screening: estimates from the European Randomized Study of Screening for Prostate Cancer. *J Natl Cancer Inst* 2003; 95:868–878.
24. Tornblom M *et al*. Lead time associated with screening for prostate cancer. *Int J Cancer* 2004; 108:122–129.

25. Epstein JI, Walsh PC, Carmichael M *et al.* Pathologic and clinical findings to predict tumor extent of nonpalpable (stage T1c) prostate cancer. *JAMA* 1994; 271:368.
26. Stamey TA, Freiha FS, McNeal JE *et al.* Localized prostate cancer. Relationship of tumor volume to clinical significance for treatment of prostate cancer. *Cancer* 1993; 71:933.
27. Epstein JI, Pizov G, Walsh PC. Correlation of pathologic findings with progression after radical retropubic prostatectomy. *Cancer* 1993; 71:3582.
28. Epstein JI, Carmichael M, Partin AW *et al.* Is tumor volume an independent predictor of progression following radical prostatectomy? A multivariate analysis of 185 clinical stage B adenocarcinomas of the prostate with 5 years of followup. *J Urol* 1993; 149:1478.
29. Epstein JI, Chan DW, Sokoll LJ *et al.* Nonpalpable stage T1c prostate cancer: prediction of insignificant disease using free/total prostate specific antigen levels and needle biopsy findings. *J Urol* 1998; 160:2407.
30. Goto Y, Ohori M, Arakawa A *et al.* Distinguishing clinically important from unimportant prostate cancers before treatment: value of systematic biopsies. *J Urol* 1996; 156:1059.
31. Kattan MW, Eastham JA, Wheeler TM *et al.* Counseling men with prostate cancer: a nomogram for predicting the presence of small, moderately differentiated, confined tumors. *J Urol* 2003; 170:1792.
32. Augustin H, Hammerer PG, Graefen M *et al.* Insignificant prostate cancer in radical prostatectomy specimen: time trends and preoperative prediction. *Eur Urol* 2003; 43:455.
33. Noguchi M, Stamey TA, McNeal JE *et al.* Relationship between systematic biopsies and histological features of 222 radical prostatectomy specimens: lack of prediction of tumor significance for men with nonpalpable prostate cancer. *J Urol* 2001; 166:104.
34. Irwin MB, Trapasso JG. Identification of insignificant prostate cancers: analysis of preoperative parameters. *Urology* 1994; 44:862–867; discussion 867–868.
35. Cupp MR, Bostwick DG, Myers RP, Oesterling JE. The volume of prostate cancer in the biopsy specimen cannot reliably predict the quantity of cancer in the radical prostatectomy specimen on an individual basis. *J Urol* 1995; 153:1543–1548.
36. Anast JW, Andriole GL, Bismar TA, Yan Y, Humphrey PA. Relating biopsy and clinical variables to radical prostatectomy findings: can insignificant and advanced prostate cancer be predicted in a screening population? *Urology* 2004; 64:544–550.
37. Bill-Axelson A, Holmberg L. Radical prostatectomy versus watchful waiting (update). *N Engl J Med* 2005; 352:1977–1984.
38. Egawa S, Arai Y, Tobisu K *et al.* Use of pretreatment prostate-specific antigen doubling time to predict outcome after radical prostatectomy. *Prostate Cancer Prostatic Dis* 2000; 3:269.
39. McLaren DB, McKenzie M, Duncan G *et al.* Watchful waiting or watchful progression? Prostate specific antigen doubling times and clinical behavior in patients with early untreated prostate carcinoma. *Cancer* 1998; 82:342.
40. D'Amico AV, Chen MH, Roehl KA, Catalona WJ. Preoperative PSA velocity and the risk of death from prostate cancer after radical prostatectomy. *N Engl J Med* 2004; 351:125–135.
41. Choo R, Klotz L, Danjoux C *et al.* Feasibility study: watchful waiting for localized low to intermediate grade prostate carcinoma with selective delayed intervention based on prostate specific antigen, histological and/or clinical progression. *J Urol* 2002; 167:1664.
42. Choo R, DeBoer G, Klotz L *et al.* PSA doubling time of prostate carcinoma managed with watchful observation alone. *Int J Radiat Oncol Biol Phys* 2001; 50:615.
43. Klotz L. Active surveillance for prostate cancer: for whom? *J Clin Oncol* 2005; 23:8165–8169.
44. Epstein JI, Walsh PC, Carter HB. Dedifferentiation of prostate cancer grade with time in men followed expectantly for stage T1c disease. *J Urol* 2001; 166:1688.
45. Steineck G, Helgesen F, Adolfsson J *et al.* Scandinavian Prostatic Cancer Group Study Number 4. Quality of life after radical prostatectomy or watchful waiting. *N Engl J Med* 2002; 347:790–796.

7

Treatment of low-risk prostate cancer

Bruce R. Kava, Alan M. Nieder, Mark S. Soloway

INTRODUCTION

Mr John Smith is a 59-year-old man referred for evaluation with recently diagnosed clinical stage T1c prostate cancer. On a routine insurance examination his prostate-specific antigen (PSA) was noted to be 6.3 ng/ml. This prompted a referral to a urologist, who examined the patient and suggested that he undergo a prostate biopsy. His digital rectal examination (DRE) demonstrated a 30-g soft prostate without any discrete nodules. A 12-core transrectal ultrasound (TRUS) biopsy demonstrated Gleason 3 + 3 prostate cancer in 2 out of 12 cores (both right-sided) with a total cancer volume of 20% in each of the cores. He is an otherwise healthy and active businessman. He has mild lower urinary tract symptoms (AUASS 7) and no complaints of erectile dysfunction (SHIM 22). He now presents with his wife for a second opinion regarding treatment options.

Counselling the newly diagnosed prostate cancer patient is one of the more formidable tasks in urology. Patients often desire an active or collaborative role in treatment decision-making [1]. As a result, the healthcare provider is expected to translate and individualize the seemingly endless and often contradictory clinical data that have emerged about this disease over the last 25 years. Uncertainty related to the variable natural history of prostate cancer, the high prevalence of autopsy prostate cancer and the lack of any clear-cut advantage of one treatment modality over another are recurring themes that characterize these data and create a sense of frustration for clinicians. More importantly, the diagnosis of prostate cancer may create distress for as many as 50% of patients, who are faced with complex and controversial decisions that may dramatically alter their quality of life (QOL) [2]. Moreover, men often initially believe that their sexual function will be terminated and are distressed over their partner's reaction, whereas the partner is often initially less concerned with the quality of life outcomes and more interested in curing the disease [3].

Risk stratification of patients with prostate cancer assists in the selection of patients who are candidates for treatment with curative intent. In addition to providing prognostic information for the individual, it also may provide insight into the urgency with which treatment is instituted. Traditionally, urologists have relied upon serum prostate-specific antigen (PSA), biopsy Gleason score and DRE to predict the final pathological stage at the time of radical prostatectomy. More recently, nomograms have been developed and validated using large cohorts of patients that attempt to predict the biochemical recurrence 5 and 10 years after radical prostatectomy in those patients with clinically localized disease. Despite this, the

Bruce R. Kava, MD, Department of Urology, University of Miami Miller School of Medicine, Miami, Florida, USA
Alan M. Nieder, MD, Department of Urology, University of Miami Miller School of Medicine, Miami, Florida, USA
Mark S. Soloway, MD, Professor and Chairman, Department of Urology, University of Miami Miller School of Medicine, Miami, Florida, USA

accuracy of these nomograms falls short of perfect, with concordance indices between 0.68 and 0.84 [4–8]. Moreover, there is evidence that they are even less accurate for that group of low-risk patients based upon favourable PSA, Gleason score and clinical stage [7].

Recently, the utilization of the triad of the serum PSA, Gleason score and T stage has categorized patients into broader prognostic categories as defined by the low, intermediate and high risk of biochemical (PSA) failure following treatment. The delineation of low-risk patients as those patients with a pretreatment serum PSA ≤10, a Gleason score of 6 or less and clinical T1c or T2a disease has been embraced by several authors [9–12] and will serve as the definition of low risk for the remainder of this chapter, unless otherwise annotated. Also, low cancer volume on biopsy (e.g. few cores and a small amount of cancer on each core) typically helps define low-risk patients. Driven by the widespread use of PSA testing, as well as the heightened public awareness of prostate cancer, it is this low-risk group of patients that now accounts for close to 50% of patients being diagnosed with prostate cancer [7]. The substantial growth of this risk group is demonstrated in an analysis of the CaPSURE (Cancer of the Prostate Strategic Urologic Research Endeavor) data, which demonstrated that between 1989–1992 and 2001–2002 the percentage of patients with low-risk disease increased from 29.5% to 46.8% [13].

TO TREAT OR NOT TO TREAT?

During Mr Smith's initial consultation a significant component of our discussion revolved around his favourable-risk prostate cancer. We told him that his low moderate Gleason score, PSA of 6 and low volume on biopsy placed him into a low-risk category for disease progression, with a high likelihood of cure with any of the treatment modalities.

PRE-PSA ERA DATA ON CONSERVATIVE MANAGEMENT OF PROSTATE CANCER

Several studies of untreated prostate cancer patients have identified the importance of tumour grade as a powerful determinant of prostate cancer progression. In a pooled analysis of 828 patients from six non-randomized studies of men with localized prostate cancer, Chodak *et al.* found that the 10-year cancer specific-survival of untreated prostate cancer patients with well and moderately differentiated tumours was 87% [14].

Twenty-year follow-up of two ongoing observational cohorts of untreated prostate cancer patients has also recently confirmed that tumours with a low histological grade may progress very slowly. Johansson provided follow-up for 223 of 306 patients that had been diagnosed with prostate cancer between 1979 and 1984 [15]. Although more than 90% of the patients died during follow-up, only 16% of these deaths were attributed to prostate cancer. For those patients with low-grade tumours, the 20-year cause-specific mortality rate was only 9%. Albertsen *et al.* recently provided 20-year follow-up of 767 men with localized prostate cancer that were treated with observation or androgen deprivation therapy alone [16]. All men were diagnosed between 1971 and 1984, and were prospectively followed by the Connecticut Tumor Registry. Although PSA values were not initially available to stage the patients, the Gleason grading system was utilized, transrectal biopsy was used to make the diagnosis and modern record-keeping was used to obtain follow-up in these patients. Using a regression model that was used to construct a competing risk analysis, they found that men with Gleason scores of 2–4 have a minimal risk of dying from prostate cancer (6 deaths per 1000 person-years) 20 years following diagnosis. These patients are rarely found today, as most patients have higher Gleason scores. For patients with Gleason scores of 5, 6 and 7, there is an intermediate risk of 12, 30 and 65 deaths per 1000 person-years respectively.

Extrapolating these data to the contemporary prostate cancer patient is difficult because the majority of the patients were diagnosed prior to the widespread use of PSA testing. In addition, a large number of patients in the Scandinavian study were diagnosed based upon the results of aspiration cytology, which has a high false-positive rate [17]. Despite these limitations, it has become clear that many, if not most, individuals with low-grade tumours will not die from prostate cancer, regardless of whether treatment is instituted or not.

CONTEMPORARY STUDIES EVALUATING CONSERVATIVE MANAGEMENT OF LOW-RISK PROSTATE CANCER

While these observational studies have provided us with important information regarding the prostate cancer patient in the pre-PSA era, a recent randomized study has questioned the role of conservative management of patients with clinically localized prostate cancer. Between 1988 and 1999 the Scandinavian Prostatic Cancer Study group randomized patients with localized prostate cancer to treatment with either radical prostatectomy ($n = 347$) or watchful waiting ($n = 348$) [18]. With a mean follow-up of 8.2 years, patients undergoing radical prostatectomy demonstrated significant advantages in terms of cancer-specific survival, development of distant metastases, local progression, the need for initiation of hormonal therapy, palliative radiation therapy and the requirement for laminectomy. Despite these compelling data, there is still no difference in overall survival between the two arms of the study. In addition, it is noteworthy that only 5% of the cancers in this study were screen-detected, more than 75% were palpable, stage T2 or greater tumours, and approximately 50% had a PSA > 10.0 ng/ml. As a result, these data cannot be extrapolated to determine the need for treatment for our low-risk prostate cancer patient.

Active surveillance with delayed intervention has only recently emerged as a very appealing treatment option for many men with low-risk prostate cancer. Several contemporary series have added to the growing body of evidence that confirms the feasibility and at least short-term low-risk for disease progression and mortality from this approach. Table 7.1 summarizes some of these studies. While follow-up is short, there are several concerns that have been raised within these studies. In two, repeat prostate biopsies were performed, which yielded a higher Gleason score than the one that had been performed prior to patient entry (Klotz and Carter) [19, 20]. In fact, prostate biopsies may undergrade the histology of prostate cancer when compared to the final radical prostatectomy histology in up to 43% of cases [21–25]. This undergrading raises concerns about the accuracy of risk assignment at the outset. A second concern raised within these series is that in the data presented by Klotz, 24 of the patients have undergone radical prostatectomy, all because of a prostate-specific antigen doubling time (PSADT) of less than 2 years [20]. The final histology demonstrated an unexpectedly high prevalence of pT3N0 and N1 prostate cancer (16 patients, 66%) for a group that was thought to be low risk. Whether a rapid PSADT is a marker for more aggressive phenotype warrants further study.

There remains a considerable amount of scepticism about active surveillance with delayed intervention on the part of medical providers. In a recent evaluation of 24 405 low-risk prostate cancer patients from 13 Surveillance, Epidemiology and End Results registries, Miller *et al.* reported that 45% of patients opted for initial expectant management [26]. Comparison with historical and comparable SEER (Surveillance Epidemiology and End Results)-based data from 1988 to 1990 demonstrates that this is a smaller percentage of patients opting for initial expectant management. Interestingly, data from CaPSURE have also confirmed this downward trend in the utilization of active surveillance for low-risk prostate cancer patients [27]. In this analysis of 5365 patients diagnosed with localized prostate cancer, there was a progressive decline in the utilization of expectant management from 9.5% of men diagnosed between 1992 and 1994, to 5.5% of men diagnosed between 1998 and 2000. Of note, the most profound decline was seen in those patients with low-risk prostate cancer. Even more interesting is that, during those years, the percentage of patients within academic centres in the CaPSURE database increased their enrolment of patients on expectant therapy from 5% to 15%. Reasons for the profound decline within the community can only be attributed to

Table 7.1 Watchful waiting for low-risk prostate cancer

Study (year)	Clinical characteristics	No. of patients	Follow-up	Five-year probability of treatment	DOD/disease-specific survival
Carter et al. (2003) [19]	T1–T2 PSA 20 or less Gleason 6 or less	313	3.8 (0.5–10.5) years	75%	2 (0.6%)/NS
Klotz (2006) [20]	Age <70 Gleason 6 or less PSA <10 (or age >70, Gleason 3+4=7 or less, PSA <15)	299	5.3 years	34% (within 8 years of follow-up)	2 (0.6%)/99.3%
Koppie et al. (2000) [67]	Gleason 6 or less, PSA <5, cT1c or cT2a Gleason 7 or less, PSA 5–15, cT1-T2	67 177	2.25 years 2.25 years	22% 49%	0 (0%)/NS 1 (0.5%)/NS
Zietman et al. (2001) [68]	T1c/T2a (65%) Gleason 6 or less (80%) PSA 10 or less (79%)	199	3.4 years	57%	2 (1)/98.6%

DOD, dead of disease; NS, not specified; PSA, prostate-specific antigen.

medicolegal issues, financial incentives and concerns regarding a lack of a uniform strategy to monitor and potentially salvage patients on watchful waiting.

IMPACT OF DELAY IN TREATMENT OF LOW-RISK PROSTATE CANCER

Mr Smith and his wife were obviously most concerned about his diagnosis and his need for emergent treatment. They had previously been counselled that he needed to undergo treatment rapidly to prevent disease progression.

A variety of factors may contribute to a delay between the time of diagnosis and the initiation of therapy in the prostate cancer patient. In some cases the patient requires time to familiarize himself with the various treatment options. Other delays may occur as a result of an already overburdened healthcare system. Finally, given the sentiment that prostate cancer has a very prolonged natural history, there is occasionally what appears to be no urgency in initiation of therapy by either the healthcare provider or the patient.

Several studies have addressed the impact of delay in radical prostatectomy. Nam *et al.* followed 645 patients who underwent radical prostatectomy between 1987 and 1998 [28]. With a median follow-up of 4 years (range 0.4–11.7 years), they found that the 10-year biochemical recurrence-free survival (BRFS) was greater in patients who underwent surgery within 3 months of diagnosis, compared with those that waited for longer than 3 months (74.6% versus 61.3%, $P = 0.05$). Two other studies, however, fail to confirm any effect of delay in surgery for up to 150 days, particularly for those patients with low-risk prostate cancer. In the first study, Khan *et al.* [29], evaluating 926 men with predominantly low-risk cancer undergoing radical prostatectomy, no negative impact was associated with delays of up to 150 days in either the final pathology or in the 5- and 10-year BRFS. In the second study, 150 patients were evaluated. There was no correlation between biochemical recurrence and the interval from biopsy to surgery, either as a continuous or a categorical variable. There were only 16 patients, however, that delayed surgery for more than 180 days. More recently, however, Freedland *et al.* retrospectively evaluated 895 patients with low-risk prostate cancer and found that, while there was no adverse association between the time from biopsy to radical prostatectomy pathological features, delays of more than 180 days were associated with a higher risk of biochemical progression [30].

CANCER CONTROL FOLLOWING PRIMARY TREATMENT OF LOW-RISK PROSTATE CANCER

After an extensive discussion regarding the different treatment modalities and the risks and benefits of active surveillance, the patient decided that he wanted to undergo treatment for his cancer. We specifically discussed the BRFS rates following surgery and radiation.

Because of the lack of prospective, head-to-head, randomized studies comparing surgery with the different forms of radiation it has been historically difficult to give patients precise data on the optimal treatment for them. Also, because of the variability of the disease and the need to personalize and individualize each patient's treatment, the urologist is rarely able to give an answer – supported by randomized clinical trials – when the patient asks 'what should I do?'.

Prostate cancer, unlike most other cancers, has the benefit of a very accurate serum tumour marker, PSA, to follow patients postoperatively. PSA, a serine protease, is an exquisitely sensitive marker of prostate cancer recurrence following radical prostatectomy. Typically, a PSA cut-off of either 0.2 ng/ml or 0.4 ng/ml defines biochemical recurrence, and thus allows for computation of the BRFS. Following radiotherapy, either external beam (EBRT) or interstitial seed placement, the PSA may not nadir to undetectable or below 0.2 ng/ml. For this reason, different authors have utilized different PSA cut-offs to analyse post-radiotherapy recurrences. The most often used criteria is the ASTRO (American Society for Therapeutic

Radiology and Oncology) criteria, which acknowledges a cancer recurrence following radiotherapy as three successive rises of PSA, and backdates the time of recurrence to the mid-
point between the nadir and the first rise of the PSA. Because of this different method of
calculating and evaluating prostate cancer recurrence, it is often difficult to directly compare
surgical and radiation series for recurrence.

The decision ultimately becomes personalized to each patient's pathological stratification
based upon their risk category. Decisions regarding different treatment modalities tend to
also consider the patient's comorbidity, such as whether the patient is a good surgical candidate or not based upon their body habitus and risk of cardiac disease [31]. Dillioglugil *et
al.* retrospectively reviewed a single surgeon database of 472 patients who underwent radical retropubic prostatectomy (RRP) and specifically evaluated the complications [32]. The
authors stratified complications by ASA category, age, operative time and year of surgery.
They found that ASA class III patients had a threefold increased risk of major complications
(21%), a greater length of stay and an increased need for intensive care unit (ICU) care, and
included both patient mortalities. Importantly, the risk of complications was related to the
presence of comorbidities and not to age or operative time. Recent studies have confirmed
minimal perioperative morbidity and mortality in well-selected patients. The overall perioperative mortality rate is less than 0.5% [11, 32, 33]. Similarly, the risk of wound complications
and rectal injuries is also less than 1%. In our own centre, with the use of venous intermittent
compression devices and early ambulation following surgery, the risk of deep vein thrombosis (DVT) is less than 1% [34].

Also factored into the decision regarding surgery versus radiation therapy is an assessment of the patient's baseline lower urinary tract voiding symptoms, sexual function and
interest in maintaining it, and general lifestyle. These QOL issues will be discussed in the
next section.

Contemporary prostate cancer series have stratified prostate cancer risk based upon the
pretreatment serum PSA, clinical stage and Gleason score. In a retrospective analysis of 1872
men treated with surgery or radiation therapy at two centres, D'Amico *et al.* validated the
significant differences in PSA-based outcome between low-, intermediate- and high-risk
patients regardless of whether patients received surgery or radiation [12]. For those men
with low-risk features (defined by a PSA of <10, T1c or T2a and Gleason score of 6 or less),
patients derived equal 5-year PSA-free survival benefit from treatment with radical prostatectomy, radiation therapy or brachytherapy. Furthermore, the addition of neoadjuvant
androgen deprivation to brachytherapy did not contribute any advantage in terms of biochemical recurrence.

There have been many single surgeon and single radiation therapy series describing good
outcomes for low-risk prostate cancer (Table 7.2). It has historically been difficult to compare
them precisely because the definition of low-risk prostate cancer has varied, the criteria for
BRFS has not been uniform, the follow-up has varied and the treatments may not have been
uniform (e.g. lack of lymph node dissection in surgery, lack of a centralized pathological
analysis, lack of standard dosimetry). Nevertheless, multiple surgical series on low-risk prostate cancer have demonstrated BRFS rates of greater than 85%. Multiple radiation therapy
series have also demonstrated excellent BRFS rates for low-risk prostate cancer in patients
treated with either XRT or brachytherapy. There have been no standard patient stratifica-
tions as in the surgical series; however, when extrapolating data regarding low-risk patients,
BRFS rates have also approached 85%. Importantly, radiation therapy efficacy is also dose
dependent.

Several features of radiation in the low-risk prostate cancer patient warrant mention. In
a retrospective study by Zelefsky *et al.*, patients treated with doses above 75 Gy had higher
biochemical-free survival (BFS) than levels below 70 Gy [35]. Other studies have demonstrated similar findings. Zietman *et al.* performed a randomized trial evaluating the use of
high-dose EBRT [36]. In this study that assessed 393 patients from two academic centres,

Table 7.2 Biochemical free survival (BFS) in contemporary series of treated patients with low-risk prostate cancer

Study (year)	Clinical characteristics	Treatment modality	No. of patients	BFS (%)
D'Amico et al.(1998) [12]	T1c–T2a PSA 10 or less Gleason score 6 or less	RRP EBRT BT alone	402 225 91	85 (5 years) 88 (5 years) 87 (5 years)
Borchers et al. (2004) [69]	T1c–T2a PSA 10 or less Gleason score 6 or less	RRP BT alone	80 52	96 (2 years) 85 (2 years)
Roehl et al. (2004) [70]	T1c–T2a PSA 10 or less Gleason score 6 or less	RRP	1774	69–77 (10 years)
Martinez et al. (2000) [71]	T1c–T2a PSA 10 or less Gleason score 6 or less	RRP EBRT (59.2–70.2 Gy)	157 225	84 (5 years) 69 (5 years)
Zelefsky et al. (2001) [35]	T1–T2 PSA 10 or less Gleason score 6 or less	EBRT (64.8–70.2 Gy) EBRT (75.6–86.4 Gy)	91 188	77 (5 years) 90 (5 years)
Zietman et al. (2005) [36]	T1c–T2a PSA 10 or less Gleason score 6 or less	EBRT (70.2 Gy) EBRT (79.2 Gy)	116 111	60 (5 years) 85 (5 years)
Grimm et al. (2001) [72]	T1c–T2b PSA 10 or less Gleason score 6 or less	I^{125} BT	75 (pre-1988) 95 (post-1988)	65 (5 years) 87 (5 years)
Potters et al. (2005) [73]	PSA 10 or less Gleason score 6 or less <50% positive Bx cores	I^{125} BT Pd^{103} BT	481	91 (5 years)
Blasko et al. (2000) [74]	T1–T2 PSA 10 or less Gleason score 6 or less	Pd^{103} BT	103	94 (5 years)
Freedland et al. (2004) [75]	T1c–T2a PSA 10 or less Gleason score 6 or less	RRP	175	80 (5 years)

Continued overleaf

Table 7.2 Continued

Study (year)	Clinical characteristics	Treatment modality	No. of patients	BFS (%)
Kupelian et al. (2004) [76]	T1–T2 70% Gleason score 6 or less 65% PSA 10 or less 21% received neoadjuvant LHRH-A	RRP EBRT <72 Gy EBRT >72 Gy Seeds Seeds+EBRT	1034 484 301 950 222	81 (5 years) 51 (5 years) 81 (5 years) 77 (5 years) 83 (5 years)
Stone et al. (2005) [77]	T1c–T2a PSA 10 or less Gleason score 6 or less	I^{125} BT	146	91 (10 years)
Sylvester et al. (2003) [78]	T1c–T2b PSA 10 or less Gleason score 6 or less	I^{125} or Pd^{103}BT+EBRT (45 Gy)	63	85 (10 years)

BT, brachytherapy; EBRT, external beam radiation therapy; PSA, prostate-specific antigen; RRP, radical retropubic prostatectomy.

eligibility included patients with T1b to T2b prostate cancer with PSA levels less than 15 ng/ml and no evidence of metastatic disease. There were 227 patients with T1c and T2a prostate cancer, PSA < 10 and a Gleason score of 6 or less who were randomized between the two arms and received conformal radiation to the prostate alone. These patients were independently analysed and found to have a 60.1% BFS at 5 years when receiving 70.2 Gy versus 80.5% BFS when 79.2 Gy was delivered.

One additional factor, pretreatment PSADT, has recently been found to be associated with BFS, prostate cancer-free survival and all cause-specific survival. In a retrospective study by D'Amico et al., 125 of the 358 patients studied had low-risk disease and were followed after EBRT [37]. PSA recurrence occurred in 16 of the 29 (%) patients with a pretreatment PSADT of > 2 compared with 31/96 patients with a PSADT < 2. This translated into a 10% risk of prostate cancer-specific mortality for the men with a PSADT > 2 compared with 0 in the other group.

HEALTH-RELATED QUALITY OF LIFE FOLLOWING PRIMARY TREATMENT OF LOW-RISK PROSTATE CANCER

Assuring Mr Smith that whichever treatment he chooses he will have a good chance of achieving a long-term BRFS, after the oncological efficacy of the treatment options was discussed the patient expressed concern regarding urinary incontinence and erectile dysfunction.

The assessment of health-related quality of life (HRQOL) following radical prostatectomy requires an evaluation of both general and disease-specific issues facing the patient with prostate cancer. Urinary function, sexual function and bowel function are prostate cancer-specific aspects of HRQOL. In addition, general HRQOL domains include one's sense of overall well-being and function in the physical, emotional and social domains. Assessment of HRQOL issues is best performed with self-administered, validated questionnaires.

Utilizing validated instruments for assessing general HRQOL following radical prostatectomy, several studies have noted relatively few alterations in general HRQOL compared with age-matched control subjects [38–40]. However, while the overall general HRQOL scores may initially decline immediately following surgery, one study demonstrated that there was a significant improvement back to baseline after the first year [41, 42]. More recently, studies have observed some subtle differences in overall HRQOL in patients with localized prostate cancer, possibly reflecting the effects of stage migration and younger patients detected in screened populations. In a comparison of 783 untreated men with incidental prostate cancer with 1928 age-matched healthy control subjects, men with prostate cancer had significantly better physical function and less bodily pain, but had worse general health, vitality, social function and role limitations as a result of physical and emotional problems [43]. This suggests that the disease itself, and not just the treatment, may affect HRQOL.

The initial impact of altered sexual and urinary function on overall HRQOL has been well documented. Prior to the advent of the anatomical nerve-sparing radical prostatectomy, virtually all patients undergoing surgery had erectile dysfunction. Early published radical prostatectomy series found that age, preoperative potency, the number of neurovascular bundles preserved and final pathological stage all influenced the preservation of erectile function in men undergoing prostate cancer [44, 45]. Studies that have utilized self-administered instruments have found that 21–50% of patients can have erections firm enough for intercourse following radical prostatectomy [46–48]. In addition, the return of potency following radical prostatectomy has been found to be a time-dependent process, in which there is a gradual return of potency in many individuals during the first 24 months [42, 47].

A few studies have compared HRQOL outcomes in men undergoing radical prostatectomy or radiation therapy. Litwin et al. evaluated urinary function and bother in 564 men undergoing either radical prostatectomy or radiation therapy using a validated questionnaire, the UCLA Prostate Cancer Index [49]. As expected, urinary function scores were significantly better immediately after treatment in men who underwent radiation therapy compared with surgery. However, after 12 months men in both groups had nearly identical urinary function scores and these scores remained relatively stable for up to 2 years. Conversely, urinary bother was significantly greater immediately after treatment in men receiving radiation therapy compared with men undergoing surgery. After 1 year, the radiation therapy groups' urinary bother scores improved; however, they always remained slightly lower than the surgery groups' scores. Interestingly, non-married men experienced more urinary bother and reported decreased urinary function than married men. The authors comment that their UCLA Prostate Cancer Index was designed to measure urinary leakage symptoms following surgery and not necessarily the irritative symptoms that men typically experience following radiation therapy.

Potosky *et al.* similarly compared HRQOL outcomes in men who underwent surgery or radiation therapy. At 5-year follow-up, the men who underwent surgery were more likely to have incontinence and erectile dysfunction, but had less bowel dysfunction [50]. McCammon *et al.* also compared men who underwent surgery with those who received radiation therapy [51]. Importantly, these authors studied men who were operated on between 1984 and 1994, and received radiation therapy between 1974 and 1994. Thus, the patient population and the surgical and radiation therapy outcomes may not be representative of what is currently seen or achieved. Nevertheless, while men who underwent surgery had a greater risk of incontinence, there was no difference in the two groups when comparing urinary bother. The risks of erectile dysfunction were similar in the two groups. As expected, those who received radiation therapy experienced a significantly greater amount of bowel dysfunction.

Wei *et al.* compared HRQOL outcomes in over 1000 men who had undergone surgery or received EBRT or brachytherapy at one centre between 1995 and 1999 [40]. The authors reported that, while each group demonstrated decreased sexual function, the cohort of men who received brachytherapy demonstrated the worst bowel, urinary and sexual HRQOL outcomes. Brandeis *et al.* compared men who underwent brachytherapy (with or without pretreatment EBRT) with those who underwent surgery, and with age-matched healthy control subjects [52]. While general HRQOL outcomes did not differ greatly between the groups, it was noted that patients who receive combined EBRT and brachytherapy demonstrated the worst HRQOL outcomes.

The advent of phosphodiesterase type-5 (PDE-5) agents has significantly benefited many men with post-prostatectomy erectile dysfunction. PDE-5 inhibitors are the first line of therapy in the management of erectile dysfunction in men who have undergone nerve-sparing radical prostatectomy. Improvements in frequency of penetration, the ability to maintain an erection, and both patient and spousal satisfaction are seen in up to 70% of cases [53]. For those men who fail PDE-5 inhibitors, intracavernous injection therapy, transurethral pharmacological therapy, vacuum erection devices and implantation of a penile prosthesis are additional options. The use of these adjunctive therapies is discussed in a recent review of management strategies when PDE-5 inhibitors fail [54].

Two large series have demonstrated continence rates of between 91% and 95% between 18 and 24 months following radical prostatectomy [55, 56]. Catalona *et al.* reported that continence (defined as no need of any pad for protection) was only found to be higher in younger men, and was independent of nerve preservation, clinical stage, pathological stage, postoperative radiation therapy or the number of prior prostatectomies performed by the surgeon [55].

Penson *et al.* utilized the SEER database and demonstrated minimal significant long-term urinary dysfunction following radical prostatectomy [57]. In this study, 25% of men reported frequent urination or lack of urinary control at 6 months. By 24 months, the proportion of men reporting this much leakage had decreased to 10.4% and by 5 years, to 13.9%. Interestingly, 40% of men at 6 months and 22% of men at 5 years still reported using one or two pads per day. Yet only 11% and 13% of men at 2 and 5 years, respectively, considered urinary incontinence a moderate or great problem. Haffner *et al.* prospectively evaluated 342 patients undergoing radical prostatectomy with the UCLA Prostate Cancer Index [58]. At 24 months, the likelihood of returning to baseline urinary function and bother was 92% or greater, irrespective of the nerve-sparing status. In another study of a large managed care population in California, 40% of patients had daily leakage of urine, 90% of patients used two or fewer pads per day, 30% claimed total urinary control and 45% considered their problem to be occasional [38].

Following radiation therapy, HRQOL assessments typically demonstrate increased urinary bother scores, mostly related in irritative voiding symptoms. Bowel dysfunction, not typically seen following surgery, is also often identified. The degree of bowel dysfunction is probably related to the type of radiation, the radiation fields and the total dose of radiation. Widmark *et al.* noted that after external radiation therapy nearly 60% of men experience bowel problems, though 90% of these were considered minor [59]. However, in another study, 25% and 11% of men reported moderate and severe bowel dysfunction [60].

BENEFITS OF RADICAL PROSTATECTOMY

While the data are relatively equivalent for long-term cancer-specific survival for men with low-risk prostate cancer undergoing radical prostatectomy or radiation therapy, we do believe that there are some benefits to surgery, especially for men who are healthy and can easily tolerate surgery. While no prospective study has ever demonstrated an increased risk of secondary pelvic malignancies in men receiving EBRT, multiple retrospective studies have raised concerns. Moon *et al.* recently retrospectively reviewed the SEER database to determine the risk of secondary malignancy in men treated with either radiation therapy or radical prostatectomy [61]. The authors demonstrated the men who received EBRT compared with men who under went surgery had a significantly increased odds ratio of developing a secondary malignancy in the bladder and rectum, 1.63 and 1.60 respectively. Furthermore, those who received EBRT had a statistically increased risk of secondary malignancies in other areas of the body. Interestingly, those men who received interstitial seed therapy did not have an increased risk of secondary malignancies. Other authors have also reported similar results: Baxter *et al.* demonstrated a significantly increased odds ratio (1.7) for rectal cancer for men who received EBRT [62].

Another benefit of surgery over radiation is the easier availability of salvage treatments for men who progress. While salvage prostatectomy is indeed a viable option for post-radiation failures, the operation does have a high risk of complications, and is often performed only in high-volume centres [63]. Conversely, it is much easier to treat a local prostatectomy failure with EBRT, and most radiation therapists are able to provide this treatment. Also, significant complications following surgery, such as global incontinence, can usually be corrected with surgical options such as an artificial urinary sphincter. Conversely, significant grade IV complications following radiotherapy, such as a contracted bladder or severe and chronic radiation cystitis and proctitis, are much more difficult to treat and do not lend themselves to a simple outpatient procedure.

Following contemporary radical prostatectomy for the treatment of low-risk prostate cancer most men are able to return to work and their baseline level of function in a very short while. A full course of EBRT encompasses 6 to 8 weeks and, while men can continue to work, there is a significant increase in fatigue and other side-effects. Moreover, the actual time to complete each daily radiation fraction dose may be considerable when considering the drive to and from the radiation centre, the waiting and the actual treatment itself. Alternatively, we have demonstrated that most men who undergo radical prostatectomy are back to their baseline level of functioning within 3 weeks [64]. Specifically, in a prospective study, we demonstrated that it takes a mean of 19 days for men to return to their baseline level of activity following prostatectomy. This can be accomplished for a number of reasons, including: short hospital stay (1–2 days), minimal risk of major bleeding, prostatectomy performed under spinal anaesthesia, a small pfannenstiel incision to decrease post-operative pain, and only a 1-week post-operative catheterization [65]. Furthermore, we do not routinely leave a drain post-operatively, which allows the patient easier and earlier ambulation [66].

CONCLUSIONS

After his extensive consultation, Mr Smith and his wife decided to defer a treatment decision for 1 week to allow them time to review options and consult the internet. At his return visit Mr Smith elected to undergo radical prostatectomy. While he was a good candidate for either surgery or radiation he felt strongly that he wanted to have the tumour 'cut out'. He was also significantly concerned with potential future irritative symptoms that he felt that surgery was the best option for him.

The decision on how to treat low-risk prostate cancer is a difficult one for both patients and physicians alike. A detailed discussion with the patient is required firstly to assess the patient's risk of disease and secondly to assess what is the best treatment option for him. As there have been no prospective, randomized, multicentre trials comparing outcomes for low-risk prostate cancer, the physician is forced to extrapolate from the best available data. Not only must the patient's other comorbidities and lifestyle factor into the decision-making analysis, but a conversation with the patient's partner often is necessary as well.

REFERENCES

1. Davison BJ, Parker PA, Goldenberg SL. Patients' preferences for communicating a prostate cancer diagnosis and participating in medical decision-making. *BJU Int* 2004; 93:47–51.
2. Gwede CK, Pow-Sang J, Seigne J *et al.* Treatment decision-making strategies and influences in patients with localized prostate carcinoma. *Cancer* 2005; 104:1381–90.
3. Soloway CT, Soloway MS, Kim SS, Kava BR. Sexual, psychological and dyadic qualities of the prostate cancer 'couple'. *BJU Int* 2005; 95:780–785.
4. Stephenson AJ, Scardino PT, Eastham JA *et al.* Preoperative nomogram predicting the 10-year probability of prostate cancer recurrence after radical prostatectomy. *J Natl Cancer Inst* 2006; 98:715–717.
5. Bianco FJ Jr, Kattan MW, Scardino PT, Powell IJ, Pontes JE, Wood DP Jr. Radical prostatectomy nomograms in black American men: accuracy and applicability. *J Urol* 2003; 170:73–76; discussion 76–77.
6. Graefen M, Karakiewicz PI, Cagiannos I *et al.* International validation of a preoperative nomogram for prostate cancer recurrence after radical prostatectomy. *J Clin Oncol* 2002; 20:3206–3212.
7. Greene KL, Meng MV, Elkin EP *et al.* Validation of the Kattan preoperative nomogram for prostate cancer recurrence using a community based cohort: results from Cancer of the Prostate Strategic Urological Research Endeavor (CaPSURE). *J Urol* 2004; 171:2255–2259.
8. Kattan MW, Eastham JA, Stapleton AM, Wheeler TM, Scardino PT. A preoperative nomogram for disease recurrence following radical prostatectomy for prostate cancer. *J Natl Cancer Inst* 1998; 90:766–771.
9. Athanasopoulos A, Gyftopoulos K, Giannitsas K, Fisfis J, Perimenis P, Barbalias G. Combination treatment with an alpha-blocker plus an anticholinergic for bladder outlet obstruction: a prospective, randomized, controlled study. *J Urol* 2003; 169:2253–2256.
10. Hull GW, Rabbani F, Abbas F, Wheeler TM, Kattan MW, Scardino PT. Cancer control with radical prostatectomy alone in 1,000 consecutive patients. *J Urol* 2002; 167:528–534.
11. Zincke H, Oesterling JE, Blute ML, Bergstralh EJ, Myers RP, Barrett DM. Long-term (15 years) results after radical prostatectomy for clinically localized (stage T2c or lower) prostate cancer. *J Urol* 1994; 152:1850–1857.
12. D'Amico AV, Whittington R, Malkowicz SB *et al.* Biochemical outcome after radical prostatectomy, external beam radiation therapy, or interstitial radiation therapy for clinically localized prostate cancer. *JAMA* 1998; 280:969–974.
13. Cooperberg MR, Lubeck DP, Mehta SS, Carroll PR: Time trends in clinical risk stratification for prostate cancer: implications for outcomes (data from CaPSURE). *J Urol* 2003; 170:S21–25; discussion S26–27.

14. Chodak GW, Thisted RA, Gerber GS *et al*. Results of conservative management of clinically localized prostate cancer. *N Engl J Med* 1994; 330:242–248.
15. Johansson JE, Andren O, Andersson SO *et al*. Natural history of early, localized prostate cancer. *JAMA* 2004; 291:2713–2719.
16. Albertsen PC, Hanley JA, Fine J. 20-year outcomes following conservative management of clinically localized prostate cancer. *JAMA* 2005; 293:2095–2101.
17. Holmberg L, Bill-Axelson A, Helgesen F *et al*. A randomized trial comparing radical prostatectomy with watchful waiting in early prostate cancer. *N Engl J Med* 2002; 347:781–789.
18. Bill-Axelson A, Holmberg L, Ruutu M *et al*. Radical prostatectomy versus watchful waiting in early prostate cancer. *N Engl J Med* 2005; 352:1977–1984.
19. Carter CA, Donahue T, Sun L *et al*. Temporarily deferred therapy (watchful waiting) for men younger than 70 years and with low-risk localized prostate cancer in the prostate-specific antigen era. *J Clin Oncol* 2003; 21:4001–4008.
20. Klotz L. Active surveillance with selective delayed intervention for favorable risk prostate cancer. *Urol Oncol* 2006; 24:46–50.
21. Sved PD, Gomez P, Manoharan M, Kim SS, Soloway MS. Limitations of biopsy Gleason grade: implications for counseling patients with biopsy Gleason score 6 prostate cancer. *J Urol* 2004; 172:98–102.
22. Bostwick DG. Grading prostate cancer. *Am J Clin Pathol* 1994; 102:S38–56.
23. Cam K, Yucel S, Turkeri L, Akdas A. Accuracy of transrectal ultrasound guided prostate biopsy: histopathological correlation to matched prostatectomy specimens. *Int J Urol* 2002; 9:257–260.
24. Chun FK, Briganti A, Shariat SF *et al*. Significant upgrading affects a third of men diagnosed with prostate cancer: predictive nomogram and internal validation. *BJU Int* 2006; 98:329–334.
25. D'Amico AV, Renshaw AA, Arsenault L, Schultz D, Richie JP. Clinical predictors of upgrading to Gleason grade 4 or 5 disease at radical prostatectomy: potential implications for patient selection for radiation and androgen suppression therapy. *Int J Radiat Oncol Biol Phys* 1999; 45:841–846.
26. Miller DC, Gruber SB, Hollenbeck BK, Montie JE, Wei JT. Incidence of initial local therapy among men with lower-risk prostate cancer in the United States. *J Natl Cancer Inst* 2006; 98:1134–1141.
27. Harlan SR, Cooperberg MR, Elkin EP *et al*. Time trends and characteristics of men choosing watchful waiting for initial treatment of localized prostate cancer: results from CaPSURE. *J Urol* 2003; 170:1804–1807.
28. Nam RK, Jewett MA, Krahn MD *et al*. Delay in surgical therapy for clinically localized prostate cancer and biochemical recurrence after radical prostatectomy. *Can J Urol* 2003; 10:1891–1898.
29. Khan MA, Mangold LA, Epstein JI, Boitnott JK, Walsh PC, Partin AW. Impact of surgical delay on long-term cancer control for clinically localized prostate cancer. *J Urol* 2004; 172(5 Pt 1):1835–1839.
30. Freedland SJ, Kane CJ, Amling CL, Aronson WJ, Presti JC Jr, Terris MK. Delay of radical prostatectomy and risk of biochemical progression in men with low risk prostate cancer. *J Urol* 2006; 175:1298–1302; discussion 1302–1303.
31. Marr PL, Elkin EP, Arredondo SA, Broering JM, DuChane J, Carroll PR. Comorbidity and primary treatment for localized prostate cancer: data from CaPSURE. *J Urol* 2006; 175:1326–1331.
32. Dillioglugil O, Leibman BD, Leibman NS, Kattan MW, Rosas AL, Scardino PT. Risk factors for complications and morbidity after radical retropubic prostatectomy. *J Urol* 1997; 157:1760–1767.
33. Lepor H, Nieder AM, Ferrandino MN. Intraoperative and postoperative complications of radical retropubic prostatectomy in a consecutive series of 1,000 cases. *J Urol* 2001; 166:1729–1733.
34. Koya MP, Manoharan M, Kim SS, Soloway MS. Venous thromboembolism in radical prostatectomy: is heparinoid prophylaxis warranted? *BJU Int* 2005; 96:1019–1021.
35. Zelefsky MJ, Fuks Z, Hunt M *et al*. High dose radiation delivered by intensity modulated conformal radiotherapy improves the outcome of localized prostate cancer. *J Urol* 2001; 166:876–881.
36. Zietman AL, DeSilvio ML, Slater JD *et al*. Comparison of conventional-dose vs high-dose conformal radiation therapy in clinically localized adenocarcinoma of the prostate: a randomized controlled trial. *JAMA* 2005; 294:1233–1239.
37. D'Amico AV, Renshaw AA, Sussman B, Chen MH. Pretreatment PSA velocity and risk of death from prostate cancer following external beam radiation therapy. *JAMA* 2005; 294:440–447.
38. Litwin MS, Hays RD, Fink A *et al*. Quality-of-life outcomes in men treated for localized prostate cancer. *JAMA* 1995; 273:129–135.
39. Madalinska JB, Essink-Bot ML, de Koning HJ, Kirkels WJ, van der Maas PJ, Schroder FH. Health-related quality-of-life effects of radical prostatectomy and primary radiotherapy for screen-detected or clinically diagnosed localized prostate cancer. *J Clin Oncol* 2001; 19:1619–1628.

40. Wei JT, Dunn RL, Sandler HM *et al.* Comprehensive comparison of health-related quality of life after contemporary therapies for localized prostate cancer. *J Clin Oncol* 2002; 20:557–566.

41. Lubeck DP, Litwin MS, Henning JM, Stoddard ML, Flanders SC, Carroll PR. Changes in health-related quality of life in the first year after treatment for prostate cancer: results from CaPSURE. *Urology* 1999; 53:180–186.

42. Litwin MS, Flanders SC, Pasta DJ, Stoddard ML, Lubeck DP, Henning JM. Sexual function and bother after radical prostatectomy or radiation for prostate cancer: multivariate quality-of-life analysis from CaPSURE. Cancer of the Prostate Strategic Urologic Research Endeavor. *Urology* 1999; 54:503–508.

43. Bacon CG, Giovannucci E, Testa M, Glass TA, Kawachi I. The association of treatment-related symptoms with quality-of-life outcomes for localized prostate carcinoma patients. *Cancer* 2002; 94:862–871.

44. Quinlan DM, Epstein JI, Carter BS, Walsh PC. Sexual function following radical prostatectomy: influence of preservation of neurovascular bundles. *J Urol* 1991; 145:998–1002.

45. Catalona WJ, Bigg SW. Nerve-sparing radical prostatectomy: evaluation of results after 250 patients. *J Urol* 1990; 143:538–543; discussion 544.

46. Talcott JA, Rieker P, Propert KJ *et al.* Patient-reported impotence and incontinence after nerve-sparing radical prostatectomy. *J Natl Cancer Inst* 1997; 89:1117–1123.

47. Stanford JL, Feng Z, Hamilton AS *et al.* Urinary and sexual function after radical prostatectomy for clinically localized prostate cancer: the Prostate Cancer Outcomes Study. *JAMA* 2000; 283:354–360.

48. Noldus J, Michl U, Graefen M, Haese A, Hammerer P, Huland H. Patient-reported sexual function after nerve-sparing radical retropubic prostatectomy. *Eur Urol* 2002; 42:118–124.

49. Litwin MS, Pasta DJ, Yu J, Stoddard ML, Flanders SC. Urinary function and bother after radical prostatectomy or radiation for prostate cancer:a longitudinal, multivariate quality of life analysis from the Cancer of the Prostate Strategic Urologic Research Endeavor. *J Urol* 2000; 164:1973–1977.

50. Potosky AL, Davis WW, Hoffman RM *et al.* Five-year outcomes after prostatectomy or radiotherapy for prostate cancer: the prostate cancer outcomes study. *J Natl Cancer Inst* 2004; 96:1358–1367.

51. McCammon KA, Kolm P, Main B, Schellhammer PF. Comparative quality-of-life analysis after radical prostatectomy or external beam radiation for localized prostate cancer. *Urology* 1999; 54:509–516.

52. Brandeis JM, Litwin MS, Burnison CM, Reiter RE. Quality of life outcomes after brachytherapy for early stage prostate cancer. *J Urol* 2000; 163:851–857.

53. Zippe CD, Kedia AW, Kedia K, Nelson DR, Agarwal A. Treatment of erectile dysfunction after radical prostatectomy with sildenafil citrate (Viagra). *Urology* 1998; 52:963–966.

54. Kava BR. Advances in the management of post-radical prostaectomy erectile dysfunction: treatment strategies when PDE-5 inhibitors don't work. *Reviews Urology* 2005; 7:s39–50.

55. Catalona WJ, Carvalhal GF, Mager DE, Smith DS. Potency, continence and complication rates in 1,870 consecutive radical retropubic prostatectomies. *J Urol* 1999; 162:433–438.

56. Bianco FJ Jr, Scardino PT, Eastham JA. Radical prostatectomy: long-term cancer control and recovery of sexual and urinary function ('trifecta'). *Urology* 2005; 66:83–94.

57. Penson DF, McLerran D, Feng Z *et al.* 5-year urinary and sexual outcomes after radical prostatectomy: results from the Prostate Cancer Outcomes Study. *J Urol* 2005; 173:1701–1705.

58. Haffner MC, Landis PK, Saigal CS, Carter HB, Freedland SJ. Health-related quality-of-life outcomes after anatomic retropubic radical prostatectomy in the phosphodiesterase type 5 ERA:impact of neurovascular bundle preservation. *Urology* 2005; 66:371–376.

59. Widmark A, Fransson P, Tavelin B. Self-assessment questionnaire for evaluating urinary and intestinal late side-effects after pelvic radiotherapy in patients with prostate cancer compared with an age-matched control population. *Cancer* 1994; 74:2520–2532.

60. Crook J, Esche B, Futter N. Effect of pelvic radiotherapy for prostate cancer on bowel, bladder, and sexual function: the patient's perspective. *Urology* 1996; 47:387–394.

61. Moon K, Stukenborg GJ, Keim J, Theodorescu D. Cancer incidence after localized therapy for prostate cancer. *Cancer* 2006; 107:991–998.

62. Baxter NN, Tepper JE, Durham SB, Rothenberger DA, Virnig BA. Increased risk of rectal cancer after prostate radiation: a population-based study. *Gastroenterology* 2005; 128:819–824.

63. Vaidya A, Soloway MS. Salvage radical prostatectomy for radiorecurrent prostate cancer: morbidity revisited. *J Urol* 2000; 164:1998–2001.

64. Sved PD, Nieder AM, Manoharan M *et al.* Evaluation of analgesic requirements and postoperative recovery after radical retropubic prostatectomy using long-acting spinal anesthesia. *Urology* 2005; 65:509–512.

65. Nieder AM, Manoharan M, Kim SS, Soloway MS. Neither alpha-blocker therapy nor cystography is required before early catheter removal after radical prostatectomy. *BJU Int* 2005; 95:323–325.

66. Araki M, Manoharan M, Vyas S, Nieder AM, Soloway MS. A pelvic drain can often be avoided after radical retropubic prostatectomy – an update in 552 cases. *Eur Urol*, 2006.

67. Koppie TM, Grossfeld GD, Miller D *et al.* Patterns of treatment of patients with prostate cancer initially managed with surveillance: results from The CaPSURE database. Cancer of the Prostate Strategic Urological Research Endeavor. *J Urol* 2000; 164:81–88.

68. Zietman AL, Thakral H, Wilson L, Schellhammer P. Conservative management of prostate cancer in the prostate specific antigen era: the incidence and time course of subsequent therapy. *J Urol* 2001; 166:1702–1706.

69. Borchers H, Kirschner-Hermanns R, Brehmer B *et al.* Permanent 125I-seed brachytherapy or radical prostatectomy: a prospective comparison considering oncological and quality of life results. *BJU Int* 2004; 94:805–811.

70. Roehl KA, Han M, Ramos CG, Antenor JA, Catalona WJ. Cancer progression and survival rates following anatomical radical retropubic prostatectomy in 3,478 consecutive patients: long-term results. *J Urol* 2004; 172:910–914.

71. Martinez AA, Gonzalez JA, Chung AK *et al.* A comparison of external beam radiation therapy versus radical prostatectomy for patients with low risk prostate carcinoma diagnosed, staged, and treated at a single institution. *Cancer* 2000; 88:425–432.

72. Grimm PD, Blasko JC, Sylvester JE, Meier RM, Cavanagh W. 10-year biochemical (prostate-specific antigen) control of prostate cancer with (125)I brachytherapy. *Int J Radiat Oncol Biol Phys* 2001; 51:31–40.

73. Potters L, Morgenstern C, Calugaru E *et al.* 12-year outcomes following permanent prostate brachytherapy in patients with clinically localized prostate cancer. *J Urol* 2005; 173:1562–1566.

74. Blasko JC, Grimm PD, Sylvester JE, Badiozamani KR, Hoak D, Cavanagh W. Palladium-103 brachytherapy for prostate carcinoma. *Int J Radiat Oncol Biol Phys* 2000; 46:839–850.

75. Freedland SJ, Aronson WJ, Kane CJ *et al.* Biochemical outcome after radical prostatectomy among men with normal preoperative serum prostate-specific antigen levels. *Cancer* 2004; 101:748–753.

76. Kupelian PA, Potters L, Khuntia D *et al.* Radical prostatectomy, external beam radiotherapy <72 Gy, external beam radiotherapy > or =72 Gy, permanent seed implantation, or combined seeds/external beam radiotherapy for stage T1-T2 prostate cancer. *Int J Radiat Oncol Biol Phys* 2004; 58:25–33.

77. Stone NN, Stock RG, Unger P. Intermediate term biochemical-free progression and local control following 125iodine brachytherapy for prostate cancer. *J Urol* 2005; 173:803–807.

78. Sylvester JE, Blasko JC, Grimm PD, Meier R, Malmgren JA. Ten-year biochemical relapse-free survival after external beam radiation and brachytherapy for localized prostate cancer: the Seattle experience. *Int J Radiat Oncol Biol Phys* 2003; 57:944–952.

8

Treatment strategies for high-risk prostate cancer

Mark R. Feneley, Heather A. Payne

INTRODUCTION

The clinical management of prostate cancer has become increasingly complex, owing to a growing armamentarium of treatments from different medical specialties becoming available. In spite of prostate-specific antigen (PSA) testing, the presentation of prostate cancer at a locally advanced stage remains common in the UK, accounting for one-third of all new cases. The term 'locally advanced prostate cancer', however, is loosely used to encompass a spectrum of disease profiles that may include any of the following:

1   clinical stage T3 or T4, N0 or N1, and M0, at diagnosis;
2   clinical stages T1 and T2 at diagnosis, where so-called 'high-risk' features indicate the likelihood of extraprostatic invasion or clinically undetectable metastatic disease;
3   clinically localised tumour giving rise to recurrent or persistent local disease, or metastatic disease, following definitive treatment with radical prostatectomy or radical radiotherapy;
4   pathological stage pT2 or pT3 disease with 'high-risk' features, where radiotherapy may be offered as adjuvant therapy following radical prostatectomy.

There is little consensus on a definition for locally advanced prostate cancer, and it is therefore unsurprising that there is tremendous variation in therapeutic practice. Patients may be offered radical radiotherapy, radical prostatectomy or androgen deprivation therapy – either alone or in combination. For other patients, a period of watchful waiting, enrolment in a clinical trial or intervention with a novel or experimental therapeutic modality may be acceptable. The optimal combination, timing and intensity of treatment continue to be strongly debated, and clinical outcomes may vary substantially between patients with apparently similar tumour characteristics. Recognizing such evident limitations of a traditional concept of 'locally advanced' disease based upon tumour stage, newer concepts of disease risk are beginning to evolve based upon growing experience of clinical outcomes following alternative treatments, and refinements in diagnosis, pathological assessment and clinical staging.

This chapter will consider the treatment of so-called 'high-risk' prostate cancer and concepts of risk categorization. During the past 20 years, the diagnosis and treatment of prostate cancer has become increasingly proactive. Concern has arisen that for many men with early-

Mark R. Feneley, MD(Cantab) FRCS(Eng) FRCS(Urol), Senior Lecturer in Urological Oncological Surgery, University College London, London, UK
Heather A. Payne, MB BS FRCP RRCR, Consultant Oncologist, Meyerstein Institute of Urorolgy, University College London, London, UK

stage disease, the adverse effects of early treatment may outweigh the disease-specific risk. But, in spite of the potential advantages of this aggressive approach, the continuing high mortality from prostate cancer focuses interest in therapeutic strategies that may improve survival for men with locally advanced disease, and in diagnostic strategies that may identify patients for whom this benefit can be most assured.

HISTORICAL BACKGROUND

The management of prostate cancer, as for any other disease, is guided by the natural history of the untreated and treated pathology as well as by the likely impact of the clinical disease on the life expectancy or quality of life of the individual patient. Therapeutic approaches are traditionally considered in relation to clinical stage as assessed by clinical examination, serum PSA levels, radiological and radioscintographic investigation.

Before the effectiveness of hormone therapy was recognized over 60 years ago [1], prostate cancer could only be treated effectively by such surgery as radical prostatectomy or radiation therapy. The pioneers of radical prostatectomy recognized that this operation was most likely to be effective when the disease was pathologically organ confined, and a form of brachytherapy was used for locally advanced disease [2]. In that era, the operation was fraught with complications [3], and clinical staging was unreliable against modern standards. In contrast, treatment with oestrogen or castration, discovered by Huggins and Hodges, was rapidly effective, and clinically evident from the dramatic response of symptomatic metastatic disease and the tumour marker serum prostate acid phosphatase (PAP) [4]. These two endocrine strategies (oestrogen or castration) were compared in a series of randomized studies by the Veterans Administration Cooperative Urological Research Group. It was shown that oestrogen was as effective as castration, but associated with cardiovascular side-effects that offset survival [5]. Therapeutic advantage therefore related principally to delayed disease progression. Over the past 30 years, many studies have attempted to determine whether and for whom androgen deprivation may improve survival. Clinical staging investigations have been refined and are now used routinely in clinical practice. PSA has been characterized as a superior serum tumour marker, and become essential for prostate cancer detection and monitoring. Consequently, clinical outcomes following alternative treatments can now be examined more critically than previously possible, particularly in relation to disease stage.

The growing number of therapeutic strategies for patients with prostate cancer invites their comparison, not least in reaching for therapeutic decisions. A patient's prospects after treatment are not adequately represented and anticipated from observational studies alone and reported disease-specific outcomes and treatment related adverse effects may appear favourable in an uncontrolled setting. This becomes more evident when outcome assessments are derived from retrospectively collated data based in non-standard, heterogeneous (selected) patient populations. The extent of observational bias can never be fully appreciated without appropriate randomized studies that evaluate meaningful outcomes as primary endpoints, by intention to treat, where the alternative interventions are allocated to specified disease characteristics in a study population that is otherwise representative of the unselected patient group. Without well-designed studies, clinical comparisons tend to be teased by witless desperation, drawing conclusions flawed through invalid deduction.

CONCEPTS IN STAGING AND DISEASE RISK: PROGNOSTIC EVALUATION

The treatment of prostate cancer has traditionally been considered in relation to clinical tumour stage. Differing benefit–risk characteristics for alternative interventions at various disease stages support this approach. Furthermore, a growing body of evidence (discussed later in this chapter) suggests that alternative treatment strategies may alter outcomes, particularly for tumours that are not pathologically organ-confined. By defining tumour risk categories, supplementary to clinical staging, it may be possible to differentiate outcome differences between treatment strategies that would apply more reliably to individual patients.

Many clinical and pathological factors have been characterized for their individual prognostic value, where they predict disease progression. Gleason grading is a historical landmark example of such achievement [6]. For clinically localized prostate cancer, a conservative approach can (still) be justified for most well-differentiated tumours – in contrast to other malignant diseases for which deferred treatment would rarely be justified. Although grade categories correlate with prognosis, within each grade category individual prognosis is not certain. Furthermore, the variable outcomes for each grade category are not discriminated by alternative interventions. Although prognostic, clinical stage and PSA have similar limitations. Other established prognostic factors, such as pathological stage and tumour volume, require surgical specimens, and categorization is only possible for appropriate patients who select surgical treatment.

Careful pathological assessment of radical prostatectomy specimens has established pathological stage as the most important predictor of progression. Tumours that appear to be organ confined on digital rectal examination (DRE) or imaging are not necessarily organ confined by histological criteria, and the extent of pathological upstaging reflects its variable dependence on clinical presentation, population exposure to screening practice and patient age. The Partin tables, initially developed in 1993, demonstrated how DRE, preoperative biopsy grade and serum PSA are important clinical predictors of pathological stage [7], and these same factors also relate to biochemical recurrence following treatment [8]. The 'tables' were updated in 1997 and further validated in 2000 [9, 10]. They have been widely used in clinical practice prior to surgery for patients with apparently localized prostate cancer. The Kattan nomogram is also commonly used to calculate the 5-year freedom from PSA-defined progression after radical prostatectomy and again has been validated in a variety of patient groups and updated [8]. Many other nomograms are now published, predicting disease behaviour and response to treatment, incorporating preoperative and postoperative factors, based on single- as well as multi-institutional experience [11, 12].

In spite of their limitations, clinical stage, serum PSA and Gleason sum score form the principal basis for therapeutic recommendations. For the individual patient, the usefulness of this approach has gradually become more limited with increasing population exposure to PSA screening. As a result of this, there has been a stage-shift towards the diagnosis of non-palpable disease and lower PSA levels, as well as less variation in Gleason grade at presentation alongside more rigorous grading criteria. Outcomes for individual patients remain uncertain in spite of alternative treatment options, particularly those with non-organ-confined cancer or Gleason grade > 6.

In comparison with the prediction of curable disease (for which any differences in outcomes between alternative therapies has not yet been demonstrated), therapeutic issues relating to treatment of locally advanced cancer are more complex. There is no agreed definition for 'locally advanced prostate cancer'. Applied purely according to disease stage, the term would be defined in terms of the measurable anatomical extent of the tumour. 'Locally advanced' cancer would include TNM stage T3 (tumour extending to the periprostatic area or into seminal vesicles), T4 (tumour invading the external sphincter, bladder neck, rectum, levator ani muscles or fixed to pelvic side wall) or N1 (regional pelvic lymph node involvement associated with any local T stage), but without evidence of distant metastases M0 [13]. This classification includes a wide spectrum of prostate cancers with widely different outcomes. In some cases, these differences may reflect the presence of undetectable micrometastatic disease. Differing efficacy between treatment modalities may also be postulated. Variability in outcomes stage for stage also relates to the inherent inaccuracies of clinical and radiological staging.

In a recent survey of over 150 specialist oncologists and urologists in the UK, respondents were asked to give their definition of locally advanced prostate cancer [14]. A total of 95 different answers were given, with various combinations of pretreatment PSA, Gleason score, TNM staging and other pathological features. These inconsistencies between physicians' responses indicate the need for a clearer definition of locally advanced prostate cancer. They also suggest that the current thinking underlying disease management is based principally on a combination of patient risk factors.

A categorization that defines three risk groups (high risk, intermediate risk and low risk) according to established prognostic factors has been described by D'Amico *et al.* [15]. High-risk patients were defined as those men with a greater than 50% chance of failure after primary therapy and included any patient with AJCC stage T2c or above, pretreatment PSA level of more than 20 ng/ml or a biopsy Gleason score of 8 or more. Other algorithms estimate the risk of recurrence after primary therapy. These risk categories not only indicate the diversity of patients with anatomical locally advanced disease but also reflect risks associated with clinical understaging or the presence of microscopic metastases either locally in the pelvis or at distant sites.

Although physicians are accustomed to assessing individual risk factors as the basis for treatment recommendations, the relative significance of any particular categorical factor may not be equivalent for all patients throughout the natural history of the disease. Disease categorization quantifying the disease-risk status of individual patients appears therefore to be a logical basis for alternative treatment recommendations. This practical application of the risk concept, however, requires identical definitions for various outcomes across all treatment options, and the deficiencies of clinical outcome measures other than survival become obvious when attempting to compare combinations of surgical, radiotherapeutic and endocrine interventions.

High-risk patients including those with locally advanced disease present two specific challenges. There is a need for local control and also a need to treat any microscopic metastases likely to be present but undetectable until disease progression. The optimal treatment approach to high-risk prostate cancer will often therefore necessitate a multimodality approach.

PROGNOSTIC EVALUATION: THE IMPACT OF TREATMENT

The current status of curative treatment for biologically significant prostate cancer would be refined if it were possible to identify prospectively those patients for whom specific therapeutic strategies would be curative (i.e. gaining long-term PSA-free survival) where cure is required. This applies particularly to patients with non-organ-confined cancer, as men with pathologically organ-confined cancer (stage pT2) detected by PSA in a screening programme can generally be cured by definitive treatment (even if this represents overtreatment for many). The problem is that for individuals with pathological stage pT3 disease, matched for Gleason score and PSA, recurrence cannot be reliably predicted, and for some treatment appears to have been too late.

Local treatment for non-metastatic prostate cancer has generally been considered to have no survival impact where cure is not achieved. This assumption however is untested, and long-term survival may include a prolonged period with biochemical recurrence before there is clinically detectable disease [16]. Patients with early biochemical recurrence (< 2 years from surgery) appear to be more likely to develop metastatic disease, compared with patients with later recurrence who may live for many years without clinical disease [16]. However, the majority of well-selected surgical patients who develop biochemical recurrence will do so at least 2 years after surgery. PSA recurrence by itself, therefore, does not preclude long-term survival with good quality of life [17]. Any advantage to be gained after definitive treatment in terms of metastatic progression or improved survival may not be realised for many years. Even outside a screening context, the survival advantage with definitive treatment intent may not be apparent for at least 10 years, along with only a very small effect on interim prostate cancer mortality [18, 19]. In this study, some patients in the surgical arm with (unanticipated) lymph node metastases were treated by androgen deprivation, and therefore an effect of earlier antiandrogen therapy cannot be excluded.

ANDROGEN DEPRIVATION

Systemic therapy with androgen deprivation monotherapy, and 'early' androgen deprivation alone has not yet been shown to improve overall survival by reducing prostate cancer specific mortality, other than in subgroup analysis [20, 21]. (Androgen deprivation in an adjuvant or neoadjuvant setting is considered below.) Early intervention with androgen deprivation has, however, been shown to offer a cancer-specific survival advantage, particularly in patients without distant metastases (Figure 8.1) [22]. In studies of early hormone therapy, there have been recurring difficulties in assessing survival that relate to case selec-

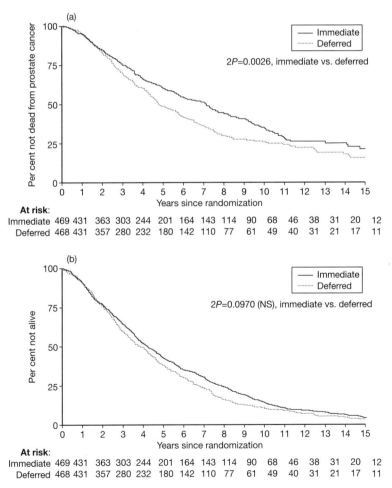

Figure 8.1 Medical Research Council (MRC) randomized study of immediate versus deferred hormone therapy. All-patient survival by immediate versus deferred hormone therapy. (a) Prostate cancer-specific survival (statistically significant difference between treatment arms). (b) Overall survival (no statistically significant difference between treatment arms) [22].

tion, statistical power and design. Where comorbidities are a major contributor to overall mortality, a clinically important and significant survival benefit from an intervention may be masked in an underpowered study where there is a non-significant difference of overall survival. Allowing for such considerations and the potential benefit of tumour debulking in other fields of oncology, it is necessary to consider that local treatment of prostate cancer may add benefit to systemic therapy, either by combination or by synergism.

One randomized study supports benefit from adjuvant androgen deprivation therapy for patients found to have lymph node metastasis at the time of radical prostatectomy (Figure 8.2) [23]. Based on pathological staging provided by this surgical option, these men would be considered to be at increased risk for disease progression [24]. This was a small study with median follow-up of 7.1 years, and patients had poorer outcomes than would be expected for this stage. Based on the rapid disease progression rate in those patients who did not receive immediate androgen deprivation therapy – 78% cancer-specific survival at 5 years – this study appears to have evaluated a select group of patients with pathological stage N1 disease and other (unknown) high-risk factors. Nevertheless, a statistically and clinically significant benefit was observed with early androgen deprivation for the study cohort. The benefit of adjuvant androgen deprivation therapy with radiotherapy is now established (discussed below).

No effect of neoadjuvant hormone manipulation on biochemical recurrence has been seen in patients having radical prostatectomy [25, 26]. It has, however, been important to observe that there may be survival benefit from combination radiation and neoadjuvant

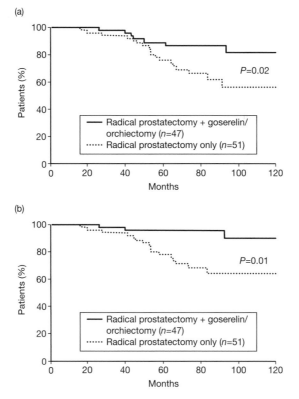

Figure 8.2 Eastern Cooperative Oncology Group (ECOG) Trial 7887. Immediate hormonal therapy compared with observation after radical prostatectomy and pelvic lymphadenectomy in men with node-positive prostate cancer. Statistically significant improvement in (a) overall survival and (b) prostate cancer-specific survival with early androgen deprivation therapy using goserelin or orchiectomy [23].

hormone manipulation in patients with high-risk prostate cancer [27, 28] (discussed below). These observations may reflect the relatively favourable prognosis of disease in most patients undergoing radical prostatectomy, with the possibility that longer follow-up may be required to observe the effect (if any) of neoadjuvant therapy in this group of patients. The magnitude of any outcome advantage, as well as the duration follow-up required to detect this advantage, both appear to relate to 'disease risk'. Concepts of disease risk are therefore becoming increasingly important for clinicians and patients. They relate therapeutic outcome to alternative therapeutic strategies.

RADICAL PROSTATECTOMY: SURGICAL MARGINS STATUS AND LYMPHADENECTOMY

Radical prostatectomy offers a local definitive treatment for early-stage prostate cancer, evaluable in relation to removal of tumour, pathological staging and prognostic assessment. It also assures total removal of the primary organ that otherwise may host new or recurrent disease. The prognostic significance of the positive surgical margin has to be considered both in association with, and independent of, other established prognostic indicators that include clinical stage, serum PSA, Gleason grade, seminal vesicle invasion and lymph node metastases.

The reported overall positive margin rate and prevalence of stage pT3 tumours at radical prostatectomy is around 10% and 35% respectively [29]. Variability in these figures in published series reflects case determination and the changing presentation and pathological stage of disease at diagnosis over the past 20 years [30, 31]. These trends may also influence the apparent prognostic significance of positive surgical margins (see below). Aside from tumour factors, positive surgical margins have been shown to relate to case selection, surgical technique and method of histopathological determination [32–35].

The prognostic significance of surgical margin status is dependent on tumour grade, with several studies emphasising little discriminatory prognostic value in patients with high Gleason grade or adverse prognostic factors [32, 36]. Clinical progression is relatively uncommon after radical prostatectomy for organ-confined tumours compared to tumours of more advanced pathological stage, and for organ-confined disease the most significant factor for recurrence again relates to tumour grade [37].

The clinical relevance of a positive margin with stage pT2 disease relates principally to prognostically independent tumour-related factors. Some studies suggest that surgical incision into organ-confined tumour has little or no prognostic significance [36, 38]; however, definition may be important as other studies suggest the converse, particularly with Gleason 7 disease [39–41]. An increased risk associated with a particular anatomical site of a positive margin may reflect technical aspects to the adequacy of prostatic excision. Blute *et al.* showed that in men with pT2 disease surgical margin status at various anatomical sites was independently significant for recurrence only at the prostate base and had no significance at the apex or urethral margin after adjusting for Gleason grade, PSA and ploidy [42]. For a positive apical margin, definition may again contribute to an apparent lack of prognostic significance [43, 44].

For stage pT3 disease, surgical margin status as well as the extent of extraprostatic invasion may be of considerable relevance for long-term disease outcomes and impact of alternative treatment strategies for disease control. Around 25% of men having radical prostatectomy for pT3 disease may be expected to have a positive surgical margin [31]. An adverse impact of a positive margin independent of Gleason grade and PSA has been shown in stage pT3 disease [41, 45, 46]. As the surgeon's usual intent is a negative margin, the importance of margin status for outcome cannot be tested prospectively. Consequently, there are inevitable difficulties in assessing the overall independent significance of positive margins, and in making valid comparisons between studies that attempt to do so.

Any significant overall impact of surgical margin status *determining* biochemical recurrence and survival would define limitations of surgery and a potential role for alternative or additional intervention. A positive surgical margin may increase the risk of PSA progression over all patients by 1.5 to 4-fold [30, 36, 46, 47]. Positive margin status is frequently associated with established and independent adverse prognostic factors for biochemical recurrence [42, 48], but has not been shown in multivariate analysis to confer independent survival disadvantage [49]. In patients with Gleason grade < 7, the extent of extracapsular penetration and surgical margin status may contribute to the (relatively low) risk of progression [47], whereas for Gleason 7 disease, negative margin status may be particularly important for surgical cure [41]. Long-term prognosis with Gleason grade 8–10 is relatively poor, although less so with organ-confined disease, and otherwise does not seem to be influenced significantly by margin status [37, 50–53] (Figure 8.3).

In the presence of metastatic disease (or the likelihood of undetectable micrometastatic disease), margin status would not be expected to contribute prognostic significance, and this has been confirmed [36]. Ohori *et al.* showed that in patients with seminal vesicle involvement or lymph node metastases, margin status does not have prognostic significance [36]. Other studies suggest margin status may be significant even with lymph node invasion, indicating the importance of tumour clearance as well as a potential therapeutic effect of lymphadenectomy [54]. Even in the absence of positive margins, high-risk features (such as

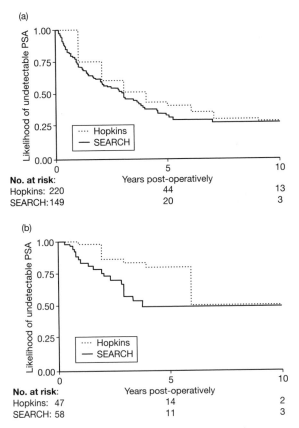

Figure 8.3 Biochemical progression-free survival in patients with biopsy Gleason score 9–10 treated by radical prostatectomy either at Johns Hopkins Hospital or within the Shared Equal Access Regional Cancer Centre Hospital (SEARCH). Database according to (a) all pathological stages and (b) organ-confined pathological stage and negative surgical margins [50]. PSA, prostate-specific antigen.

high Gleason grade tumour) may be present that are not necessarily associated with the size of the dominant tumour [55] or elevated PSA [56].

Tumour volume has been clearly correlated with positive surgical margins, and many studies indicate that tumour volume is prognostic [37, 51, 52, 57]. The recent study by Nelson *et al.* suggests that the prognostic significance for both tumour volume and margin status remains significant after considering other established prognostic indicators, including pre-operative PSA, Gleason grade, seminal vesicle invasion and nodal metastases [58].

The oncological concern with a positive margin relates to the presence (or otherwise) of residual local disease opposite a positive margin, and whether residual local disease represents a treatable sole nidus for biochemical or clinical recurrence. The primary intent of surgery is total removal of all prostatic tissue and containment of the tumour within the surgical specimen. As a secondary aim, the surgeon endeavours to preserve the neurovascular bundle where this will not compromise oncological control. These factors must be considered together, in relation to surgical technique and tumour pathology. The importance of complete dissection of the prostate base and prostate apex, as well as their careful pathological assessment has been previously discussed.

A positive surgical margin at radical prostatectomy does not imply that PSA will remain detectable following surgery or that biochemical recurrence is inevitable. It is therefore apparent that a positive surgical margin does not imply residual malignancy. With follow-up, the majority of men with positive margins remain free of recurrence [51, 59]. In a recent study where a nerve bundle was resected based on positive frozen section findings, only 14% had tumour in adjacent resected tissue [60]. The need for adjuvant therapy for patients with adverse prognostic factors remains controversial, and an indication based on surgical margin status alone would not confer benefit for the majority. The effect of prior careful case selection in this surgical cohort limits extrapolation to patients presenting with higher risk tumours.

Surgical criteria recommended to indicate the need for wide local excision of periprostatic tissue have traditionally related to tumour volume and position [61]. There is no doubt that extracapsular neurovascular bundle involvement is associated with adverse prognosis [62], and that wide excision of the bundle may reduce the likelihood of a positive margin and risk of progression [63]. While neurovascular infiltration in preoperative biopsies may have some independent adverse prognostic value [64], it may not be a significant independent of other prognostic factors after radical prostatectomy [65]. Excision of the neurovascular bundles contributes to surgical morbidity and should be avoided unless it confers therapeutic advantage. The indications for excision may include pathology findings (tumour position, grade, perineural invasion), preoperative clinical findings (palpable tumour, particularly at the apex), and operative findings (induration involving the bundle at operation) [66]. Walsh and colleagues have demonstrated that palpable tumour, extracapsular invasion and biopsy perineural invasion do not necessarily infer the need for neurovascular bundle excision [67, 68], and this has been confirmed by others [69]. Furthermore, excision of the bundle does not ensure negative margins elsewhere [68, 70]. Predictive models have been proposed for predicting presence and side of extracapsular invasion [71], and for nerve sparing [72]. With nerve sparing in appropriately selected patients, oncological outcomes do not appear to be compromised [73]. Use of frozen section where extracapsular extension is suspected in cases of palpable tumour may allow bundle preservation without compromise of surgical margin, and confirms that palpable tumour alone does not imply stage pT3 disease [60].

Lymphadenectomy is the most reliable means of assessing the presence of metastatic disease in the regional and pelvic lymph nodes [74]. In patients with lymph node metastases, an obturator fossa dissection may not be sufficient for the detection of lymph node involvement and accurate pathological staging, owing to metastases skipping this sentinel node group [75]. The presence of nodal metastases may influence further treatment, and the use of adjuvant hormone therapy following surgery has been discussed elsewhere in this chapter. But even without adjuvant treatment, a significant proportion of patients will remain disease-free for many years, particularly those with microscopic nodal disease and favourable risk features; therefore immediate hormone therapy may not be justified for all patients [11, 76]. Based on the extended disease-free survival observed in these patients following radical prostatectomy and pelvic node dissection, lymphadenectomy *may* have some therapeutic benefit in *some* patients [77, 78]. This hope is further supported where a more extensive lymph node dissection assures better disease-free survival [79]. Conversely, in those patients with regional metastases and therefore potentially adverse prognosis, the extent of lymph excision may not relate linearly to the risk of recurrence; but for those without metastases a low risk of recurrence can be assured more reliably by a more extensive lymph node dissection [80]. Lymphadenectomy may not be warranted in all patients having radical prostatectomy for screen detected cancer, owing to the low prevalence of metastatic disease; where it is carried out selectively, it should be recommended for patients with intermediate or high-risk disease. For some patients with high-risk disease, staging lymphadenectomy without radical prostatectomy may be undertaken before definitive treatment is recommended.

The value of adjuvant radiotherapy following radical prostatectomy where margins are positive is often debated. The overall low risk of progression associated with a positive surgical margin does not warrant adjuvant therapy and its potential morbidity in all patients, particularly in the absence of other adverse prognostic risk factors (as described above). Therapeutic concern relates to the presence of undetected micrometastatic disease where further local treatment would be unlikely to offer significant prognostic advantage, particularly as risk factors for PSA recurrence after adjuvant radiotherapy for positive surgical margins are the same as those shown by other studies to predict positive margins [81]. No survival benefit from adjuvant radiotherapy to the prostate bed after radical prostatectomy has yet been demonstrated. In the EORTC (European Organisation for Research and Treatment of Cancer) 22911 study, men with pT3 disease or positive surgical margins were randomized to receive either immediate adjuvant radiotherapy or delayed intervention. Adjuvant radiotherapy significantly improved biochemical progression-free survival, clinical progression-free survival and reduced locoregional failure at 5 years [82].

Androgen deprivation therapy may be given alongside adjuvant radiotherapy based on its advantage with primary radiation therapy. The combination of surgery, radiotherapy and hormone therapy is under investigation in current clinical trials. By comparison, the combination of radiotherapy with adjuvant antiandrogen therapy (without radical prostatectomy) for high-risk patients is favourable (discussed below).

Salvage radiotherapy after PSA recurrence may be effective, for controlling local disease particularly when given early after biochemical failure, but again no survival benefit has been shown. The optimal strategy, dose and timing of radiotherapy and/or systemic therapies following radical prostatectomy, and their long term benefit, have not been sufficiently evaluated in clinical trials.

RADIOTHERAPY

Treatment has traditionally included external beam radiotherapy (EBRT) but many patients experience disease progression within 5 years of this treatment modality alone [83]. The results of EBRT are poorer for patients with locally advanced or high-risk prostate cancer than for those with localized, low-risk disease. Gleason score, T stage and pathological lymph node status have been described as major independent predictors of death due to prostate cancer in men treated with EBRT. Roach *et al.* used these three prognostic factors to analyse the outcomes of 1557 men entered into Radiation Therapy Oncology Group (RTOG) clinical trials between 1975 and 1992 who received radiotherapy alone [84]. They identified four prognostic subgroups. The 5-, 10- and 15-year disease-specific survival was 96%, 86% and 72% for group 1; 94%, 75% and 61% for group 2; 83%, 62% and 39% for group 3; and 64%, 34% and 27% for group 4.

Zagars *et al.* also showed that the risk of progression or relapse after radical radiotherapy increases with poor prognostic factors such as initial PSA level ≥10 and any single Gleason score ≥4 on biopsy [85]. These studies demonstrate the fact that conventional radiotherapy alone is an inadequate treatment for high-risk prostate cancer.

The radiotherapy treatment fields can include the prostate gland and seminal vesicles. There is controversy regarding irradiation of the pelvic lymph nodes; advocates propose an advantage in local control, while others believe it just adds to morbidity. Several studies have looked to see if whole pelvic radiotherapy with a prostate boost is advantageous compared to prostate gland radiotherapy alone. The results are conflicting with some suggesting improved local control/survival and others increased toxicity without benefit. The RTOG 9413 prospective randomized controlled trial has published preliminary results suggesting a significant improvement in progression-free survival in the whole pelvis radiotherapy arm without increased toxicity. Further results are awaited. Intensity modulated radiotherapy (IMRT) is being assessed as a method of irradiating pelvic nodes in patients with a high risk of involvement, with progressive dose escalation while avoiding significant radiation dose to the bowel. Results are awaited.

There is evidence that for prostate cancer, increased radiation dose is associated with increased cancer cell kill. However, the traditional two-dimensional (2-D) technique of treatment planning and delivery is limited by the normal tissue toxicity of the surrounding structures (bladder, rectum and bowel), such that the dose that can be safely delivered to the prostate by EBRT is around 65 Gy. New technological advances such as three-dimensional conformal radiotherapy (3-D-CRT) have improved the precision of EBRT and have permitted the delivery of higher doses by limiting the doses to the surrounding normal tissues. 3-D-CRT at conventional doses reduces side-effects. A study of 225 men randomized to conventional vs. conformal techniques for a treatment dose of 64 Gy demonstrated that significantly fewer men developed radiation-induced proctitis and bleeding in the conformal group than in the conventional group (37% versus 56% ≥RTOG grade 1, $P = 0.004$; 5% versus 15% ≥RTOG grade 2, $P = 0.01$). There were no differences between groups in bladder function after treatment (53% versus 59% ≥RTOG grade 1, $P = 0.34$; 20% versus 23% ≥RTOG grade 2, $P = 0.61$) with historical controls. The 3-D-CRT approach therefore reduces the dose-limiting late side-effect of proctitis and has allowed for dose escalation to the whole prostate to 78 Gy.

More recently a further development has been IMRT. This is an advanced form of 3-D-CRT, which uses sophisticated computer-assisted technology to modify and shape the intensity of multiple radiotherapy beams during treatment to deliver very precise coverage of the target area whilst sparing surrounding sensitive tissues. This has allowed doses of greater than 80 Gy to be used in prostate cancer treatment.

The advantages of higher doses of radiotherapy have been shown in clinical studies. Pollack *et al.* [86] demonstrated the benefits of dose escalation for men with T1 to T3 prostate cancer in a phase III randomized study at the MD Anderson Hospital. A total of 305 men were randomized between 1993 and 1998 to compare the efficacy of 70 Gy vs. 78 Gy with a median follow-up of 60 months. The primary endpoint was freedom from failure (FFF), including biochemical failure, which was defined as three rises in PSA. The FFF rates for the 70 Gy and 78 Gy arms at 6 years were 64% and 70% respectively ($P = 0.03$). Dose escalation to 78 Gy preferentially benefited those with a pretreatment PSA > 10. For this higher risk group the FFF rate was 62% for the 78 Gy arm vs. 43% for those who received 70 Gy ($P = 0.01$). For patients with a pretreatment PSA ≤10, no significant dose response was found, with an average 6-year FFF rate of about 75%. Although no difference occurred in overall survival, the freedom from distant metastasis rate was higher for those with PSA levels > 10 who were treated to 78 Gy (98% versus 88% at 6 years, $P = 0.056$) (Figure 8.4).

In a further study of dose escalation, Zelefsky and colleagues have shown that increasing the dose delivered beyond 70 Gy in men with intermediate and high-risk disease improved

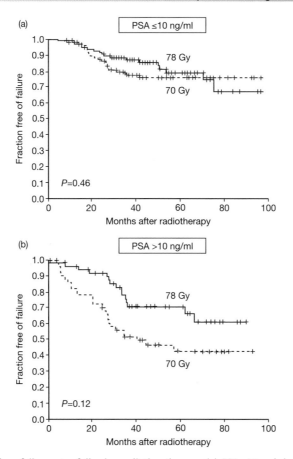

Figure 8.4 Freedom from failure rates following radiation therapy. (a) PSA < 10 ng/ml, (b) PSA > 10 ng/ml. Statistically significant difference with dose escalation from 70 to 78 Gy for PSA > 10 ng/ml [86].

the 5-year actuarial PSA relapse-free survivals from 50% to 70% and 21% to 47% respectively [87]. Furthermore, this group of high-risk patients have shown a progressive reduction in positive biopsies at 2 or more years in these patients, with increasing dose.

Dearnaley and colleagues in the UK have looked at results of 5-year actuarial PSA control rates in patients who received the standard dose of 64 Gy compared with those escalated to 74 Gy [88]. Patients receiving the conventional dose had 5-year control rates of 59% vs. 71% in the patients who were treated at 74 Gy.

Further developments in radiotherapy for prostate cancer have included studies investigating different fractionation schedules. There is increasing evidence that hypofractionated schedules, involving a smaller number of larger doses per fraction of radiation, may be optimal for prostate cancer. This reflects the fact that it has recently been recognized that the alpha/beta ratio for prostate cancer is low [89]. The alpha/beta ratio is a radiobiological term describing the shape of the cell survival curve for individual tissues. Conventionally, radiobiology states that the alpha/beta ratios for tumours are higher than those for surrounding normal late-reacting tissue. Tissues with a lower alpha/beta ratio will undergo greater cell killing by larger doses per fraction of radiotherapy than tissues with a higher ratio. The use of a smaller number of larger sized fractions may therefore be a more effective treatment. This type of regime is the subject of ongoing clinical studies.

A further method of dose escalation is with a high-dose-rate (HDR) brachytherapy boost in combination with external beam irradiation. HDR brachytherapy consists of placing hollow needles into the prostate under ultrasound guidance. Dose conformity is enhanced by generation of a steep dose gradient between the prostate and normal tissues and by controlling the length of time the radioactive iridium-192 source temporarily dwells at each position within the hollow needles. This allows large doses of radiation to be delivered within a few minutes to the prostate, seminal vesicles and periprostatic tissues. This technique allows for the administration of a truly conformal and optimized treatment which also takes account of organ movement. The results of a HDR boost in combination with EBRT are encouraging for those high-risk patients who have been shown to benefit from dose escalation. A recent study by Martinez $et\ al.$ reports pooled results from their institutions of 1260 men with intermediate to high-risk prostate cancer (PSA ≥ 10 ng/ml, GS ≥ 7 or $\geq$ cT2b) treated with a HDR boost (dose escalated from 5.5 Gy×3 to 15 Gy×2) and EBRT (36–50 Gy + 1.8–2 Gy daily, five times per week). At 4.4 years median follow-up, the 8-year biochemical no evidence of disease (bNED) status was 81% [90].

These studies demonstrate a wide variety of different methods of radiotherapy dose delivery and clearly demonstrate the advantages of dose escalation, especially for those men with high-risk tumours. However, the optimal delivery of therapy, dose and fractionation schedules is yet to be determined and remains the subject of multiple ongoing clinical studies.

RADIOTHERAPY IN COMBINATION WITH HORMONE TREATMENT

A further challenge in treating high-risk prostate cancer is the concurrent treatment of microscopic metastases at distant sites. This means that despite improved local treatment many men will ultimately progress to metastatic disease, which can cause debilitating morbidity including bone pain, fracture, spinal cord compression and urinary dysfunction. There is considerable evidence that the addition of systemic treatment in the form of hormone therapy with androgen suppression is superior to radiotherapy alone in patients with high-risk disease. This combination therapy has been shown to improve survival and increase time to progression.

Neoadjuvant hormone therapy in the form of gonadotrophin hormone-releasing hormone agonists (GnRHa) prior to definitive radiotherapy is commonly used. Neoadjuvant hormonal therapy (NHT) is therapy given prior to definitive local treatment with curative intent. The aims of NHT are to reduce tumour bulk and to potentially treat microscopic metastases together with the primary tumour. The advantages are that this can cause, on average, a 25–30% cytoreduction of the prostate [91, 92], and potentially allow smaller fields of radiotherapy to be used with sparing of the rectum and bladder. There have also been reports that there may be a sensitizing effect between hormone therapy and radiation treatment. There are several theories as to the mechanism of this including that reduction of tumour bulk improves oxygenation and therefore increases radiation sensitivity [93, 94]. Also, if hormone responsive cells move to a resting phase during neoadjuvant treatment, this could reduce repopulation rate and enhance tumour cell death (increased apoptosis). There is also clinical evidence to support this treatment approach. The RTOG 86–10 investigated the addition of hormone therapy (goserelin and flutamide) for 2 months before and 2 months during radiotherapy compared with radiation treatment alone in 456 men with locally advanced prostate cancer [27]. At 6.7 years median follow-up (8.6 years for surviving patients), the patients in the combined arm had a significantly improved 5-year cause-specific survival of 90% vs. 85%. A subgroup analysis showed that those with Gleason sum 6 tumours had an overall survival advantage at 5 years of 70% vs. 52%.

Adjuvant androgen suppression immediately after radical radiotherapy has been shown to significantly increase overall survival, progression-free survival, and significantly reduce local progression, distant metastases and biochemical progression in several large randomized studies using goserelin.

The EORTC 22863 trial evaluated the effectiveness of adjuvant therapy with Zoladex (goserelin) 3.6 mg initiated at the onset of radiotherapy and continued for 3 years in patients with high-risk non-metastatic prostate cancer [95]. Four hundred and fifteen patients were randomized to receive either radiotherapy with immediate goserelin 3.6 mg therapy (every 4 weeks for 3 years, $n = 207$) or radiotherapy alone ($n = 208$) with hormonal treatment given for disease progression. Results reported after a median follow-up of 5.5 years demonstrated a significant improvement in overall survival (78% vs. 62%) and disease-free survival (74% vs. 40%) in favour of immediate adjuvant hormone treatment as opposed to radiotherapy alone with hormone therapy at relapse (Figure 8.5).

Further data is available from the RTOG 85–10 where a total of 977 patients were randomized to receive either pelvic radiation plus goserelin 3.6 mg (started during the last week of radiotherapy to be continued indefinitely every month or until relapse) or radiotherapy alone (goserelin started at relapse) [28]. At a median follow-up of 7.6 years, adjuvant goserelin significantly improved absolute survival compared with radiation monotherapy (estimated 10-year survival rate 49 vs. 39%, $P = 0.002$). The largest benefits were seen in the subgroups with high Gleason grades (Gleason 8–10). The RTOG 85–31 is the largest and longest study of its kind and confirms data from previous trials with shorter duration of follow-up (Figure 8.6). The results of this highly significant study demonstrate important overall survival benefits. Patients with high Gleason scores have the greatest risk of disease progression and most significant risk of metastases and this group (Gleason 8–10) demonstrated the largest benefits from combined modality therapy on subgroup analysis.

There remain uncertainties regarding the optimal timing and duration of hormone therapy. Timing has varied between different trials. Goserelin was added during the final week of RTOG 85–31, and the first week of EORTC 22863. There were also differences in the duration of adjuvant goserelin therapy between the studies with hormone therapy administered indefinitely (RTOG 85–31) or for 3 years (EORTC 22863). Patient quality of life is an important issue when deciding on the duration of therapy and any long-term side-effects must also be considered. We await further results of these and other studies to determine the optimal duration of hormone treatment. The introduction of new radiotherapy techniques, as described above, have allowed dose escalation beyond that delivered in RTOG 85–31 and again this combination may lead to even greater improvement in outcome.

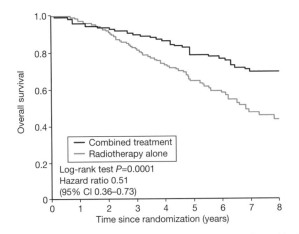

Figure 8.5   EORTC Trial 22863. Radiotherapy with and without adjuvant gonadotrophin hormone-releasing agonist in patients with locally advanced prostate cancer. Statistically significant difference in overall survival between treatment arms [95].

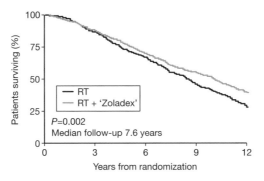

Figure 8.6 RTOG 85–31. Radiotherapy with and without adjuvant androgen deprivation therapy. Statistically significant difference in overall survival between treatment arms [28].

Data from the third analysis of the Early Prostate Cancer (EPC) study have shown that bicalutamide 150 mg adjuvant to radiotherapy significantly improved overall survival compared with radiotherapy alone [hazard ratio (HR) 0.65, $P = 0.03$] for men with locally advanced prostate cancer at a median follow-up of 7.4 years [96]. The prostate cancer mortality for this subgroup was 24% for patients treated with radiotherapy alone compared with 16% for those treated with combined modality therapy. This represents the first evidence of a significant overall survival benefit for any non-castration-based hormonal therapy given as adjuvant treatment to prostate cancer patients. These results compare favourably with those discussed for RTOG 85–31 and now allow clinicians and patients a choice of which adjuvant hormone therapy to use without concerns of reducing the efficacy of treatment. This choice is very important with regards to side-effects of treatment. Potential quality of life advantages [97] have been demonstrated with bicalutamide 150 mg with regards to potency, libido, physical capacity and preservation of bone mineral density [98] at the cost of an increase in breast symptoms (gynaecomastia and nipple tenderness). The choice of treatment allows men to tailor side-effects of therapy to their own particular needs and lifestyles.

CONCLUSION

There is a growing body of evidence to suggest that combination modality treatment may improve disease-specific outcomes and overall survival over single modalities for select patient groups. The appropriate timing of combination modality interventions may relate to concepts of disease risk rather than stage alone, in contrast to the established importance of pathological stage in predicting long-term disease-free survival (cure) after definitive treatment. Interest in synergistic or multimodality treatments is likely to grow with the promise of targeted therapies and new chemotherapy regimens supplementing endocrine manipulation for systemic therapy. Randomized studies are essential to assess outcomes following therapeutic interventions, and they need to be carefully designed to demonstrate meaningful cancer-specific and overall advantage in patients in whom comorbidities may also significantly influence quality of life and survival.

REFERENCES

1. Huggins C, Stevens RE Jr, Hodges CW. Studies on prostatic cancer: effects of castration on advanced carcinoma of the prostate gland. *Arch Surg* 1941; 43:209.
2. Young HH, Davis DM. Neoplasms of the Urogenital Tract. In: *Young's Practice of Urology*. WB Saunders, Philadelphia 1926, pp. 653–654.
3. Chute R. Radical retropubic prostatectomy for cancer. *J Urol* 1954; 71:347–372.

4. Huggins C, Hodges CV. Studies on prostatic cancer: I. The effect of castration, of estrogen and of androgen injection on serum phosphatases in metastatic carcinoma of the prostate. *J Urol* 2002; 168:9–12.
5. Byar DP, Corle DK. Hormone therapy for prostate cancer: results of the Veterans Administration Cooperative Urological Research Group studies. *NCI Monogr* 1988; 7:165–170.
6. Gleason DF, Mellinger GT. Prediction of prognosis for prostatic adenocarcinoma by combined histological grading and clinical staging. *J Urol* 1974; 111:58–64.
7. Partin AW, Yoo J, Carter HB *et al*. The use of prostate specific antigen, clinical stage and Gleason score to predict pathological stage in men with localized prostate cancer. *J Urol* 1993; 150:110–114.
8. Kattan MW, Eastham JA, Stapleton AM, Wheeler TM, Scardino PT. A preoperative nomogram for disease recurrence following radical prostatectomy for prostate cancer. *J Natl Cancer Inst* 1998; 90:766–771.
9. Partin AW, Kattan MW, Subong EN *et al*. Combination of prostate-specific antigen, clinical stage, and Gleason score to predict pathological stage of localized prostate cancer. A multi-institutional update. *JAMA* 1997; 277:1445–1451.
10. Blute ML, Bergstralh EJ, Partin AW *et al*. Validation of Partin tables for predicting pathological stage of clinically localized prostate cancer. *J Urol* 2000; 164:1591–1595.
11. Kattan MW, Wheeler TM, Scardino PT. Postoperative nomogram for disease recurrence after radical prostatectomy for prostate cancer. *J Clin Oncol* 1999; 17:1499–1507.
12. Kattan MW, Shariat SF, Andrews B *et al*. The addition of interleukin-6 soluble receptor and transforming growth factor beta1 improves a preoperative nomogram for predicting biochemical progression in patients with clinically localized prostate cancer. *J Clin Oncol* 2003; 21:3573–3579.
13. American Joint Committee on Cancer. *Prostate. AJCC Cancer Staging Manual.* Springer, New York, 2002, pp. 309–316.
14. Payne H, Gillatt D. Differences and commonalities in the management of locally advanced prostate cancer: results from a survey of oncologists and urologists in the UK. *BJU Int* 2007; 99: 545–553.
15. D'Amico AV, Whittington R, Malkowicz SB *et al*. Biochemical outcome after radical prostatectomy, external beam radiation therapy, or interstitial radiation therapy for clinically localized prostate cancer. *JAMA* 1998; 280:969–974.
16. Pound CR, Partin AW, Eisenberger MA, Chan DW, Pearson JD, Walsh PC. Natural history of progression after PSA elevation following radical prostatectomy. *JAMA* 1999; 281:1591–1597.
17. Ward JF, Blute ML, Slezak J, Bergstralh EJ, Zincke H. The long-term clinical impact of biochemical recurrence of prostate cancer 5 or more years after radical prostatectomy. *J Urol* 2003; 170:1872–1876.
18. Bill-Axelson A, Holmberg L, Ruutu M *et al*. Radical prostatectomy versus watchful waiting in early prostate cancer. *N Engl J Med* 2005; 352:1977–1984.
19. Holmberg L, Bill-Axelson A, Helgesen F *et al*. A randomized trial comparing radical prostatectomy with watchful waiting in early prostate cancer. *N Engl J Med* 2002; 347:781–789.
20. Medical Research Council Prostate Cancer Working Party Investigators Group. Immediate versus deferred treatment for advanced prostatic cancer: initial results of the Medical Research Council Trial. *Br J Urol* 1997; 79:235–246.
21. Studer UE, Whelan P, Albrecht W *et al*. Immediate or deferred androgen deprivation for patients with prostate cancer not suitable for local treatment with curative intent: European Organisation for Research and Treatment of Cancer (EORTC) Trial 30891. *J Clin Oncol* 2006; 24:1868–1876.
22. Kirk D. Hormone therapy for prostate cancer: optimization and timing. In: Kirby RS, Partin AW, Feneley MR, Parsons JK, eds. *Prostate Cancer: Principles and Practice.* Taylor and Francis, London, 2005, pp. 959–966.
23. Messing EM, Manola J, Sarosdy M, Wilding G, Crawford ED, Trump D. Immediate hormonal therapy compared with observation after radical prostatectomy and pelvic lymphadenectomy in men with node-positive prostate cancer. *N Engl J Med* 1999; 341:1781–1788.
24. Kattan MW, Wheeler TM, Scardino PT. Postoperative nomogram for disease recurrence after radical prostatectomy for prostate cancer. *J Clin Oncol* 1999; 17:1499–1507.
25. Soloway MS, Sharifi R, Wajsman Z, McLeod D, Wood DPJ, Puras-Baez A. Randomized prospective study comparing radical prostatectomy alone versus radical prostatectomy preceded by androgen blockade in clinical stage B2 (T2bNxM0) prostate cancer. The Lupron Depot Neoadjuvant Prostate Cancer Study Group. *J Urol* 1995; 154(2 Pt 1):424–428.
26. Soloway MS, Pareek K, Sharifi R *et al*. Neoadjuvant androgen ablation before radical prostatectomy in cT2bNxMo prostate cancer: 5-year results. *J Urol* 2002; 167:112–116.

27. Pilepich MV, Winter K, John MJ et al. Phase III radiation therapy oncology group (RTOG) trial 86–10 of androgen deprivation adjuvant to definitive radiotherapy in locally advanced carcinoma of the prostate. Int J Radiat Oncol Biol Phys 2001; 50:1243–1252.

28. Pilepich MV, Winter K, Lawton CA et al. Androgen suppression adjuvant to definitive radiotherapy in prostate carcinoma – long-term results of phase III RTOG 85–31. Int J Radiat Oncol Biol Phys 2005; 61:1285–1290.

29. Khan MA, Partin AW, Mangold LA, Epstein JI, Walsh PC. Probability of biochemical recurrence by analysis of pathologic stage, Gleason score, and margin status for localized prostate cancer. Urology 2003; 62:866–871.

30. Swindle P, Eastham JA, Ohori M et al. Do margins matter? The prognostic significance of positive surgical margins in radical prostatectomy specimens. J Urol 2005; 174:903–907.

31. Han M, Partin AW, Chan DY, Walsh PC. An evaluation of the decreasing incidence of positive surgical margins in a large retropubic prostatectomy series. J Urol 2004; 171:23–26.

32. Epstein JI. Incidence and significance of positive margins in radical prostatectomy specimens. Urol Clin N Am 1996; 23:651–663.

33. Stamey TA, Villers AA, McNeal JE, Link PC, Freiha FS. Positive surgical margins at radical prostatectomy: importance of the apical dissection. J Urol 1990; 143:1166–72; discussion.

34. Eastham JA, Kattan MW, Riedel E et al. Variations among individual surgeons in the rate of positive surgical margins in radical prostatectomy specimens. J Urol 2003; 170(6 Pt 1):2292–2295.

35. Sehdev AE, Pan CC, Epstein JI. Comparative analysis of sampling methods for grossing radical prostatectomy specimens performed for nonpalpable (stage T1c) prostatic adenocarcinoma. Hum Pathol 2001; 32:494–499.

36. Ohori M, Wheeler TM, Kattan MW, Goto Y, Scardino PT. Prognostic significance of positive surgical margins in radical prostatectomy specimens. J Urol 1995; 154:1818–1824.

37. Palisaar RJ, Graefen M, Karakiewicz PI et al. Assessment of clinical and pathologic characteristics predisposing to disease recurrence following radical prostatectomy in men with pathologically organ-confined prostate cancer. Eur Urol 2002; 41:155–161.

38. Barocas DA, Han M, Epstein JI et al. Does capsular incision at radical retropubic prostatectomy affect disease-free survival in otherwise organ-confined prostate cancer? Urology 2001; 58:746–751.

39. Freedland SJ, Aronson W, Presti JC Jr et al. Should a positive surgical margin following radical prostatectomy be pathological stage T2 or T3? Results from the SEARCH database. J Urol 2003; 169:2142–2146.

40. Shuford MD, Cookson MS, Chang SS et al. Adverse prognostic significance of capsular incision with radical retropubic prostatectomy. J Urol 2004; 172:119–123.

41. Epstein JI, Pound CR, Partin AW, Walsh PC. Disease progression following radical prostatectomy in men with Gleason score 7 tumor [see comments]. J Urol 1998; 160:97–100.

42. Blute ML, Bostwick DG, Bergstralh EJ et al. Anatomic site-specific positive margins in organ-confined prostate cancer and its impact on outcome after radical prostatectomy. Urology 1997; 50:733–739.

43. van den Ouden D, Bentvelsen FM, Boeve ER, Schroder FH. Positive margins after radical prostatectomy: correlation with local recurrence and distant progression. Br J Urol 1993; 72:489–494.

44. Fesseha T, Sakr W, Grignon D, Banerjee M, Wood DP Jr, Pontes JE. Prognostic implications of a positive apical margin in radical prostatectomy specimens. J Urol 1997; 158:2176–2179.

45. Kausik SJ, Blute ML, Sebo TJ et al. Prognostic significance of positive surgical margins in patients with extraprostatic carcinoma after radical prostatectomy. Cancer 2002; 95:1215–1219.

46. Karakiewicz PI, Eastham JA, Graefen M et al. Prognostic impact of positive surgical margins in surgically treated prostate cancer: multi-institutional assessment of 5831 patients. Urology 2005; 66:1245–1250.

47. Epstein JI, Partin AW, Sauvageot J, Walsh PC. Prediction of progression following radical prostatectomy. A multivariate analysis of 721 men with long-term follow-up. Am J Surg Pathol 1996; 20:286–292.

48. Wieder JA, Soloway MS. Incidence, etiology, location, prevention and treatment of positive surgical margins after radical prostatectomy for prostate cancer. J Urol 1998; 160:299–315.

49. Porter CR, Kodama K, Gibbons RP et al. 25-year prostate cancer control and survival outcomes: a 40-year radical prostatectomy single institution series. J Urol 2006; 176:569–574.

50. Bastian PJ, Gonzalgo ML, Aronson WJ et al. Clinical and pathologic outcome after radical prostatectomy for prostate cancer patients with a preoperative Gleason sum of 8 to 10. Cancer 2006; 107:1265–1272.

51. Vis AN, Schroder FH, van der Kwast TH. The actual value of the surgical margin status as a predictor of disease progression in men with early prostate cancer. Eur Urol 2006; 50:258–265.

52. Stamey TA, McNeal JE, Yemoto CM, Sigal BM, Johnstone IM. Biological determinants of cancer progression in men with prostate cancer. *JAMA* 1999; 281:1395–1400.
53. Mian BM, Troncoso P, Okihara K *et al.* Outcome of patients with Gleason score 8 or higher prostate cancer following radical prostatectomy alone. *J Urol* 2002; 167:1675–1680.
54. Karakiewicz PI, Eastham JA, Graefen M *et al.* Prognostic impact of positive surgical margins in surgically treated prostate cancer: multi-institutional assessment of 5831 patients. *Urology* 2005; 66:1245–1250.
55. Epstein JI, Carmichael MJ, Partin AW, Walsh PC. Small high grade adenocarcinoma of the prostate in radical prostatectomy specimens performed for nonpalpable disease: pathogenetic and clinical implications. *J Urol* 1994; 151:1587–1592.
56. D'Amico AV, Chen MH, Malkowicz SB *et al.* Lower prostate specific antigen outcome than expected following radical prostatectomy in patients with high grade prostate and a prostatic specific antigen level of 4 ng/ml or less. *J Urol* 2002; 167:2025–2030.
57. Graefen M, Noldus J, Pichlmeier U *et al.* Early prostate-specific antigen relapse after radical retropubic prostatectomy: prediction on the basis of preoperative and postoperative tumor characteristics. *Eur Urol* 1999; 36:21–30.
58. Nelson BA, Shappell SB, Chang SS *et al.* Tumour volume is an independent predictor of prostate-specific antigen recurrence in patients undergoing radical prostatectomy for clinically localized prostate cancer. *BJU Int* 2006; 97:1169–1172.
59. Simon MA, Kim S, Soloway MS. Prostate specific antigen recurrence rates are low after radical retropubic prostatectomy and positive margins. *J Urol* 2006; 175:140–144.
60. Eichelberg C, Erbersdobler A, Haese A *et al.* Frozen section for the management of intraoperatively detected palpable tumor lesions during nerve-sparing scheduled radical prostatectomy. *Eur Urol* 2006; 49:1011–1016.
61. Aus G, Abbou CC, Bolla M *et al.* EAU guidelines on prostate cancer. *Eur Urol* 2005; 48:546–551.
62. Partin AW, Borland RN, Epstein JI, Brendler CB. Influence of wide excision of the neurovascular bundle(s) on prognosis in men with clinically localized prostate cancer with established capsular penetration. *J Urol* 1993; 150:142–146.
63. Smith RC, Partin AW, Epstein JI, Brendler CB. Extended followup of the influence of wide excision of the neurovascular bundle(s) on prognosis in men with clinically localized prostate cancer and extensive capsular perforation. *J Urol* 1996; 156(2 Pt 1):454–457.
64. de la Taille A, Rubin MA, Bagiella E *et al.* Can perineural invasion on prostate needle biopsy predict prostate specific antigen recurrence after radical prostatectomy? *J Urol* 1999; 162:103–106.
65. O'Malley KJ, Pound CR, Walsh PC, Epstein JI, Partin AW. Influence of biopsy perineural invasion on long-term biochemical disease-free survival after radical prostatectomy. *Urology* 2002; 59:85–90.
66. Shah O, Robbins DA, Melamed J, Lepor H. The New York University nerve sparing algorithm decreases the rate of positive surgical margins following radical retropubic prostatectomy. *J Urol* 2003; 169:2147–2152.
67. Walsh PC. Radical prostatectomy, preservation of sexual function, cancer control. The controversy. *Urol Clin N Am* 1987; 14:663–673.
68. Holmes GF, Walsh PC, Pound CR, Epstein JI. Excision of the neurovascular bundle at radical prostatectomy in cases with perineural invasion on needle biopsy. *Urology* 1999; 53:752–756.
69. Sofer M, Hamilton-Nelson KL, Schlesselman JJ, Soloway MS. Risk of positive margins and biochemical recurrence in relation to nerve-sparing radical prostatectomy. *J Clin Oncol* 2002; 20:1853–1858.
70. Walsh PC, Epstein JI, Lowe FC. Potency following radical prostatectomy with wide unilateral excision of the neurovascular bundle. *J Urol* 1987; 138:823–827.
71. Ohori M, Kattan MW, Koh H *et al.* Predicting the presence and side of extracapsular extension: a nomogram for staging prostate cancer. *J Urol* 2004; 171:1844–1849.
72. Graefen M, Haese A, Pichlmeier U *et al.* A validated strategy for side specific prediction of organ confined prostate cancer: a tool to select for nerve sparing radical prostatectomy. *J Urol* 2001; 165:857–863.
73. Palisaar RJ, Noldus J, Graefen M, Erbersdobler A, Haese A, Huland H. Influence of nerve-sparing (NS) procedure during radical prostatectomy (RP) on margin status and biochemical failure. *Eur Urol* 2005; 47:176–184.
74. Burkhard FC, Bader P, Schneider E, Markwalder R, Studer UE. Reliability of preoperative values to determine the need for lymphadenectomy in patients with prostate cancer and meticulous lymph node dissection. *Eur Urol* 2002; 42:84–90.

75. McLaughlin AP, Saltzstein SI, McCollough DL, Gittes RF. Prostatic carcinoma incidence and location of unsuspected lymphatic metastases. *J Urol* 1976; 115:89–94.
76. Han M, Partin AW, Zahurak M, Piantadosi S, Epstein JI, Walsh PC. Biochemical (prostate specific antigen) recurrence probability following radical prostatectomy for clinically localized prostate cancer. *J Urol* 2003; 169:517–523.
77. Joslyn SA, Konety BR. Impact of extent of lymphadenectomy on survival after radical prostatectomy for prostate cancer. *Urology* 2006; 68:121–125.
78. Pagliarulo V, Hawes D, Brands FH *et al*. Detection of occult lymph node metastases in locally advanced node-negative prostate cancer. *J Clin Oncol* 2006; 24:2735–2742.
79. Bader P, Burkhard FC, Markwalder R, Studer UE. Disease progression and survival of patients with positive lymph nodes after radical prostatectomy. Is there a chance of cure? *J Urol* 2003; 169:849–854.
80. Masterson TA, Bianco FJ Jr, Vickers AJ *et al*. The association between total and positive lymph node counts, and disease progression in clinically localized prostate cancer. *J Urol* 2006; 175:1320–1324.
81. Kamat AM, Babaian K, Cheung MR *et al*. Identification of factors predicting response to adjuvant radiation therapy in patients with positive margins after radical prostatectomy. *J Urol* 2003; 170:1860–1863.
82. Bolla M, Van Poppel H, Collette L *et al*. Postoperative radiotherapy after radical prostatectomy: a randomised controlled trial (EORTC trial 22911). *Lancet* 2005; 366(9485):572–578.
83. Shipley WU, Thames HD, Sandler HM *et al*. Radiation therapy for clinically localized prostate cancer: a multi-institutional pooled analysis. *JAMA* 1999; 281:1598–1604.
84. Roach M, Lu J, Pilepich MV *et al*. Four prognostic groups predict long-term survival from prostate cancer following radiotherapy alone on Radiation Therapy Oncology Group clinical trials. *Int J Radiat Oncol Biol Phys* 2000; 47:609–615.
85. Zagars GK, Pollack A, Von Eschenbach AC. Management of unfavorable locoregional prostate carcinoma with radiation and androgen ablation. *Cancer* 1997; 80:764–775.
86. Pollack A, Zagars GK, Starkschall G *et al*. Prostate cancer radiation dose response: results of the M. D. Anderson phase III randomized trial. *Int J Radiat Oncol Biol Phys* 2002; 53:1097–1105.
87. Zelefsky MJ, Fuks Z, Hunt M *et al*. High dose radiation delivered by intensity modulated conformal radiotherapy improves the outcome of localized prostate cancer. *J Urol* 2001; 166:876–881.
88. Dearnaley DP, Hall E, Lawrence D *et al*. Phase III pilot study of dose escalation using conformal radiotherapy in prostate cancer: PSA control and side-effects. *Br J Cancer* 2005; 92:488–498.
89. Bentzen SM, Ritter MA. The alpha/beta ratio for prostate cancer: what is it, really? *Radiother Oncol* 2005; 76:1–3.
90. Martinez AA, Demanes DJ, Galalae R *et al*. Lack of benefit from a short course of androgen deprivation for unfavorable prostate cancer patients treated with an accelerated hypofractionated regime. *Int J Radiat Oncol Biol Phys* 2005; 62:1322–1331.
91. Henderson A, Langley SE, Laing RW. Is bicalutamide equivalent to goserelin for prostate volume reduction before radiation therapy? A prospective, observational study. *Clin Oncol (R Coll Radiol)* 2003; 15:318–321.
92. Zelefsky MJ, Leibel SA, Burman CM *et al*. Neoadjuvant hormonal therapy improves the therapeutic ratio in patients with bulky prostatic cancer treated with three-dimensional conformal radiation therapy. *Int J Radiat Oncol Biol Phys* 1994; 29:755–761.
93. Linberg R, Conover CD, Shum KL, Shorr RG. Increased tissue oxygenation and enhanced radiation sensitivity of solid tumors in rodents following polyethylene glycol conjugated bovine hemoglobin administration. *In Vivo* 1998; 12:167–173.
94. Hara I, Miyake H, Yamada Y *et al*. Neoadjuvant androgen withdrawal prior to external radiotherapy for locally advanced adenocarcinoma of the prostate. *Int J Urol* 2002; 9:322–328.
95. Bolla M, Collette L, Blank L *et al*. Long-term results with immediate androgen suppression and external irradiation in patients with locally advanced prostate cancer (an EORTC study): a phase III randomised trial. *Lancet* 2002; 360(9327):103–106.
96. McLeod DG, Iversen P, See WA, Morris T, Armstrong J, Wirth MP. Bicalutamide 150 mg plus standard care vs standard care alone for early prostate cancer. *BJU Int* 2006; 97:247–254.
97. Iversen P, Tyrrell CJ, Kaisary AV *et al*. Bicalutamide monotherapy compared with castration in patients with nonmetastatic locally advanced prostate cancer: 6.3 years of followup. *J Urol* 2000; 1645:1579–1582.
98. Sieber PR, Keiller DL, Kahnoski RJ, Gallo J, McFadden S. Bicalutamide 150 mg maintains bone mineral density during monotherapy for localized or locally advanced prostate cancer. *J Urol* 2004; 171(6 Pt 1):2272–6.

9

Treatment strategies for biochemical recurrence of prostate cancer

Vincent Khoo, Anita Mitra

INTRODUCTION

Widespread use of prostate-specific antigen (PSA) testing has led to an increase in the number of men being diagnosed with prostate cancer and stage-shift towards earlier stage disease. PSA testing is also used extensively for monitoring of patients during follow-up. Within 10 years of radical treatment with either prostatectomy or radiotherapy, 20–40% of men are reported have a biochemical recurrence [1]. Identifying biochemical relapse can present a clinical dilemma as there remains considerable debate as to what threshold of PSA represents true biochemical recurrence in the context of alternative primary treatment regimens. Furthermore, ultrasensitive assays may be used providing measurements to 0.01 ng/ ml or below and giving rise to false-positives [2]. Any rising level of PSA can cause patient anxiety even if currently recommended thresholds for biochemical relapse have not been exceeded.

There are many factors that need to be taken into consideration when a patient has developed biochemical relapse. Performance status and comorbidities influence treatment options. Besides total PSA, PSA kinetics may be determined such as time to PSA relapse, PSA velocity and PSA doubling time (PSADT). It is important to establish whether or not there is clinically detectable local and/or systemic disease, as this will also influence treatment recommendations. Staging investigations may include repeat prostate biopsies, bone scan, magnetic resonance imaging (MRI) of the pelvis and computed tomography (CT) of the abdomen and pelvis. The range of salvage treatments available and their profile of side-effects must be considered and discussed with the patient, as the patient's preference will play an important part in the decision-making process.

The management and treatment strategies for biochemical recurrence of prostate cancer are complex. This chapter will review the definitions of biochemical relapse, natural history, diagnosis and management options available for a variety of different clinical settings of biochemical PSA relapse.

DEFINITION OF BIOCHEMICAL RELAPSE

Various definitions of biochemical relapse have been proposed for each definitive treatment. Validating a suitable threshold that represents true biochemical relapse is important to per-

Vincent Khoo, MBBS FRACR FRCR MD, Consultant and Honorary Senior Lecturer in Clinical Oncology, Department of Radiotherapy and Oncology, Royal Marsden Hospital & Institute of Cancer Research, London, UK
Anita Mitra, MBBS MRCP FRCR, Clinical Research Fellow, Institute of Cancer Research, Sutton, UK

mit timing of appropriate treatment, to avoid undue distress to the patient and to avoid overtreatment. Uniformity of definitions would also allow comparisons among different institutions and different treatment modalities. Summaries of the key issues are reviewed following primary surgical and radiotherapy treatments.

PSA RECURRENCE AFTER RADICAL PROSTATECTOMY

Following successful radical prostatectomy, serum PSA should fall to undetectable levels within 1 month [3]. A large number of laboratories currently utilize PSA assays that can detect levels as low as 0.01 ng/ml. Any detectable levels of PSA (defined as greater than 0.01 ng/ml) could be falsely construed as residual malignant prostatic tissue or relapse were it not for the large disparity between this finding and the progression to clinical disease. Some patients in whom PSA remains detectable after radical prostatectomy do not experience a continuing increase in PSA. In this situation, it can be speculated that this represents residual benign prostate gland, and expectant management with serial PSA testing is a reasonable management option.

Current recommendations for post-prostatectomy thresholds have ranged from 0.2 to 0.5 ng/ml [1–8]. Amling *et al.* [5] reported on 2783 men treated by radical prostatectomy in a single institution. In this study group, pathological stages were pT2 (68%), pT3a/b (21%) and pT3c (11%), and Gleason sum scores were Gleason 5–6 (61%), Gleason 7 (23%) and Gleason 8–10 (4%). They found that the percentage of men experiencing disease progression was dependent on the PSA threshold used. Nearly 50% of patients with PSA ≤0.29 ng/ml (773 men) never experienced disease progression, either clinical or biochemical. A PSA level of ≥0.4 ng/ml (1086 men) was most strongly associated with ongoing progression. In 70% of men with this level of PSA, the disease subsequently progressed, and most of these required treatment. Although the median follow-up in the study was 6.3 years, it is important to note that the cohort follow-up for those men with PSA < 0.4 ng/ml was more limited, at only 3 years.

Freedland *et al.* [6] proposed a PSA threshold of 0.2 ng/ml based on their retrospective study of 358 post-radical prostatectomy patients. They observed that if PSA exceeded > 0.21– 0.3 ng/ml the chance of further PSA progression at 1 and 3 years was 86% and 100% respectively. In addition, initial PSA levels and Gleason scores were also predictive of biochemical recurrence. Unlike the previous study, this one included clinical stage T3 and T4 disease cases.

The optimal definition of biochemical relapse after radical surgery is far from resolved as some patients with detectable postoperative PSA may not progress beyond 0.4–0.5 ng/ml. Currently, the data support a PSA threshold level of between 0.2–0.4 ng/ml. It may be reasonable to use the lower limit of 0.2 ng/ml, especially in cases where PSADT and velocity are suggestive of more aggressive disease. One European Consensus statement in 2004 recommended that a PSA threshold of 0.2 ng/ml with one subsequent rise be used to define relapse status, but suggested that salvage treatment only be commenced when the PSA reached 1–1.5 ng/ml [9]. Recently, the Working Group on the 'state of rising PSA' for clinical trials have recommended that a cut-off threshold of 0.4 ng/ml is used as eligibility criteria in clinical trials [10]. Issues regarding the interval for PSA testing in a 'rising state' are also not defined. It is reasonable to consider repeating PSA levels 2- to 4-monthly if the PSA is rising and salvage treatment is being considered, but this depends on initial PSA level and clinical parameters as well as the PSA dynamics as outlined above.

Natural History of Biochemical Recurrence After Radical Prostatectomy
PSA-free survival rates following radical prostatectomy vary substantially and depend on several factors such as initial PSA levels, pathological stage, Gleason grade, margin status and individual centre experience. Approximately 25–53% of men will suffer biochemical PSA

failure within 10 years following radical retropubic prostatectomy [7, 11]. Preliminary data from one large laparoscopic radical prostatectomy series suggests that recurrences rates are similar to retropubic prostatectomy [12].

In a retrospective review of 1997 post-prostatectomy men at the Johns Hopkins Hospital in Baltimore, there were 304 cases of biochemical recurrence that were not treated with hormones [7]. Of these patients, 34% developed metastases with a mean time to development of 8 years from the time of PSA rise (defined as greater than 0.2 ng/ml). The median actuarial time to death from the development of metastases was 5 years (a total of 13 years from the time of PSA rise). Time to biochemical progression post-surgery, Gleason score and PSADT were predictive of the time to development of metastatic disease. When grouped by tumour grade, of those with Gleason combined score 5–7, 79% were free of metastases 5 years after prostatectomy and 50% at 10 years. With Gleason combined score of 8–10, metastatic disease-free survival was 50% post prostatectomy but dropped to 18% at 10 years.

The Mayo Clinic's review of 3903 radical prostatectomy patients with a mean follow-up of 8.8 years reported that 33% of men experienced biochemical recurrence, and one-third of these men progressed to clinical disease [8]. In this study, biochemical failure was defined as a PSA of 0.4 ng/ml and clinical failure as demonstrable metastatic disease on radionuclide bone scan or histological evidence of failure (lymph node biopsy or prostate bed biopsy). The majority of relapses (73%) occurred 30 days to 5 years after prostatectomy with 27% occurring ≥5 years afterwards. The progression to clinical disease was at a rate similar to that in men who experienced biochemical recurrence within 5 years of surgery.

These data demonstrate that clinical progression to metastasis and subsequent death can be variable and lengthy. Again the challenge for the oncologist is to select those men who have more aggressive disease and warrant earlier management as well as to be aware of prognostic factors that predict for poor outcomes. PSA kinetics and other clinical prognostic variables as outlined previously can be helpful indicators in this assessment.

PSA RECURRENCE AFTER RADICAL IRRADIATION

There remains considerable controversy over the optimal definition of biochemical relapse following irradiation. In this setting, PSA levels can decline gradually and often do not reach undetectable levels with irradiation alone. Decrease in serum PSA following treatment depends not only on tumour eradication, but also on the cellular effects of radiation on normal prostate tissue and its radiosensitivity. Other factors include prostate size and the type of irradiation (external beam and/or brachytherapy). The median time to PSA nadir is 18–36 months following external beam radiotherapy (EBRT) alone and this may be longer after brachytherapy [13, 14]. In up to one-third of cases, 'transient' and benign elevation of PSA levels can occur within 12–18 months post-irradiation although PSA 'bounces' can also occur at similar rates between 2 and 5 years following radiotherapy [14–16]. In addition, the use of hormones in the adjuvant setting in high-risk disease suppresses PSA values to undetectable levels and on their withdrawal, the PSA values usually rise. Distinguishing biochemical progression from these benign PSA elevations in the early stages can be difficult. Sensible caution and serial PSA determinations are needed in this situation.

In 1997, the American Society for Therapeutic Radiology and Oncology (ASTRO) Consensus Panel agreed on guidelines (Table 9.1) for the use of PSA following radiotherapy [13]. It was also recommended that PSA determinations should be made at 3- to 4-monthly intervals for 2 years following radiotherapy and every 6 months thereafter. One European Consensus statement in 2004 endorsed the ASTRO definition of biochemical PSA relapse [9]. Although the ASTRO definition of biochemical recurrence appears to be a robust endpoint, it has weaknesses. It lacks specificity when androgen deprivation treatment is used, causing miscalculation because the PSA level can transiently increase after the completion of androgen deprivation therapy (ADT). Kaplan–Meier estimates of biochemical failure are

Table 9.1 ASTRO consensus agreement for guidelines on PSA use following radiation therapy

Biochemical failure is not justification per se to initiate additional treatment. It is not equivalent to clinical failure. It is, however, an appropriate early endpoint for clinical trials
Three consecutive increases in PSA is a reasonable definition of biochemical failure after radiotherapy. For clinical trials the date of failure should be the midpoint between the post-irradiation nadir PSA and the first of the three consecutive rises
No definition of PSA failure has as yet been shown to be a surrogate for clinical progression or survival
Nadir PSA is a strong prognostic factor but there is no absolute level that is a valid cut-off point for separating successful and unsuccessful treatments. The nadir PSA is similar in prognostic value to pretreatment PSA

Ref. 13.

inaccurate when the follow-up period is short because of backdating, as biochemical failure is assigned a date earlier than the PSA level used to declare/diagnose it [17, 18]. Reports suggest that the ASTRO definition overestimates biochemical disease survival by introducing lead time bias [19, 20]. In addition, there is no consideration of assay inconsistency, no specification of how much of a magnitude of a rise is significant, no account taken of the PSA 'bounce' phenomenon, difficulty in addressing 'tied or same' values over a period, the time taken to document three consecutive PSA rises and the slope of the PSA rise.

The biochemical failure misclassification rate of the ASTRO definition has been estimated in men with extended follow-up after radiotherapy alone and radiotherapy plus ADT to be 6% and 23% respectively [21]. As a consequence, a modification of the ASTRO definition was proposed. This modification requires two additional consecutive rises in PSA when a decline has occurred immediately after three consecutive rises and better predicts for a continued rise in PSA after radiotherapy plus ADT. The date of failure for the modified definition is backdated similar to the original ASTRO definition.

A multi-institutional review from nine centres was undertaken assessing 102 definitions of biochemical relapse after radical radiotherapy alone to a minimum dose of 60 Gy in 4839 men with a median follow-up of 6.3 years [22]. All patients had clinically localized disease (stage T1b–T2, N0, M0) and no ADT was used either before or after radiotherapy. Four definitions were found to be superior to the others in terms of sensitivity, specificity, positive and negative predictive values and hazard of clinical failure after biochemical recurrence. These are listed in Table 9.2. Whilst this study provides a useful evaluation of the utility of the different definitions for biochemical PSA failure, this review is limited by the treatment parameters of its study cohort. It is difficult to generalize to current radiotherapeutic practices that treat men with more advanced disease stages, higher radiation doses ≥70 Gy and with radiotherapy regimes using neoadjuvant/adjuvant ADT.

A more recent study based on current radiotherapeutic practices was reported from the Fox Chase Cancer Centre. This retrospective study assessed 586 men who received radiotherapy alone and 102 men treated with radiotherapy and ADT [23]. The median radiation dose delivered for both groups was > 70 Gy. Three definitions of biochemical recurrence were evaluated: ASTRO, modified ASTRO and the PSA nadir plus 2 ng/ml. The PSA nadir plus 2 ng/ml definition was found to have the highest sensitivity and specificity, and consequently outperformed the ASTRO and modified ASTRO definitions in terms of the predictive power for clinical failure (Table 9.3).

The optimal definition of biochemical relapse post-irradiation continues to be refined. Currently the 'PSA nadir plus 2 ng/ml' definition appears to be relatively robust and would be a sensible definition to use in the clinical setting in the absence of more conclusive data. However, it must be recognized that current radiotherapy trials may apply several other

Table 9.2 Definitions for biochemical PSA recurrence following radical radiotherapy

Two PSA rises backdated with each rise ≥0.5 ng/ml
PSA at or greater than the absolute nadir plus 2
PSA at or greater than the current nadir plus 2
PSA at or greater than the current nadir plus 3
Ref. 22.

Table 9.3 Assessment of PSA biochemical failure definition

	EBRT + ADT			RT alone		
Variable (%)	ASTRO	Modified ASTRO	Nadir + 2 ng/ml	ASTRO	Modified ASTRO	Nadir + 2 ng/ml
Sensitivity	88	88	100	92	92	92
Specificity	56	71	75	74	76	80
PPV	15	19	25	30	31	36
NPV	98	99	100	99	99	99
OA	59	68	77	76	77	81

EBRT, external beam radiotherapy; ADT, androgen deprivation therapy; ASTRO, American Society for Therapeutic Radiology and Oncology; PPV, positive predictive value; NPV, negative predictive value; OA, overall accuracy. Modified from ref. 23.

definitions as described above. In these settings, PSA assessments should be taken 3- to 4-monthly within the first 2 years and 6-monthly thereafter. For those undergoing ADT, 3- to 4-monthly PSA should be undertaken during ADT and the above guideline instituted following completion of ADT.

Natural History of Biochemical Recurrence After Radical Irradiation

It has been estimated that up to 59–66% can experience biochemical PSA recurrence at 5 years following EBRT [24, 25]. One long-term study with a minimum follow-up of 22.9 years reported relapses after both 10 and 20 years' follow-up, with relapses occurring steadily throughout the study period [26]. Although the 60 Gy dose used in this study is now considered suboptimal, it should be appreciated that in prostate cancer, long-term follow-up is necessary in order to fully quantify the true probability of biochemical recurrence.

The clinical utility of PSA in the post-irradiation setting relates to the premise that PSA is an early surrogate for clinical failure and disease-specific survival. This is supported by a multi-institutional, EBRT study of 1159 patients with organ-confined T1–2 disease using the ASTRO definition [25]. In those who did not undergo ADT until clinical failure, the 5-year clinical disease-free survival rate was 78%, 66% and 49% for low-, intermediate- and high-risk cases and the 10-year clinical disease-free survival was 58%, 56% and 46% respectively. This patient group was biased by the fact patients pretreated with ADT were excluded from the study and it is these patients that have the most aggressive disease. However, the authors argue that their estimates are similar to the surgical series reported by Pound et al. [7] apart from a better 10-year response in high-grade disease.

SALVAGE TREATMENT APPROACHES

The management approach to a patient with biochemical recurrence is complex and requires an understanding that relates the rising PSA levels to the behaviour of local, distant or both local and distant disease, as well as other prognostic factors, initial treatment, therapeutic ratio of the potential salvage therapies, appropriate timing of the treatment and finally the preference of the patient. Furthermore, both physician and patient need to appreciate that there are currently no data to support the notion that salvage therapies will improve cancer-specific survival. In general, if subclinical or clinical metastatic disease is suspected, standard management involves initiation of (some form of) ADT. This is discussed in more detail in Chapter 11. However, if only local disease is anticipated, then potential salvage local therapies may be used such as salvage radiotherapy, salvage prostatectomy, cryotherapy, brachytherapy and high intensity focused ultrasound. These latter treatment salvage options will now be addressed in this chapter.

SALVAGE RADIOTHERAPY

Following radical prostatectomy and biochemical recurrence, salvage radiotherapy may be considered if local recurrence only is anticipated. In 1999, the ASTRO Consensus Panel outlined that there was no particular subset of patients that had a better prognosis with salvage radiotherapy [27]. It was recommended that a minimum dose of radiotherapy of 64–65 Gy be delivered to the prostate bed when the PSA is < 1.5 ng/ml. On the assumption that radiotherapy results in a logarithmic reduction of cell numbers, it is expected that lower PSA values should produce better results [28–30]. Some studies have reported better outcomes following salvage radiotherapy when patients have PSA < 1.0 ng/ml [28, 31, 32]. However, it is more difficult to extrapolate outcomes to PSA levels ≤0.2 ng/ml.

More recently, the European Organisation for Research and Therapeutic Oncology (EORTC) reported their randomized results on the issue of immediate postoperative radiotherapy versus observation in the setting of positive surgical margins or pathological T3 disease [33]. With a median follow-up of 5 years, both biochemical and clinical progression-free survival was significantly improved in the irradiated group treated at 60 Gy compared with the observation group (74.0% vs. 52.6% respectively). This study does not address the value of 'true' adjuvant postoperative or salvage postoperative irradiation in other clinical settings. A randomized trial in the UK given the acronym RADICALS (Radiotherapy and Androgen Deprivation In Combination After Local Surgery) will soon be open to address this question. This study aims to address two questions: (1) the issue of adjuvant radiotherapy versus observation with early salvage radiotherapy for rising PSA; and (2) the use of postoperative radiotherapy with and without two different durations of ADT.

Unfortunately durable reported response rates after salvage radiotherapy have been disappointing. Although initial lowering of PSA values to undetectable levels may be achieved in 60–90% of cases, the 3–5 year actuarial PSA recurrence-free rates only range from 10% to 50% [28, 30, 32, 34–36]. It is important to note that older radiotherapy series may have used radiation doses that may be considered subtherapeutic today and the patient cohort often included high-risk disease cases that may have already had occult metastases.

Prognostic Factors in Salvage Radiotherapy
It is important but difficult to distinguish local from systemically recurrent disease when PSA values rise from undetectable levels after radical prostatectomy. There are a variety of prognostic factors used in this assessment. Pathology factors have been reported to relate to outcomes. Cases with Gleason combined score of > 7 have been reported to be associated with a higher incidence of systemic disease [37, 38]. Resection margins may also be prognostic with post-prostatectomy biochemical recurrence, where complete resection and negative margins may reflect systemic disease in contrast to positive surgical margins that could indicate local residual disease for which salvage radiotherapy would be effective [38]. Palpable prostatic fossa mass, seminal vesicle involvement and radiotherapy doses < 65 Gy have also been reported as poor prognostic features with worse freedom from biochemical failure [36].

PSA thresholds for treatment have already been discussed but PSA kinetics remains an important consideration. It has been suggested that more than 180 days to first detectable PSA value predicts for greater success in the use of salvage radiotherapy [39]. The time to rising PSA after prostatectomy has also been shown to be an independent predictor of metastases [7]. Men with a delayed rise in PSA are generally thought to be better candidates for salvage radiotherapy compared with those with persistently detectable PSA post prostatectomy. There are conflicting reports with others suggesting otherwise [28, 30].

One of the largest multi-institutional analyses of 8669 patients reported that PSA velocity > 2 ng/ml/year, an interval to PSA failure < 3 years and a post-radical prostatectomy PSADT < 3 months places men at increased risk of metastases, and these individuals are poor candidates for local salvage treatment [40]. Based on this, the authors proposed that the optimal candidate for local salvage treatment is a man whose PSA velocity was 2 ng/ml/year or less, interval to PSA failure exceeds 3 years, post-treatment PSADT is at least 12 months and who did not have a Gleason score of 8–10 or seminal vesicle or lymph node involvement.

Side-effects of Salvage Radiotherapy

Since radical prostatectomy tends to pull the bladder neck into the prostatic fossa, salvage radiotherapy may expose more of the normal bladder to irradiation. Although one would expect genitourinary side-effects to be more severe than seen with primary radiotherapy, the incidence of acute urinary toxicity is mild to moderate and not more severe than primary radiotherapy. Rectal irritation is common but rarely severe. The incidence of rectal bleeding is similar to that of patients treated with an intact prostate, with 10–20% risk of mild intermittent rectal spotting and less than 5% requiring intervention. The incidence of new onset post-radiotherapy urinary incontinence requiring a pad and/or dilatation is low and does not seem to be increased with adjuvant radiotherapy post-prostatectomy [41]. The absolute increase over prostatectomy alone in major incontinence is < 1%, haematuria is < 5%, major rectal bleeding is 2–6% and this is usually transient, and bowel urgency and incontinence is < 5 % [41–43]. Another important side-effect is erectile dysfunction. The data recorded are often limited, but an absolute increase in erectile impotence of approximately 30% for salvage radiotherapy over prostatectomy alone is reported [44]. In general, men receiving salvage radiotherapy do not seem to experience increase treatment-related morbidity.

ADT IN SALVAGE RADIOTHERAPY

There is little data on the utility of either neoadjuvant or adjuvant ADT in salvage radiotherapy. If post-prostatectomy biochemical recurrence is thought to represent a more aggressive disease category, then it may be argued from the published data on neoadjuvant or adjuvant ADT in high-risk primary prostate cancer that the improvement in disease-free and survival benefit seen in this situation [45, 46] may also be translated across to the salvage radiotherapy situation. One small retrospective, single-centre study reported on 81 patients who received salvage radiotherapy (60 Gy) and 3 months of neoadjuvant ADT [47]. The actuarial biochemical PSA-free recurrence rate at 3 and 5 years was 75% and 50% respectively, but median follow-up remains short at 38 months. Another retrospective case series reported a benefit of adjuvant ADT (median duration of 24 months) following salvage radiotherapy with 81% of men in this group being free of PSA relapse at 5 years compared with 54% in those not receiving ADT [48]. However, other investigators have reported similar control rates for men receiving salvage radiotherapy with or without ADT [28].

The use of ADT in salvage radiotherapy remains a controversial area but will shortly be the subject of a randomized trial (RADICALS). Outside of a study, neoadjuvant ADT would generally only be recommended if erectile function were not a concern. The impact of ADT on potency may be modified by the use of non-steroidal antiandrogens rather than luteinizing hormone-releasing hormone (LHRH) agonists.

SALVAGE PROSTATECTOMY

Long-term PSA control from salvage prostatectomy can be achieved in 30–43% of patients, data which may support the use of salvage therapy after radiation failure [49, 50]. It has been reported that stage-specific 5-year progression-free survival rates of salvage prostatectomy resemble those of standard prostatectomy, provided patients are referred early, with 5-year progression-free survival of 77%, 71% and 24% in patients with organ-confined disease, extracapsular extension and SV invasion and/or LN involvement respectively [51].

Currently a multicentre phase II study is being conducted under the auspices of the Cancer and Leukemia Group B (CALGB) Genitourinary Committee to examine the role of salvage prostatectomy in T1–2NxM0 prostate cancer cases with PSA ≤30 ng/ml prior to radiotherapy and ≥18 months following radiotherapy.

Prognostic Factors for Salvage Prostatectomy

Three parameters have been consistently identified as predictors of local failure after primary (radiotherapy) treatment: PSA nadir, time to nadir and PSADT. Whilst it is believed that the lower the PSA nadir the better the outcome, there is no absolute level of PSA nadir that predicts for success or failure. For clinically staged T1–2 disease, it was reported that a PSA nadir of ≤0.5 ng/ml was associated with a 5-year freedom from biochemical PSA progression of 90% and was an independent prognostic factor on multivariate analysis to Gleason score or initial presenting PSA [52]. Other investigators have suggested that in addition to the PSA nadir, both the rate of PSA decline and rise are predictive of outcomes [53]. Men with post-treatment PSA nadirs of 1–4 ng/ml were five times more likely to experience local failure compared to PSA nadirs < 1 ng/ml ($P = 0.0002$). A rapid rate of rise [i.e. $> 1.4 \log(\text{ng/ml})/\text{year}$, or PSADT < 6 months] was the most significant independent predictor of metastatic failure. These factors can be used to assess appropriate surgical salvage candidates.

Value of Prostate Biopsy After Radiation Therapy

Some investigators recommend that salvage treatment after radiotherapy failure should be given early before the PSA exceeds 10 ng/ml and when it is rising within 1–2 years of radiotherapy [51]. These investigators argued that the case is strengthened if a positive biopsy is found during this period, particularly if no histological treatment effect is observed in the biopsy specimen. However, it is important to note that histological clearance of tumour cells after radiotherapy may be prolonged as up to one-third of patients with a positive result within 2 years of treatment will later convert to a negative biopsy [54]. This information argues against the previous recommendation. Furthermore it has been reported that the rate of PSA progression after radiotherapy is only 50% at 7 years in those patients with stable PSA levels and a positive prostate biopsy at 2 years [55]. It could be argued that 50% of men with radiation failure would therefore not require salvage treatment and could be spared any potential attendant complications of salvage surgery. In this study, PSA progression occurred after 7 years, thus, for an individual patient approaching 75 years or beyond, other medical comorbidities may be more clinically relevant. Given the uncertainty, it is not surprising that the ASTRO Consensus Panel does not recommend routine biopsy at present as they argue that positive biopsy results less than 2 years after treatment correlate poorly with disease progression [27].

Side-effects of Salvage Prostatectomy

In one small early-salvage prostatectomy series of 40 cases, the rate of major complications was 33% with incontinence rates of 58% and rectal injury in 15% [56]. A recent series has reported a substantially lower major complication rate of 13% and rectal injury in only 2%, but urinary incontinence and anastomotic stricture rates remained high at 68% and 32% respectively [57]. The high complication rates in earlier series were observed mainly in patients who had undergone pre-radiotherapy pelvic lymph node dissection and/or ret-ropubic interstitial radiotherapy, which frequently caused extensive pelvic fibrosis. Now that these procedures are infrequently performed, complications of salvage operations may approach that of primary radical prostatectomy.

It is important to note that patient selection and operator experience may signifi-cantly influence the rate of treatment-related morbidity. This issue has been reviewed by Stephenson *et al.* [57] when they compared the complication rates of salvage prostatectomy in 100 patients treated from 1993 to the rates published prior to 1993. The major complication rate decreased significantly from 33% to 13% ($P = 0.02$) and the rectal injury rate from 15% to 2% ($P = 0.01$). Up to 39% of patients were dry and 68% required one pad daily or less at 5 years. The 5-year potency rate was reported to be 28% following unilateral or bilateral nerve-sparing prostatectomies. This rate varies widely and will largely be dependent on institution and operator expertise.

SALVAGE CRYOTHERAPY

Cryotherapy is an established technique for *in situ* ablation of tissue by freezing. When intro-duced in the 1980s as an alternative primary treatment for prostate cancer, high local failure rates due to limited techniques and equipment led to its disfavour. More recently, techno-logical advances of 'third generation' probe design, accurate probe placement under direct transrectal ultrasound guidance and utilization of multiple freeze-thaw cycles, provide bet-ter control and more uniform application of the 'freeze', leading to its resurgence. It is mainly used for post-radiotherapy failures. One of its main limitations is the need to spare the ure-thra from the full 'freeze' effect by a warming device; the degree of warming can be variable and sparing of the urethra may underexpose prostatic tissue especially at the apex and limit its success [58, 59]. Operative technique and methodology are crucial to successful outcome. The MD Anderson group reported incomplete cryoablation in 59% of cases and a positive biopsy rate of 23% post-cryosurgery with the number of cryoprobes used and freeze-thaw cycles used correlating with inadequate cryotherapy [59].

Overexposure of the prostate–rectal/bladder interfaces to freezing can result in significant morbidity. Complication rates can be high with reports of urinary incontinence in 7–73% of cases, obstructive urinary symptoms in 55–67%, impotence in up to 72%, severe perineal pain in up to 8%, rectourethral fistula in 0–3% and significant altered quality of life in up to 40% [58, 60–62]. It is clear that complication rates vary substantially and will depend on operator experience and expertise.

Again, there is no clear definition for biochemical failure after salvage cryotherapy and so the reported rates of PSA progression vary widely. It may be sensible to use the same definition of failure as post-radiotherapy failure. The 2-year biochemical relapse-free rate following salvage cryotherapy ranges between 55–74%, using PSA thresholds for failure that range from 0.3–4 ng/ml [58, 60, 62]. There have been few longer-term studies. One series of 131 cases reported a 5-year biochemical relapse-free rate of 40% in which PSA failure was defined as 2 ng/ml above nadir [63]. In this series, the 5-year disease specific was 87% in those with Gleason combined score ≤8 compared to 63% in those with Gleason ≥9 and 57% in those with pre-salvage PSA of ≤10 ng/ml compared to 23% in those with PSA > 10 ng/ml. As with other forms of salvage treatment, pre-salvage PSA, Gleason pattern and stage remain predictors of a sustained response.

SALVAGE BRACHYTHERAPY AFTER EBRT

Brachytherapy is an interstitial technique of transperineal implantation of either low or high-dose rate radiation sources under direct ultrasound guidance. Data remain limited, with most being from case series. One small retrospective series of 17 salvage low-dose-rate brachytherapy cases reported a 5-year PSA freedom from second relapse of 53% [64]. In this study, patients with ≤PSA 10 ng/ml at the time of salvage had a freedom from second relapse rate of 67% compared with 25% for men with PSA > 10 ng/ml. Similarly, low-grade tumours fared better than high-grade tumours, with a freedom from second relapse rate of 83% compared with 30%. Long-term complications were limited to a 24% risk of incontinence at 5 years.

Another retrospective series of 49 salvage brachytherapy cases with 64-month median follow-up reported 3- and 5-year disease-specific survival of 89% and 79% respectively, with actuarial biochemical disease-free survival of 48% and 34% respectively [65]. Post-treatment PSA nadir was noted to be prognostic and 47% of cases achieved a threshold of < 0.5 ng/ml. For post-brachytherapy PSA nadirs of < 0.5 ng/ml, the 3- and 5-year actuarial biochemical disease-free survival was 77% and 56% respectively. The incidence of serious complications was low, with post-salvage pain in 6%, persistent haematuria in 4% and rectal ulcers in 4%. This salvage technique remains investigational and again depends on appropriate selection of cases and adequate operator experience.

SALVAGE HIGH-INTENSITY FOCUSED ULTRASONOGRAPHY (HIFU)

This relatively new technique uses an endorectal ultrasound probe that focuses and emits high-intensity ultrasound waves, causing local increases in tissue temperature to between 70°C and 100°C and thereby destroying tissue. A cooling balloon protects the rectal mucosa from high temperatures.

There are limited data for salvage HIFU. One salvage HIFU series of 71 cases following radical radiotherapy reported encouraging results, with 61% of cases having a PSA nadir of < 0.5 ng/ml after a mean follow-up of 14.8 months (range 6–86) [66]. In this series, the 80% had negative post-salvage biopsies and 44% had no evidence of disease progression at last follow-up. This study is difficult to assess for a number of reasons including the use of ADT prior to HIFU in 30% of cases, use of ADT for rising PSA post-HIFU or positive post-salvage biopsy. The additional ADT therapy affects PSA nadir results and affects the estimates for disease-free survival. Serious complications in this HIFU salvage series were bladder neck stenosis in 17%, grade 3 incontinence in 7% and rectourethral fistula in 6%. Nevertheless, the preliminary results are encouraging and this form of salvage is currently being investigated at a number of centres in Europe.

CONCLUSION

The treatment of biochemical recurrence is a challenging area and one that both oncologists and urologists are likely to be faced with more often in the future. The reflex use of ADT as standard therapy is being challenged as it is clear that there are a proportion of men who relapse only with localized disease and these patients are candidates for local salvage opportunities. However, it is important to stage and select potential salvage candidates carefully. Recognition of biochemical PSA relapse is important. There are many current definitions for biochemical PSA relapse depending on the initial primary therapy, and these will continue to be refined. There are a large number of prognostic factors that may be used for patient selection including local tumour stage, Gleason grade, PSA levels and PSA kinetics. Finally, the potential benefits of salvage need to be carefully balanced with the likely complications of the treatment for the individual patient as the profile of side-effects needs to be considered in the context of his life, hopes and tolerances.

Awareness and comprehensive evaluation of biochemical relapses with better imaging techniques such as endorectal MRI and spectroscopy for staging will be helpful advances in this situation. Furthermore the developments in robotic surgery, improvements in radiotherapy such as intensity modulated radiotherapy, image-guided radiotherapy, and other salvage techniques such as HIFU, promise exciting future advances for the salvage opportunities for isolated non-metastatic biochemical PSA relapse. However, it is important to ensure that studies in these areas are conducted carefully and prospectively with attention not only to delivery techniques and appropriate local control evaluations but also to assessments of quality of life, progression of clinical disease and survival, to ensure that the results do comprehensively reflect outcomes relevant to the individual patient.

REFERENCES

1. Djavan B, Moul JW, Zlotta A, Remzi M, Ravery V. PSA progression following radical prostatectomy and radiation therapy: new standards in the new Millennium. *Eur Urol* 2003; 43:12–27.
2. Swindle PW, Kattan MW, Scardino PT. Markers and meaning of primary treatment failure. *Urol Clin N Am* 2003; 30:377–401.
3. Walsh PC, Oesterling JE, Epstein JI, Bruzek DJ, Rock RC, Chan DW. The value of prostate-specific antigen in the management of localized prostatic cancer. *Prog Clin Biol Res* 1989; 303:27–33.
4. Zincke H, Oesterling JE, Blute ML, Bergstralh EJ, Myers RP, Barrett DM. Long-term (15 years) results after radical prostatectomy for clinically localized (stage T2c or lower) prostate cancer. *J Urol* 1994; 152(5 Pt 2):1850–1857.
5. Amling CL, Bergstralh EJ, Blute ML, Slezak JM, Zincke H. Defining prostate specific antigen progression after radical prostatectomy: what is the most appropriate cut point? *J Urol* 2001; 165:1146–1151.
6. Freedland SJ, Sutter ME, Dorey F, Aronson WJ. Defining the ideal cutpoint for determining PSA recurrence after radical prostatectomy. Prostate-specific antigen. *Urology* 2003; 61:365–369.
7. Pound CR, Partin AW, Eisenberger MA, Chan DW, Pearson JD, Walsh PC. Natural history of progression after PSA elevation following radical prostatectomy. *JAMA* 1999; 281:1591–1597.
8. Ward JF, Blute ML, Slezak J, Bergstralh EJ, Zincke H. The long-term clinical impact of biochemical recurrence of prostate cancer 5 or more years after radical prostatectomy. *J Urol* 2003; 170:1872–1876.
9. Boccon-Gibod L, Djavan WB *et al*. Management of prostate-specific antigen relapse in prostate cancer: a European Consensus. *Int J Clin Pract* 2004; 58:382–390.
10. Scher HI, Eisenberger M, D'Amico AV *et al*. Eligibility and outcomes reporting guidelines for clinical trials for patients in the state of a rising prostate-specific antigen: recommendations from the Prostate-Specific Antigen Working Group. *J Clin Oncol* 2004; 22:537–556.
11. Lu-Yao GL, Potosky AL, Albertsen PC, Wasson JH, Barry MJ, Wennberg JE. Follow-up prostate cancer treatments after radical prostatectomy: a population-based study. *J Natl Cancer Inst* 1996; 88:166–173.
12. Guillonneau B, el-Fettouh H, Baumert H *et al*. Laparoscopic radical prostatectomy: oncological evaluation after 1,000 cases at Montsouris Institute. *J Urol* 2003; 169:1261–1266.
13. Consensus statement: guidelines for PSA following radiation therapy. American Society for Therapeutic Radiology and Oncology Consensus Panel. *Int J Radiat Oncol Biol Phys* 1997; 37:1035–1041.
14. Stock RG, Stone NN, Cesaretti JA. Prostate-specific antigen bounce after prostate seed implantation for localized prostate cancer: descriptions and implications. *Int J Radiat Oncol Biol Phys* 2003; 56:448–453.
15. Ragde H, Elgamal AA, Snow PB *et al*. Ten-year disease free survival after transperineal sonography-guided iodine-125 brachytherapy with or without 45-gray external beam irradiation in the treatment of patients with clinically localized, low to high Gleason grade prostate carcinoma. *Cancer* 1998; 83:989–1001.
16. Hanlon AL, Pinover WH, Horwitz EM, Hanks GE. Patterns and fate of PSA bouncing following 3D-CRT. *Int J Radiat Oncol Biol Phys* 2001; 50:845–849.
17. Vicini FA, Kestin LL, Martinez AA. The importance of adequate follow-up in defining treatment success after external beam irradiation for prostate cancer. *Int J Radiat Oncol Biol Phys* 1999; 45:553–561.
18. Horwitz EM, Uzzo RG, Hanlon AL, Greenberg RE, Hanks GE, Pollack A. Modifying the American Society for Therapeutic Radiology and Oncology definition of biochemical failure to minimize the influence of backdating in patients with prostate cancer treated with 3-dimensional conformal radiation therapy alone. *J Urol* 2003; 169:2153–2157; discussion 2157–2159.
19. Gretzer MB, Trock BJ, Han M, Walsh PC. A critical analysis of the interpretation of biochemical failure in surgically treated patients using the American Society for Therapeutic Radiation and Oncology criteria. *J Urol* 2002; 168(4 Pt 1):1419–1422.
20. Critz FA. A standard definition of disease freedom is needed for prostate cancer: undetectable prostate specific antigen compared with the American Society of Therapeutic Radiology and Oncology consensus definition. *J Urol* 2002; 167:1310–1313.

21. Buyyounouski MK, Hanlon AL, Horwitz EM, Uzzo RG, Pollack A. Biochemical failure and the temporal kinetics of prostate-specific antigen after radiation therapy with androgen deprivation. *Int J Radiat Oncol Biol Phys* 2005; 61:1291–1298.

22. Thames H, Kuban D, Levy L *et al*. Comparison of alternative biochemical failure definitions based on clinical outcome in 4839 prostate cancer patients treated by external beam radiotherapy between 1986 and 1995. *Int J Radiat Oncol Biol Phys* 2003; 57:929–943.

23. Buyyounouski MK, Hanlon AL, Eisenberg DF *et al*. Defining biochemical failure after radiotherapy with and without androgen deprivation for prostate cancer. *Int J Radiat Oncol Biol Phys* 2005; 63:1455–1462.

24. Shipley WU, Thames HD, Sandler HM *et al*. Radiation therapy for clinically localized prostate cancer: a multi-institutional pooled analysis. *JAMA* 1999; 281:1598–1604.

25. Kuban DA, Thames HD, Levy LB *et al*. Long-term multi-institutional analysis of stage T1-T2 prostate cancer treated with radiotherapy in the PSA era. *Int J Radiat Oncol Biol Phys* 2003; 57:915–928.

26. Swanson GP, Riggs MW, Earle JD. Long-term follow-up of radiotherapy for prostate cancer. *Int J Radiat Oncol Biol Phys* 2004; 59:406–411.

27. Cox JD, Gallagher MJ, Hammond EH, Kaplan RS, Schellhammer PF. Consensus statements on radiation therapy of prostate cancer: guidelines for prostate re-biopsy after radiation and for radiation therapy with rising prostate-specific antigen levels after radical prostatectomy. American Society for Therapeutic Radiology and Oncology Consensus Panel. *J Clin Oncol* 1999; 17:1155.

28. Song DY, Thompson TL, Ramakrishnan V *et al*. Salvage radiotherapy for rising or persistent PSA after radical prostatectomy. *Urology* 2002; 60:281–287.

29. Liauw SL, Webster WS, Pistenmaa DA, Roehrborn CG. Salvage radiotherapy for biochemical failure of radical prostatectomy: a single-institution experience. *Urology* 2003; 61:1204–1210.

30. Macdonald OK, Schild SE, Vora SA *et al*. Radiotherapy for men with isolated increase in serum prostate specific antigen after radical prostatectomy. *J Urol* 2003; 170:1833–1837.

31. Nudell DM, Grossfeld GD, Weinberg VK, Roach M, III, Carroll PR. Radiotherapy after radical prostatectomy: treatment outcomes and failure patterns. *Urology* 1999; 54:1049–1057.

32. Koppie TM, Grossfeld GD, Nudell DM, Weinberg VK, Carroll PR. Is anastomotic biopsy necessary before radiotherapy after radical prostatectomy? *J Urol* 2001; 166:111–115.

33. Bolla M, van Poppel H, Collette L *et al*. Postoperative radiotherapy after radical prostatectomy: a randomised controlled trial (EORTC trial 22911). *Lancet* 2005; 366(9485):572–578.

34. Cadeddu JA, Partin AW, DeWeese TL, Walsh PC. Long-term results of radiation therapy for prostate cancer recurrence following radical prostatectomy. *J Urol* 1998; 159:173–177; discussion 177–178.

35. Leventis AK, Shariat SF, Kattan MW, Butler EB, Wheeler TM, Slawin KM. Prediction of response to salvage radiation therapy in patients with prostate cancer recurrence after radical prostatectomy. *J Clin Oncol* 2001; 19:1030–1039.

36. Katz MS, Zelefsky MJ, Venkatraman ES, Fuks Z, Hummer A, Leibel SA. Predictors of biochemical outcome with salvage conformal radiotherapy after radical prostatectomy for prostate cancer. *J Clin Oncol* 2003; 21:483–489.

37. Partin AW, Pearson JD, Landis PK *et al*. Evaluation of serum prostate-specific antigen velocity after radical prostatectomy to distinguish local recurrence from distant metastases. *Urology* 1994; 43:649–659.

38. Stephenson AJ, Shariat SF, Zelefsky MJ *et al*. Salvage radiotherapy for recurrent prostate cancer after radical prostatectomy. *JAMA* 2004; 291:1325–1332.

39. Anscher MS, Clough R, Dodge R. Radiotherapy for a rising prostate-specific antigen after radical prostatectomy: the first 10 years. *Int J Radiat Oncol Biol Phys* 2000; 48:369–375.

40. Lee AK, D'Amico AV. Utility of prostate-specific antigen kinetics in addition to clinical factors in the selection of patients for salvage local therapy. *J Clin Oncol* 2005; 23:8192–8197.

41. Van Cangh PJ, Richard F, Lorge F *et al*. Adjuvant radiation therapy does not cause urinary incontinence after radical prostatectomy: results of a prospective randomized study. *J Urol* 1998; 159:164–166.

42. Choo R, Hruby G, Hong J *et al*. (IN)-efficacy of salvage radiotherapy for rising PSA or clinically isolated local recurrence after radical prostatectomy. *Int J Radiat Oncol Biol Phys* 2002; 53:269–276.

43. Duchesne GM, Dowling C, Frydenberg M *et al*. Outcome, morbidity, and prognostic factors in postprostatectomy radiotherapy: an Australian multicenter study. *Urology* 2003; 61:179–183.

44. Formenti SC, Lieskovsky G, Skinner D, Tsao-Wei DD, Groshen S, Petrovich Z. Update on impact of moderate dose of adjuvant radiation on urinary continence and sexual potency in prostate cancer patients treated with nerve-sparing prostatectomy. *Urology* 2000; 56:453–458.

45. Bolla M, Collette L, Blank L *et al*. Long-term results with immediate androgen suppression and external irradiation in patients with locally advanced prostate cancer (an EORTC study): a phase III randomised trial. *Lancet* 2002; 360(9327):103–106.

46. Denham JW, Steigler A, Lamb DS *et al*. Short-term androgen deprivation and radiotherapy for locally advanced prostate cancer: results from the Trans-Tasman Radiation Oncology Group 96.01 randomised controlled trial. *Lancet Oncol* 2005; 6:841–850.

47. Tiguert R, Rigaud J, Lacombe L, Laverdiere J, Fradet Y. Neoadjuvant hormone therapy before salvage radiotherapy for an increasing post-radical prostatectomy serum prostate specific antigen level. *J Urol* 2003; 170(2 Pt 1):447–450.

48. Taylor N, Kelly JF, Kuban DA, Babaian RJ, Pisters LL, Pollack A. Adjuvant and salvage radiotherapy after radical prostatectomy for prostate cancer. *Int J Radiat Oncol Biol Phys* 2003; 56:755–763.

49. Bianco FJ Jr, Scardino PT, Stephenson AJ, Diblasio CJ, Fearn PA, Eastham JA. Long-term oncologic results of salvage radical prostatectomy for locally recurrent prostate cancer after radiotherapy. *Int J Radiat Oncol Biol Phys* 2005; 62:448–453.

50. Ward JF, Sebo TJ, Blute ML, Zincke H. Salvage surgery for radiorecurrent prostate cancer: contemporary outcomes. *J Urol* 2005; 173:1156–1160.

51. Stephenson AJ, Eastham JA. Role of salvage radical prostatectomy for recurrent prostate cancer after radiation therapy. *J Clin Oncol* 2005; 23:8198–8203.

52. Zietman AL, Tibbs MK, Dallow KC *et al*. Use of PSA nadir to predict subsequent biochemical outcome following external beam radiation therapy for T1–2 adenocarcinoma of the prostate. *Radiother Oncol* 1996; 40:159–162.

53. Sartor CI, Strawderman MH, Lin XH, Kish KE, McLaughlin PW, Sandler HM. Rate of PSA rise predicts metastatic versus local recurrence after definitive radiotherapy. *Int J Radiat Oncol Biol Phys* 1997; 38:941–947.

54. Crook J, Malone S, Perry G, Bahadur Y, Robertson S, Abdolell M. Postradiotherapy prostate biopsies: what do they really mean? Results for 498 patients. *Int J Radiat Oncol Biol Phys* 2000; 48:355–367.

55. Pollack A, Zagars GK, Antolak JA, Kuban DA, Rosen II. Prostate biopsy status and PSA nadir level as early surrogates for treatment failure: analysis of a prostate cancer randomized radiation dose escalation trial. *Int J Radiat Oncol Biol Phys* 2002; 54:677–685.

56. Rogers E, Ohori M, Kassabian VS, Wheeler TM, Scardino PT. Salvage radical prostatectomy: outcome measured by serum prostate specific antigen levels. *J Urol* 1995; 153:104–110.

57. Stephenson AJ, Scardino PT, Bianco FJ Jr, DiBlasio CJ, Fearn PA, Eastham JA. Morbidity and functional outcomes of salvage radical prostatectomy for locally recurrent prostate cancer after radiation therapy. *J Urol* 2004; 172(6 Pt 1):2239–2243.

58. Chin JL, Pautler SE, Mouraviev V, Touma N, Moore K, Downey DB. Results of salvage cryoablation of the prostate after radiation: identifying predictors of treatment failure and complications. *J Urol* 2001; 165(6 Pt 1):1937–1941; discussion 1941–1942.

59. Izawa JI, Morganstern N, Chan DM, Levy LB, Scott SM, Pisters LL. Incomplete glandular ablation after salvage cryotherapy for recurrent prostate cancer after radiotherapy. *Int J Radiat Oncol Biol Phys* 2003; 56:468–472.

60. Bales GT, Williams MJ, Sinner M, Thisted RA, Chodak GW. Short-term outcomes after cryosurgical ablation of the prostate in men with recurrent prostate carcinoma following radiation therapy. *Urology* 1995; 46:676–680.

61. Izawa JI, Ajam K, McGuire E *et al*. Major surgery to manage definitively severe complications of salvage cryotherapy for prostate cancer. *J Urol* 2000; 164:1978–1981.

62. Ghafar MA, Johnson CW, De La Taille A *et al*. Salvage cryotherapy using an argon based system for locally recurrent prostate cancer after radiation therapy: the Columbia experience. *J Urol* 2001; 166:1333–1337; discussion 1337–1338.

63. Izawa JI, Madsen LT, Scott SM *et al*. Salvage cryotherapy for recurrent prostate cancer after radiotherapy: variables affecting patient outcome. *J Clin Oncol* 2002; 20:2664–2671.

64. Beyer DC. Permanent brachytherapy as salvage treatment for recurrent prostate cancer. *Urology* 1999; 54:880–883.

65. Grado GL, Collins JM, Kriegshauser JS *et al*. Salvage brachytherapy for localized prostate cancer after radiotherapy failure. *Urology* 1999; 53:2–10.

66. Gelet A, Chapelon JY, Poissonnier L *et al*. Local recurrence of prostate cancer after external beam radiotherapy: early experience of salvage therapy using high-intensity focused ultrasonography. *Urology* 2004; 63:625–629.

Section III

Advanced prostate cancer – distant metastases

10

Advanced prostate cancer – distant metastases: endpoints for clinical trials

Kim N. Chi, Martin E. Gleave

INTRODUCTION

Patients that develop recurrent metastatic prostate cancer have a poor prognosis. Although hormonal therapy in the form of medical or surgical castration can induce significant long-term remissions, development of castration-resistant disease, also termed castration-adapted, androgen-independent, or hormone-refractory prostate cancer (HRPC), is inevitable. Systemic therapy for metastatic prostate cancer is remarkable for the relatively few options that have been developed. Other than hormonal therapy, most treatments that have been approved for use have been for symptomatic benefit, such as mitoxantrone chemotherapy [1], the bisphosphonate zoledronic acid [2] and radioactive isotopes [3]. Despite multiple trials of cytotoxic chemotherapy in patients with metastatic HRPC, only docetaxel has been shown to improve overall survival [4, 5]. Part of the problem of a lack of therapeutic options is due to the prolonged natural history of prostate cancer and the patient population that it affects: generally older patients with concomitant medical problems and a higher risk of death from other causes [6]. This can make accrual to clinical trials more difficult [7] and create difficulties with detecting effects of a new therapy on overall survival.

Compounding the difficulties in the development of systemic therapy for prostate cancer is the lack of reliable intermediate endpoints in order to assess the activity of a new treatment, and in turn to judge and plan whether or not to proceed with large randomized comparative studies. In HRPC, objective disease progression may be lacking, and rising serum prostate-specific antigen (PSA) may be the only quantifiable measure of disease progression. Also, patients generally do not present with measurable tumour masses; when they do occur, they tend to be within lymph nodes, of small size and uncertain significance [8]. Bone is the predominant site of metastases in HRPC but determining whether a response or progression has occurred can be difficult. Post-therapy decreases in serum PSA are frequently used to assess activity; however, PSA 'response' has not been established as a surrogate for a clinical benefit [9]. Even defining when progression has occurred is problematic as it can be discordant between symptoms, measurable disease criteria, bone scan and PSA changes.

Over the past decade, our understanding of the molecular mechanisms of cancer progression has greatly expanded and a plethora of new targets based on these mechanisms have emerged. Novel therapeutics directed against these targets have closely followed; however,

Kim N. Chi, MD FRCP[C], Assistant Professor, Department of Medicine, Division of Medical Oncology, University of British Columbia, Medical Director-Vancouver Centre Clinical Trials Unit, BC Cancer Agency, Vancouver, British Columbia, Canada

Martin E. Gleave, MD FRCS[C], Professor, Department of Urological Sciences, University of British Columbia, Director of Research, The Prostate Centre, Vancouver General Hospital, Vancouver, British Columbia, Canada

the development of these agents in prostate cancer has been a challenge for the reasons discussed above and the sheer volume of agents and drug combinations available for testing. This emphasizes the importance of clinical trial design and choice of appropriate endpoints when testing these agents in order to identify early those most promising to move forward, but also to not prematurely discard potentially useful treatments. This chapter will review the endpoints that have been utilized in recent clinical trials for men with prostate cancer with an emphasis on those with HRPC.

MOLECULAR CORRELATIVE ENDPOINTS

Generally, the primary objective of a phase I trial is to identify a dose for phase II testing. In cancer trials, this was traditionally designed around cytotoxic chemotherapy, where the intent is to give as much of the cytotoxic agent as possible to identify the 'maximum tolerated dose' based on the proportion of patients that develop severe 'dose-limiting toxicity'. With the development of novel targeted therapeutics, dose limiting toxicity may not be as relevant, as the dose of a drug that induces severe toxicity may far exceed what is actually required to suppress the molecular pathway in question [10, 11]. Thus, many early phase I and II clinical trial designs are now incorporating some measure of pharmacodynamic effect on the molecular pathway being targeted, using either cancer tissue or other surrogate tissues such as skin or peripheral blood mononuclear cells. Clearly, it is also desirable to ensure that the molecular pathway being disrupted by the targeted therapy is in fact present or relevant within the patient population included in the study. This latter point is well exemplified in lung cancer, where patients most likely to respond to small molecule tyrosine kinase inhibitors are those that have tumours with activating mutations in the epidermal growth factor receptor [12], and in breast cancer, where amplification of HER2 is required in order to see benefit from trastuzumab therapy [13].

In patients with prostate cancer, obtaining the relevant tissues to evaluate target expression and pharmacodynamic effect is difficult. Use of the original prostate pathology specimens to evaluate a particular molecular target and then extrapolating the expression to the HRPC is perilous because of the shift in gene expression that occurs with changes in disease states and androgen-independent progression [14]. In terms of recurrent disease, bone is the primary site of disease and bone biopsies are invasive and painful, and when nodal disease is present it is most often retroperitoneal and thus difficult to access. Methods to enrich for malignant cells in bone marrow or in the circulation have been developed using immunomagnetic techniques [15, 16]; however, the significance of these cells and their usefulness to profile molecular changes has not been established as of yet.

One study design that has been used effectively to evaluate pharmacodynamic endpoints in patients with prostate cancer is with a presurgery ('neoadjuvant') approach. A phase I study used a neoadjuvant design to evaluate OGX-011, an antisense inhibitor of the clusterin gene which has antiapoptotic function [17]. Patients with localized prostate cancer and high-risk features were enrolled on the study and treated with OGX-011 for 1 month, which was then followed by prostatectomy. The study incorporated a dose escalation, meaning that successive cohorts of patients were given higher doses of OGX-011. Prostatectomy specimens were then used to evaluate for clusterin expression for both inter- and intrapatient comparisons to baseline. In this way, changes in expression of clusterin could be correlated to the dose of drug received and drug levels within the prostate tissue itself could be determined. Treatment was well tolerated and significant dose-dependent effects of OGX-011 on suppressing clusterin expression and increasing apoptosis were observed. With this design and the use of a molecular endpoint, an optimal biological dose (OBD) was established for OGX-011 not based on its ability to induce severe toxicity, but rather its biological effectiveness to suppress its target. Several other studies are utilizing a similar approach with agents including viral gene therapy [18] and other small molecule inhibitors in order to determine their biological effectiveness.

Assessing the effects of treatments on bone metabolism, whether the treatments have been specifically bone directed or not, has been of great interest given the predilection of prostate cancer to metastasize to bone, as well as the incidence of treatment-induced osteopenia and osteoporosis in prostate cancer patients leading to complications [19]. In patients with bone metastases, altered bone remodelling activity can be assessed indirectly by analyzing metabolic products released from the bone matrix associated with bone formation, bone resorption and osteoclastogenesis. In patients with prostate cancer specifically, several markers of bone formation have been evaluated including bone-specific alkaline phosphatase (BAP), amino-terminal procollagen propeptides of type I collagen and osteocalcin. There has been greater interest in the evaluation of bone resorption markers as most solid tumours produce a predominantly osteolytic process and therapies for bone metastases are primarily anti-resorptive by action (i.e. bisphosphonates). Bone resorption markers that have been studied in patients with prostate cancer include bone sialoprotein, the breakdown products of type I bone collagen, and tartrate-resistant acid phosphatase (TAP). Type 1 collagen forms the basic fabric and tensile strength of bone tissue. Cross-linked C-terminal (CTX) and cross linked N-terminal (NTX) telopeptides are produced from type I collagen by cathepsin K and matrix metalloproteases, respectively, during bone resorption. Earlier studies have evaluated urine NTX normalized to creatinine, however, serum levels of NTX have been shown to correlate well with urine ratios. TAP is highly expressed in osteoclasts which specifically secrete the 5b form as an active enzyme that is rapidly cleared from the circulation, and reflects the intensity of bone resorption over the preceding 24 h independent of hepatic and renal function. Another important factor that has been identified in the pathogenesis of bone metastases is osteoclastogenesis, which determines the balance between osteoblastic and osteoclastic activity in bone. Osteoclastogenesis is regulated by osteoprotegerin (OPG), and receptor activator of NFκB (RANK) and its ligand (RANKL). Acquisition and activation of the osteoclast phenotype depends on interaction between RANKL and RANK, which is expressed on the cell surface of osteoclast precursors. OPG is a dimeric glycoprotein of the tumour necrosis factor (TNF) receptor family that controls excessive bone resorption by acting as a soluble decoy receptor for RANKL, thereby neutralizing its interaction with RANK and thus preventing osteoclast activation.

In the control arm of a study that evaluated zoledronic acid in patients with bone-metastatic hormone-refractory prostate cancer [20], elevated urinary NTX (normalized to urinary creatinine levels) and BAP have been found to be predictive for negative clinical outcomes (i.e. skeletal-related event, disease progression and death). These associations also held up for patients on bisphosphonate therapy [21]. Another study evaluated 10 serum bone turnover markers in 187 men [22], including a control group and men with varying stages of prostate cancer and treatment. From the 10 markers, logistic regression analysis identified OPG and TAP as variables that predicted bone metastases. In addition, BAP, NTX, TAP, and OPG were increased in patients with bone metastases and higher levels were associated with shorter survival, with OPG remaining significant on a multivariate analysis which included only limited clinical factors. Although all of the above markers can be measured in patients, there are no clear recommendations for which of the markers that should be used and especially which to use in prostate cancer. The inter- and intrapatient variability, stability (especially in urine) and differing assays and methods that have been used contribute to this difficulty.

PHASE II TRIAL ENDPOINTS

The objective of phase II trials is to determine whether there is sufficient clinical activity of a treatment to justify bringing it forward for further testing such as in a large-scale randomized comparative trial. Traditionally, activity has been defined as shrinkage of tumour in measurable disease sites. Various criteria have been established as to what constitutes a response in progression within clinically detectable disease with the most recently internationally accepted being that of RECIST (Response Evaluation Criteria in Solid Tumors), which is based on the unidimensional measurement of lesions [23]. The problems with applying the RECIST criteria to patients with prostate cancer are that it was developed without specifically considering the clinical presentation of patients with prostate cancer (lack of measurable disease, predominantly bone involvement) and did not include trials of prostate cancer in its inception. Methods to quantify response to therapy in bone metastases using magnetic resonance imaging are promising, but have not been validated [24].

Decreases in serum PSA have been associated with improved survival in retrospective studies [25, 26] and thus the majority of phase II trials have used post-therapy changes in PSA for the primary endpoint as a measure of antitumour activity of a new treatment. After a consensus conference, recommendations were published in 1999 outlining eligibility and response criteria as a means of standardizing methods and reporting of results from prostate cancer trials [9] (Table 10.1). For eligibility, it was considered that, in the absence of objective disease progression, a rising PSA on two separate occasions taken at last 1 week apart would be acceptable. For post-therapy PSA decline, the emphasis for reporting was on a 50% or greater decrease from baseline, which had to be confirmed by a second value at least 4 weeks later. Progression, as defined on PSA alone, was considered as a rise of 50% from nadir in those achieving a PSA 'response' and a 25% increase in those that had not.

Questions continue as to whether a PSA response is a surrogate for a clinical benefit. To evaluate this question, post-therapy PSA data were analysed from the Southwest Oncology Group Protocol (SWOG) 99–16, which was a randomized study of mitoxantrone vs. docetaxel-estramustine that demonstrated a survival benefit in favour of the docetaxel arm [5]. Various post-therapy PSA declines were evaluated for surrogacy for survival using three statistical tests [27]: Prentice's criteria, the proportion of treatment effect explained and the proportion of variation explained. The optimal post-therapy PSA decline parameter surrogate for survival was found to be a 30% PSA decline at 3 months after treatment initiation. Although promising, this data-driven result remains to be prospectively validated in future trials. Interestingly, the commonly reported 50% decrease in PSA did not meet the criteria for surrogacy (although just barely). This finding is similar to PSA data from a randomized study that evaluated docetaxel chemotherapy vs. mitoxantrone [4], which demonstrated superior overall survival benefit for those patients treated with docetaxel (often referred to as the TAX-327 study). In a further analysis, only approximately half the treatment effect on overall survival could be accounted for by the PSA 'response', which was defined as a 50% decrease from baseline [28]. Additionally, it was found that in this trial, PSA 'response' was associated

Table 10.1 PSA eligibility and response and reporting recommendations from the Prostate-Specific Antigen Working Group

Criteria	Definition
Eligibility	Two consecutive rises in PSA over a reference value. The first rising PSA must be taken at least 1 week after the reference value. A third PSA is required to show further increase; if not, a subsequent PSA must show further increase. PSA must be $\geq 5\,\mu g/l$
Post-therapy change	PSA decline of $\geq 50\%$, which must be confirmed by a second PSA value ≥ 4 weeks later
Duration of post-therapy change	Commences on the date of the first $\geq 50\%$ decline in PSA Ends when the PSA value increases by 50% above the nadir (minimum rise of $5\,\mu g/l$ or back to the baseline) confirmed by a second value
Progression	In patients whose PSA has not decreased, progressive disease is a $\geq 25\%$ increase over the baseline or nadir (minimum rise of $5\,\mu g/l$) confirmed by a second value

Adapted from ref. 9.

with pain and quality of life improvements [29], suggesting post-therapy PSA declines may be potential surrogates for important clinical benefits other than survival.

Another problem with interpretation of PSA responses is the heterogeneity of the patient population and the effect on response in single-arm phase II trials. As an example, in a single-arm, single-centre phase II trial of high-dose calcitriol plus docetaxel, the PSA response rate (defined as a 50% or more post-therapy decrease) was 81% [30], notably higher than in reported phase II and III studies of single agent docetaxel which consistently reported PSA response rates of 40–50%. However, when this regimen was taken into a multi-institutional setting in a randomized phase II study against placebo plus docetaxel, the PSA response rate was lower at 58% and not statistically different from the placebo control [31]. What was observed was a difference in overall survival, a secondary endpoint of the trial and this result has led to a randomized phase III trial which is currently in progress. This further emphasizes that intermediate response endpoints such as PSA are currently insufficient surrogates of clinical benefit and the need to exercise caution in prematurely discarding drugs based on this measure of activity alone.

Indeed, many of the new targeted therapies (and some of the currently approved agents) may not be expected to induce responses, either in measurable disease or in PSA, but still may improve other aspects of the disease such as time to disease progression, incidence of skeletal-related events, pain and other disease-related symptoms, and overall survival. An example of a new agent with a low response rate but significant clinical benefit is sorafenib, a small molecule tyrosine kinase inhibitor of the vascular endothelial growth factor receptor. In phase II and III trials in patients with kidney cancer, RECIST-defined response rates were less than 5%; however, treatment with sorafenib was associated with a significant lengthening of the time to disease progression and improved overall survival leading to the drug being approved for use [32, 33]. Intermediate endpoints, however, are subject to extensive variability in single-arm phase II trials which makes cross-trial comparison difficult. This variability is due to issues such as differing patient eligibility criteria, patient selection, endpoint definitions and interobserver variability in assessments. Although an overall survival endpoint is most appropriately left for study in large comparative randomized phase III trials, smaller randomized phase II studies may be useful for assessing these other endpoints. Traditionally, the randomized phase II design does not incorporate a formal rigorous comparison of the treatment arms but does provide an internal control to reduce the variability in the study population and investigator actions.

An intermediate endpoint that has been assessed in several trials is time to disease progression. Yet defining when progression has occurred for patients with HRPC can be as challenging as defining response for all the same reasons already discussed: bone disease is not measurable and nuclear bone scan imaging may be equivocal with many different definitions of what constitutes progression having been used and may even falsely show progression [34]. Although rising PSA is associated with poor outcome in HRPC [35, 36], what has not been established is what degree of rise is really clinically significant in the context of a post-therapy change. Furthermore, asymptomatic progression on imaging and rising PSA may not be of any particular clinical consequence or relevance in patients with HRPC. When considering progression then, disease-related symptoms should also be factored into the criteria as often symptoms can worsen in the absence of definitive evidence of objective or PSA progression. Although a subjective variable, pain and quality of life can be made qualitative through use of validated scales [1]. The need for use of increasing analgesics, radiation, surgery and/or chemotherapy to treat symptomatic disease has also been included as part of the definition of progression as these are clinically relevant and readily identifiable endpoints. In addition to problems with defining progression, using time to progression as a surrogate for overall survival is also problematic. Even if a lengthening of time to progression is seen, if relatively small then the impact on overall survival is likely to be negligible. Furthermore, therapy after progression may also have a substantial impact negating any benefit of prior interventions.

An example of the challenge of assessing progression endpoints comes from the TAX-327 study [4] where progression was defined on objective disease criteria, PSA increase and increase in pain as assessed by a validated scoring system. Progression was a composite endpoint and a patient was mandated to stop protocol therapy for any one of the criteria. As a result many patients came off the trial for one progression criteria but not the others. Because of this, a high level of censoring occurred and a time to progression analyses could not be performed. In the SWOG 99–16 study [5], progression was defined on objective disease or PSA criteria [9] and the median time to progression was 6.3 months for the docetaxel-estramustine-treated patients. What was not reported was the type of progression that occurred and at what rate (i.e. objective disease progression vs. PSA rise only) and disease-related worsening of symptoms was not considered.

Another example of the difficulty with defining and interpreting progression, especially when used as a primary endpoint, is in the clinical development of atrasentan, an endothelin receptor-A antagonist. In a randomized phase II study of atrasentan, patients with HRPC were randomized to three arms: low dose, high dose and placebo [37]. The primary endpoint was time to progression, with progression defined as the development of new lesions in the bone or soft tissue; the requirement of palliative treatment with an opioid analgesic for new disease-related pain; the occurrence of new disease-related symptoms that required intervention such as treatment with chemotherapy, radiation or surgery; the occurrence of a clinical event determined by the investigator to represent disease progression; or death occurring while the patient was receiving the study drug. The intention-to-treat analyses did not reveal a statistical difference between the arms, although in 'assessable' patients a statistical difference was found (excluding patients who did not meet study-defined PSA or antiandrogen withdrawal inclusion criteria, who were taking excluded medications, or received less than 50% of scheduled doses or fewer than 20 total doses). When atrasentan was tested in a phase III study, progression on bone scan defined as two or more new lesions resulted in protocol-mandated withdrawal from therapy in over half the patients at the first 3 month assessment, despite stable or improved symptoms or PSA in many patients. This large withdrawal reduced study power and resulted in a negative trial. Although potentially a true negative result, because of the way progression was defined and acted upon, a potential problem is that the bone scan changes at 3 months may not have taken into account the lag time between baseline investigations, start of treatment and the treatment effect, especially given the mechanism of the drug and the expectations of it to delay progression only.

Another trial which used progression as the primary endpoint was a study of sipuleucel-T (APC8015), an investigational immunotherapy product designed to stimulate T-cell immunity against prostate acid phosphatase [38]. Progression was defined as progressive disease on serial radiographic imaging tests; new cancer-related pain associated with a radiographic anatomical correlation; or other clinical events consistent with progression, such as spinal cord compression, nerve root compression or pathological fracture. No difference was detected between the experimental and placebo-treated arms (median time to progression 11.7 vs. 10.0 weeks). However, patients were followed for overall survival and a statistically significant difference favouring the experimental arm emerged. As in the atrasentan study, the results of this trial demonstrate the difficulties in using a time to progression endpoint with a therapy that is supposed to slow progression as some patients may have developed progressive disease before the treatment achieved its biological effects. Further, it raises the question of whether progression, which in this study used very practical definitions, has any real clinical relevance and bearing on overall survival in HRPC.

To summarize, when considering progression, all aspects of the disease should be accounted for including objective measurable and non-measurable disease, PSA parameters and disease-related symptoms. These must also be carefully defined within a protocol taking into account the nature of the disease, the expectations of the desired effect of the particular treatment, and the consequence on protocol-directed treatment decisions and analysis of outcomes.

PHASE III ENDPOINTS

The major purpose of a comparative phase III trial is the detection and quantitation of a clinically significant difference between two treatments. In trials of HRPC, the primary endpoint generally should be overall survival, given the importance of this endpoint for patients, that the median survival for patients with metastatic HRPC is only in the 1.5–2 year range making adequately powered phase III studies feasible, and the problems with using intermediate endpoints as discussed previously.

Of course, it should be recognized that from the patient perspective the other important clinical benefit to achieve is the management of symptoms and maintenance of quality of life, especially so in patients with HRPC who are generally of advanced age and faced with a disease that is uniformly fatal. Recognizing this, there have been two important phase III studies that used non-survival endpoints successfully.

The first was a study in patients with symptomatic HRPC who were randomized to mitoxantrone chemotherapy and prednisone vs. prednisone alone [1]. The primary study endpoint was pain response, defined as a 2-point reduction in the 6-point present pain intensity of the McGill Melzack Pain Questionnaire [39], maintained on two separate occasions at least 3 weeks apart and without an increase in analgesic score. The primary pain response was observed in 29% of patients in the mitoxantrone–prednisone arm and 12% in the prednisone alone arm. Duration of pain response was also longer in the mitoxantrone arm (43 vs. 18 weeks). The effects of treatment on health-related quality of life were assessed using the European Organization for Research and Treatment of Cancer Quality-of-Life Questionnaire C30 (EORTC QLQ-C30) [40]. After 6 weeks, patients taking prednisone showed no improvement in quality of life scores, whereas those taking mitoxantrone plus prednisone showed significant improvements in global quality of life, four functioning domains and nine symptoms, and the improvement (> 10 unit improvement on a scale of 0 to 100) lasted longer than in the prednisone-alone group [41]. On the basis of these findings, mitoxantrone was approved for the palliative treatment of patients with metastatic HRPC despite the absence of any significant difference in overall survival. As a secondary endpoint, the TAX-327 study also incorporated a similar assessment of pain and evaluated health-related quality of life with the Functional Assessment of Cancer Therapy–Prostate (FACT–P) Questionnaire [42]. Improvements in both pain and quality of life scores were observed with docetaxel therapy [4]. Data such as this showing improvements in symptoms and quality of life parameters can potentially assist both patients and physicians with treatment decision-making for therapies that, although considered effective, may have relatively modest benefits on overall survival and the potential to induce serious toxicity.

The other trial that has used a non-survival primary endpoint was a randomized trial of zoledronic acid vs. placebo for patients with bone metastases [2]. For this trial the primary endpoint was the occurrence of a skeletal-related event. Skeletal-related events were defined as pathological bone fractures (vertebral or non-vertebral), spinal cord compression, surgery to bone, radiation therapy to bone (including the use of radioisotopes) or a change of antineoplastic therapy to treat bone pain. A greater proportion of patients who received placebo had skeletal-related events than those who received zoledronic acid at 4 mg (44.2% vs. 33.2%). On the basis of this finding, zoledronic acid was approved for use in patients with HRPC metastatic to bone. There was no general improvement in pain scores, analgesic use, quality of life scores or overall survival, although the design of the trial did not lend itself to an assessment of a response in these parameters.

ENDPOINTS IN TRIALS IN HORMONE-NAIVE METASTATIC OR RISING PSA ONLY DISEASE

The challenges with conducting studies in patients with hormone-naïve or earlier stages of prostate cancer relate to the long natural history of the disease, the older age of the patient population and the risk of death from competing causes. Despite these difficulties and the logistics required to complete trials in early prostate cancer with survival endpoints, overall survival determination has been critical for establishing the effectiveness of the current standard of therapies, including adjuvant hormone therapy after radiotherapy [43] and the benefits of radical prostatectomy [44]. Studies in earlier disease using survival endpoints can also be accomplished more readily by ensuring enrolment of high-risk patients through the use of risk models and nomograms in study eligibility criteria. Not only is it clinically appropriate to focus our attention on the high-risk patient, but doing so also allows for a smaller sample size to detect the same relative benefit.

Clearly, determining the effect on overall survival of an intervention early in the disease is important especially when subsequent therapy can still have enough impact to negate improvement in a time to progression endpoint (e.g. hormone therapy [45]) or when the intervention itself can have a potentially negative impact. This latter point is emphasized by results from the Early Prostate Cancer Trial Programme, in which patients with localized non-metastatic prostate cancer were randomized to receive bicalutamide 150 mg daily or placebo. In this study, there was a trend for worse overall survival for those patients with low-risk localized prostate cancer who received treatment with bicalutamide, but a reverse trend towards prolonged survival in men with high-risk localized disease treated with bicalutamide [46].

As we bring novel therapies into earlier stages of disease and try to build upon our current treatments of local therapy and hormone therapy, use of intermediate endpoints is required for activity screening purposes given that designing trials powered to detect clinically meaningful overall survival differences for every new agent or combination therapy is not realistically feasible or accomplished in reasonable timeframes. Although intermediate endpoints may not necessarily be established surrogates for overall survival, criteria such as PSA recurrence after local therapy have implications for patients as they often lead to further therapy such as hormones or salvage radiation and, thus, can be clinically meaningful endpoints for phase III trials. PSA recurrence as an endpoint can also be refined by incorporating the rate of rise as a factor, as rapid PSA doubling times have been associated with a higher risk of metastases and death [47].

With the widespread use of frequent PSA monitoring after definitive local therapy, the vast majority of identification of recurrence in patients is based on a rising PSA alone. Furthermore, these patients are often receiving castration therapy in the absence of clinically detectable metastases and, thus, an increasing proportion of patients are also now presenting with castration-resistant disease also based on a rising PSA alone. The natural history can be prolonged in both these groups of patients (i.e. non-castrate-resistant and castrate-resistant), however, subsets of patients have a poor prognosis especially those with a rapid PSA doubling time [35, 37]. For trials involving these patients, incorporating time to development of clinical metastases as an endpoint would be an appropriate, readily definable and clinically relevant endpoint.

SUMMARY

Designing clinical trials for patients with prostate cancer can be a challenge because of both patient and disease factors. For these reasons and with the move towards molecularly targeted therapeutics, the simple study paradigms of maximum tolerated dose in phase I trials, measurable disease activity in phase II trials and overall survival in phase III trials are not necessarily appropriate or easily applied. Instead, a multifaceted approach needs to be taken, with the inclusion of biochemical, measurable tumour and disease-related symptom assessments (Table 10.2). Study endpoints need to be carefully considered and defined according to the agent being tested and its understood mechanism of action, and be relevant to the needs and clinical considerations of the patient population being studied.

Table 10.2   Endpoints in clinical trials of prostate cancer

Phase of trial	Purpose	Endpoints
Phase I	Define dose	Toxicity/adverse events
		Pharmacokinetics
		Molecular correlates
Phase II	Define activity	PSA
		Measurable disease/RECIST
		Toxicity/adverse events
		Molecular correlates
		Validated symptom scores
		Progression (trial-specific definition)
Phase III	Define efficacy	Overall survival
		Progression (trial-specific definition)
		PSA
		Validated symptom scores
		Skeletal-related events
		Measurable disease/RECIST
		Toxicity/adverse events
		Molecular correlates

REFERENCES

1.   Tannock IF, Osoba D, Stockler MR *et al.* Chemotherapy with mitoxantrone plus prednisone or prednisone alone for symptomatic hormone-resistant prostate cancer: a Canadian randomized trial with palliative end points. *J Clin Oncol* 1996; 14:1756–1764.
2.   Saad F, Gleason DM, Murray R *et al.* A randomized, placebo-controlled trial of zoledronic acid in patients with hormone-refractory metastatic prostate carcinoma. *J Natl Cancer Inst* 2002; 94:1458–1468.
3.   Serafini AN, Houston SJ, Resche I *et al.* Palliation of pain associated with metastatic bone cancer using samarium-153 lexidronam: a double-blind placebo-controlled clinical trial. *J Clin Oncol* 1998; 16:1574–1581.
4.   Tannock IF, de Wit R, Berry WR *et al.* Docetaxel plus prednisone or mitoxantrone plus prednisone for advanced prostate cancer. *N Engl J Med* 2004; 351:1502–1512.
5.   Petrylak DP, Tangen CM, Hussain MH *et al.* Docetaxel and estramustine compared with mitoxantrone and prednisone for advanced refractory prostate cancer. *N Engl J Med* 2004; 351:1513–1520.
6.   Albertsen PC, Hanley JA, Gleason DF, Barry MJ. Competing risk analysis of men aged 55 to 74 years at diagnosis managed conservatively for clinically localized prostate cancer. *JAMA* 1998; 280:975–980.
7.   Murthy VH, Krumholz HM, Gross CP. Participation in cancer clinical trials: race-, sex-, and age-based disparities. *JAMA* 2004; 291:2720–2726.
8.   Scher HI, Morris MJ, Kelly WK, Schwartz LH, Heller G. Prostate cancer clinical trial end points: 'RECIST'ing a step backwards. *Clin Cancer Res* 2005; 11:5223–5232.
9.   Bubley GJ, Carducci M, Dahut W *et al.* Eligibility and response guidelines for phase II clinical trials in androgen-independent prostate cancer: recommendations from the Prostate-Specific Antigen Working Group. *J Clin Oncol* 1999; 17:3461–3467.
10.   Baselga J, Rischin D, Ranson M *et al.* Phase I safety, pharmacokinetic, and pharmacodynamic trial of ZD1839, a selective oral epidermal growth factor receptor tyrosine kinase inhibitor, in patients with five selected solid tumor types. *J Clin Oncol* 2002 ; 20:4292–4302.
11.   Gordon MS, Margolin K, Talpaz M *et al.* Phase I safety and pharmacokinetic study of recombinant human anti-vascular endothelial growth factor in patients with advanced cancer. *J Clin Oncol* 2001; 19:843–850.
12.   Lynch TJ, Bell DW, Sordella R *et al.* Activating mutations in the epidermal growth factor receptor underlying responsiveness of non-small-cell lung cancer to gefitinib. *N Engl J Med* 2004; 350:2129–2139.
13.   Slamon DJ, Leyland-Jones B, Shak S *et al.* Use of chemotherapy plus a monoclonal antibody against HER2 for metastatic breast cancer that overexpresses HER2. *N Engl J Med* 2001; 344:783–792.

14. Bubendorf L, Kolmer M, Kononen J *et al.* Hormone therapy failure in human prostate cancer: analysis by complementary DNA and tissue microarrays. *J Natl Cancer Inst* 1999; 91:1758–1764.
15. Ellis WJ, Pfitzenmaier J, Colli J, Arfman E, Lange PH, Vessella RL. Detection and isolation of prostate cancer cells from peripheral blood and bone marrow. *Urology* 2003; 61:277–281.
16. Moreno JG, Miller MC, Gross S, Allard WJ, Gomella LG, Terstappen LW. Circulating tumor cells predict survival in patients with metastatic prostate cancer. *Urology* 2005; 65:713–718.
17. Chi KN, Eisenhauer E, Fazli L *et al.* A phase I pharmacokinetic and pharmacodynamic study of OGX-011, a 2'-methoxyethyl antisense oligonucleotide to clusterin, in patients with localized prostate cancer. *J Natl Cancer Inst* 2005; 97:1287–1296.
18. Ayala G, Satoh T, Li R *et al.* Biological response determinants in HSV-tk + ganciclovir gene therapy for prostate cancer. *Mol Ther* 2006 ; 13:716–728.
19. Krupski TL, Smith MR, Lee WC *et al.* Natural history of bone complications in men with prostate carcinoma initiating androgen deprivation therapy. *Cancer* 2004; 101:541–549.
20. Brown JE, Cook RJ, Major P *et al.* Bone turnover markers as predictors of skeletal complications in prostate cancer, lung cancer, and other solid tumors. *J Natl Cancer Inst* 2005; 97:59–69.
21. Coleman RE, Major P, Lipton A *et al.* Predictive value of bone resorption and formation markers in cancer patients with bone metastases receiving the bisphosphonate zoledronic acid. *J Clin Oncol* 2005; 23:4925–4935.
22. Jung K, Lein M, Stephan C *et al.* Comparison of 10 serum bone turnover markers in prostate carcinoma patients with bone metastatic spread: diagnostic and prognostic implications. *Int J Cancer* 2004; 111:783–791.
23. Therasse P, Arbuck SG, Eisenhauer EA *et al.* New guidelines to evaluate the response to treatment in solid tumors. European Organization for Research and Treatment of Cancer, National Cancer Institute of the United States, National Cancer Institute of Canada. *J Natl Cancer Inst* 2000; 92:205–216.
24. Tombal B, Rezazadeh A, Therasse P, Van Cangh PJ, Vande Berg B, Lecouvet FE. Magnetic resonance imaging of the axial skeleton enables objective measurement of tumor response on prostate cancer bone metastases. *The Prostate* 2005; 65:178–187.
25. Kelly WK, Scher HI, Mazumdar M, Vlamis V, Schwartz M, Fossa SD. Prostate-specific antigen as a measure of disease outcome in metastatic hormone-refractory prostate cancer. *J Clin Oncol* 1993; 11:607–615.
26. Smith DC, Dunn RL, Strawderman MS, Pienta KJ. Change in serum prostate-specific antigen as a marker of response to cytotoxic therapy for hormone-refractory prostate cancer. *J Clin Oncol* 1998; 16:1835–1843.
27. Petrylak DP, Ankerst DP, Jiang CS *et al.* Evaluation of prostate-specific antigen declines for surrogacy in patients treated on SWOG 99-16. *J Natl Cancer Inst* 2006; 98:516–521.
28. Roessner M, de Wit R, Tannock IF *et al.* Prostate-specific antigen (PSA) response as a surrogate end-point for overall survival (OS): Analysis of the TAX 327 Study comparing docetaxel plus prednisone with mitoxantrone plus prednisone in advanced prostate cancer. *J Clin Oncol* 2005; 23:4554.
29. Berthold DR, Pond G, De Wit R, Eisenberger MA, Tannock IF. Association of pain and quality of life (QOL) response with PSA response and survival of patients (pts) with metastatic hormone refractory prostate cancer (mHRPC) treated with docetaxel or mitoxantrone in the TAX-327 study. *J Clin Oncol* 2006; 24:4516.
30. Beer TM, Eilers KM, Garzotto M, Egorin MJ, Lowe BA, Henner WD. Weekly high-dose calcitriol and docetaxel in metastatic androgen-independent prostate cancer. *J Clin Oncol* 2003; 21:123–128.
31. Beer TM, Ryan CW, Venner PM *et al.* Interim results from ASCENT: A double-blinded randomized study of DN-101 (high-dose calcitriol) plus docetaxel vs. placebo plus docetaxel in androgen-independent prostate cancer (AIPC). *J Clin Oncol* 2005; 23:4516.
32. Escudier B, Szczylik C, Eisen T *et al.* Randomized Phase III trial of the Raf kinase and VEGFR inhibitor sorafenib (BAY 43–9006) in patients with advanced renal cell carcinoma (RCC). *J Clin Oncol* 2005; 23:4510.
33. Ratain MJ, Eisen T, Stadler WM *et al.* Phase II placebo-controlled randomized discontinuation trial of sorafenib in patients with metastatic renal cell carcinoma. *J Clin Oncol* 2006; 24:2505–2512.
34. Smith PH, Bono A, Calais da Silva F *et al.* Some limitations of the radioisotope bone scan in patients with metastatic prostatic cancer. A subanalysis of EORTC trial 30853. The EORTC Urological Group. *Cancer* 1990; 66(5 Suppl):1009–1016.
35. Smith MR, Kabbinavar F, Saad F *et al.* Natural history of rising serum prostate-specific antigen in men with castrate nonmetastatic prostate cancer. *J Clin Oncol* 2005; 23:2918–2925.

36. Scher HI, Kelly WM, Zhang ZF *et al*. Post-therapy serum prostate-specific antigen level and survival in patients with androgen-independent prostate cancer. *J Natl Cancer Inst* 1999; 91:244–251.

37. Carducci MA, Padley RJ, Breul J *et al*. Effect of endothelin-A receptor blockade with atrasentan on tumor progression in men with hormone-refractory prostate cancer: a randomized, phase II, placebo-controlled trial. *J Clin Oncol* 2003; 21:679–689.

38. Small EJ, Schellhammer PF, Higano CS *et al*. Placebo-controlled phase III trial of immunologic therapy with sipuleucel-T (APC8015) in patients with metastatic, asymptomatic hormone refractory prostate cancer. *J Clin Oncol* 2006; 24:3089–3094.

39. Melzack R. The McGill Pain Questionnaire: major properties and scoring methods. *Pain* 1975; 1:277–299.

40. Aaronson NK, Ahmedzai S, Bergman B *et al*. The European Organization for Research and Treatment of Cancer QLQ-C30: a quality-of-life instrument for use in international clinical trials in oncology. *J Natl Cancer Inst* 1993; 85:365–376.

41. Osoba D, Tannock IF, Ernst DS, Neville AJ. Health-related quality of life in men with metastatic prostate cancer treated with prednisone alone or mitoxantrone and prednisone. *J Clin Oncol* 1999; 17:1654–1663.

42. Esper P, Mo F, Chodak G, Sinner M, Cella D, Pienta KJ. Measuring quality of life in men with prostate cancer using the functional assessment of cancer therapy-prostate instrument. *Urology* 1997; 50:920–928.

43. Bolla M, Gonzalez D, Warde P *et al*. Improved survival in patients with locally advanced prostate cancer treated with radiotherapy and goserelin. *N Engl J Med* 1997; 337:295–300.

44. Bill-Axelson A, Holmberg L, Ruutu M *et al*. Radical prostatectomy versus watchful waiting in early prostate cancer. *N Engl J Med* 2005; 352:1977–1984.

45. Kirk D. Timing and choice of androgen ablation. *Prostate Cancer Prostatic Dis* 2004; 7:217–222.

46. McLeod DG, Iversen P, See WA, Morris T, Armstrong J, Wirth MP. Bicalutamide 150 mg plus standard care vs standard care alone for early prostate cancer. *BJU Int* 2006; 97:247–254.

47. Zhou P, Chen MH, McLeod D, Carroll PR, Moul JW, D'Amico AV. Predictors of prostate cancer-specific mortality after radical prostatectomy or radiation therapy. *J Clin Oncol* 2005; 23:6992–6998.

11

Hormonal therapy

David Gillatt

The androgen dependence of prostatic adenocarcinoma was first established more than 60 years ago by Huggins and Hodges [1]. The authors described both the effect of castration and oestrogens on advanced carcinoma of the prostate and on serum levels of acid phosphatase. Oral oestrogens and surgical castration subsequently became the standard primary treatments for advanced prostate cancer. It later became apparent that oestrogens may be associated with an increase in cardiovascular morbidity and mortality [2, 3]. As a result bilateral orchidectomy became the 'gold standard' against which other therapies were judged. Surgical castration results in a rapid reduction in circulating testosterone to $< 2\,nmol/l$ within 12 h. This defines the necessary reduction in circulating androgens to achieve therapeutic castration. Thus, achieving castrate levels of testosterone became the prime and only therapeutic strategy for advanced prostate cancer for several decades (Figure 11.1).

These early insights into the hormonal control of prostate cells, both benign and malignant, led to further developments in the understanding of the mechanisms by which endogenous androgens stimulate cellular metabolism. Circulating androgens, either testosterone or adrenal androgens, are converted to dihydrotestosterone (DHT) in the cytoplasm by the enzyme 5-alpha-reductase. DHT binds to the androgen receptor which, under the influence of a number of cytoplasmic and nuclear factors, results in protein production and cell proliferation. Prostatic growth, and therefore prostate cancer growth, is mediated by this process and can be slowed or reversed by blocking the pathway at one of several points. As a result, a number of strategies for the hormonal control of prostate cancer have been developed.

The aim of this chapter is to examine contemporary approaches to the hormonal manipulation of prostate cancer. Developments of primary hormonal therapies and the evidence for antiandrogen monotherapy, luteinizing hormone-releasing hormone agonists (LHRHa) and maximal androgen blockade (MAB) will be addressed. The chapter will examine the timing of therapy and its value used as an adjunct to local 'curative' treatments. The length of therapy and the evidence for continual versus intermittent treatment will be examined. When hormonal therapy appears to be failing, there may still be androgen dependence and therefore an argument for second- and third-line hormonal manoeuvres.

THE TIMING OF HORMONAL THERAPY

The perceived wisdom until a decade or so ago was that the timing of hormonal intervention was irrelevant in influencing survival. This led to hormonal manoeuvres often being delayed until the disease was either metastatic and/or symptomatic. Evidence emerged during the last decade in favour of the earlier use of hormonal therapy. This evidence was twofold; the Medical Research Council (MRC) study of immediate versus delayed hormonal therapy for

David Gillatt, ChM FRCS, Consultant Urologist, The Cotswold Centre, Southmead, Bristol, UK

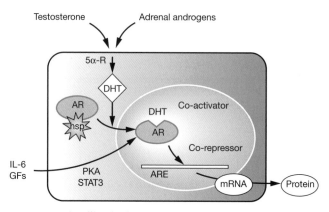

Figure 11.1 Androgen receptor signalling in the prostate. 5α-R, 5α-reductase; DHT, dihydrotestosterone; AR, androgen receptor; hsp, heat shock protein; IL-6, interleukin 6; GFs, growth factors; PKA, protein kinase A; STAT 3, signal transducers and activators of transcription 3; ARE, androgen response element.

advanced prostate cancer and a group of studies investigating the use of hormones as an adjunct to local radiation or surgery [4].

The MRC (PRO3) study randomized 934 men with either locally advanced (M0) or metastatic (M1) prostate cancer to either surgical castration or LHRHa at diagnosis, or when clinical progression occurred. Its findings are set out in Tables 11.1–11.3. There was evidence in the M0 group of a small overall survival in favour of the immediate treatment arm. What was more striking was the significant difference in tumour-associated morbidity (Table 11.3) between the groups with those men having delay in therapy being at higher risk of pathological fracture, spinal cord compression, ureteric obstruction and the development of extraskeletal metastases. These findings give backing to instituting hormonal therapy prior to symptomatic or metastatic progression.

There have been criticisms of this series because of perceived flaws in the definition and documentation of disease progression. This may have resulted in bias in the survival data; however, the marked difference in tumour morbidity in favour of early therapy is still striking.

Table 11.1 MRC study of immediate versus delayed hormone therapy: number of patients by stage and treatment arm [4]

	Immediate	*Deferred*	*Total*
M0	256	244	500
MX	83	90	173
M1	130	131	261
Total	469	465	934

Table 11.2 MRC study of immediate versus delayed hormone therapy: summary findings [4]

The MRC trial favours *immediate* hormonal therapy
Of the 469 patients in the immediate treatment group, significantly fewer patients:

- died from prostate cancer ($2P < 0.001$)
- died of any cause ($2P = 0.02$)

Significantly fewer M0 patients in the immediate treatment group developed metastases or died from prostate cancer ($2P < 0.001$)
5% of treatment-deferred patients ($n = 465$) died from prostate cancer prior to starting therapy

Table 11.3 MRC study of immediate versus delayed hormone therapy: number of major prostate cancer-related complications in each treatment arm [4]

	Immediate	Deferred
Pathological fractures	11	21
Cord compression[1]	9	23
Ureteric obstruction[1]	33	55
Extraskeletal metastases[1]	37	55

[1]$2P<0.05$, immediate vs. deferred treatment

Two European trials appear to confirm the MRC findings. Studer *et al.* [5] randomized 197 men with prostate cancer unsuitable for local therapy to immediate orchidectomy or to be deferred until symptomatic progression. The study showed longer time to progression (2.8 years increase) and better disease-specific survival in the immediate group with no impact on overall survival. The EORTC 30846 study randomized 234 N+ patients to immediate or deferred therapy [6]. There was a 23% trend towards improved survival in the immediate therapy group, although this did not reach significance.

A variety of studies [7–11] have investigated the role of adjuvant hormonal therapy in men with T1–4–N0/1–M0 prostate cancer treated with radical radiation or prostatectomy. In many studies the addition of a period of hormonal therapy improved progression-free, cancer-specific and, in some overall, survival. Of most significance are studies by Bolla *et al.* [7], Pilepich *et al.* [8, 9] and Messing *et al.* [11]. All these studies were randomized and used prolonged hormonal therapy. Each one confirms a survival advantage in favour of adjuvant hormonal therapy at up to 10 years.

In addition a randomized trial of the antiandrogen bicalutamide 150 mg versus placebo as adjunct to standard therapy (the Early Prostate Cancer, EPC, trial) showed a progression-free survival advantage in locally advanced cancers treated with radiation, surgery or watchful waiting in favour of the hormonally treated group [12, 13]. This in later analyses translated into an overall survival advantage in the radiation group [14].

These studies point to a hormonal effect which is most marked in high-risk non-metastatic but locally advanced prostate cancers. Hormonal therapy used earlier in the course of the disease will delay progression and may indeed prolong survival. This comes with a cost both financial and in terms of morbidity. The side-effects of hormonal therapy have been discussed already; however, these may in a small group of patients translate into a negative effect on mortality. It is well recognized that manipulating a man's hormones may impact upon cardiovascular risk with this being most marked with higher dose oestrogens. The EPC trial also found a small, non-statistically significant, increase in mortality in those low-risk cancers in the bicalutamide arm. This combined with no clear clinical advantage suggests that the use of hormonal manipulation in early or low-risk prostate cancer offers no benefit and indeed a small risk of harm. Identifying those at high risk of progression should allow us to target those who have most to gain from earlier hormonal therapy.

Many of the published studies showing benefit to immediate hormonal therapy have stratified their patient groups. Stratification suggests that high-risk groups benefit most from early intervention. High risk is usually based on stage (T3, pT3, LN+) or Gleason score. One strategy would be to offer all high-risk patients long-term LHRHa or antiandrogen monotherapy. A different approach in some groups would be to watch the serum PSA and treat according to its rate of rise. Certainly, in patients undergoing local 'curative' therapy, the risk of failure, metastatic progression or prostate cancer-specific death (PCSD) is closely related to prostate-specific antigen doubling time (PSADT).

In conclusion, any hormonal therapeutic strategy should include an assessment of optimum timing for the intervention. In patients with advanced metastatic disease, earlier intervention may affect survival but will certainly reduce the risk of unpleasant tumour-related morbidity. In non-metastatic disease there is evidence that early hormonal therapy will improve survival in high-risk groups. Unless the hormones are to be used in an adjuvant setting, it may be appropriate to closely monitor PSA levels and intervene if the individual has a rapid PSADT.

THE CHOICE OF PRIMARY HORMONAL THERAPY

LHRH AGONISTS

LHRH agonists (LHRHa) have become the standard method of achieving hormonal control by producing medical castration. Endogenous LHRH is produced by the neuroendocrine cells of the hypothalamus in a pulsatile fashion. Its structure was first described in 1971 by Schally *et al.* [15]. Various potent synthetic analogues are commercially available, including goserelin, leuprolide and triptorelin. LHRH normally causes the anterior pituitary to release luteinizing hormone (LH), which in turn acts upon the Leydig cells of the testes to produce testosterone. Administration of a potent agonist will cause an initial rise in testosterone [16]. Chronic administration results in pituitary depletion of LH and down-regulation of LHRH receptors within the pituitary. This insensitivity of the pituitary to LHRH results in a reduction in LH, and therefore testosterone, to castrate levels.

The initial testosterone surge following the first exposure to LHRHa may theoretically result in a tumour flare and could precipitate potentially harmful events such as spinal cord compression [17]. Any strategy utilizing LHRHa must allow for the potential of flare, particularly in those with spinal metastases or impending ureteric obstruction. This flare can be dampened by preloading the patient with either a steroidal (cyproterone acetate, CPA) or non-steroidal (bicalutamide) antiandrogen commenced prior to the first LHRHa injection and continuing to cover the period of flare (maximal at 8–14 days).

LHRHa were initially delivered by nasal spray or daily subcutaneous injection. Depot injections are now the standard, with 4- or 12-weekly applications available. Longer-acting depots are available lasting for up to 1 year but have, as yet, made little impact.

LHRHa are effective agents for producing medical castration. Initial studies confirmed their equivalence to surgical castration in terms of both disease control and testosterone suppression [18]. These agents are the most frequently used method of obtaining hormonal control in prostate cancer [19].

The morbidity of LHRHa is almost exclusively that of castration and is often underestimated (Figure 11.2). Castration will reduce libido and therefore affect sexual function. Weight gain can occur and may be difficult to reverse. Hot flushes affect up to 70% of men and, whilst usually tolerable, may be disabling in a minority. There is a significant loss of bone mineral density which over a year or more may be sufficient to increase the risk of pathological fracture (Figure 11.3).

When using LHRHa, strategies should be developed to minimize morbidity.

1   Hot flushes: explain to the patient that they are common and usually manageable. Consider a low dose of CPA (50 mg b.d.) or megestrol acetate.
2   Sexual function: counsel the patient and his partner. Phosphodiesterase-5 (PDE-5) inhibitors may help erections to return and should be considered, although loss of libido will mean that most men will not be motivated to pursue therapy.
3   Bone loss: baseline assessment using dual energy X-ray absorptiometry (DEXA) scanning is advocated by some, monitoring bone mineral density loss with yearly scans. Bisphosphonates may protect some from an increased fracture risk.

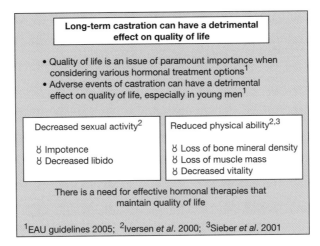

Figure 11.2   Physiological changes and quality of life following castration.

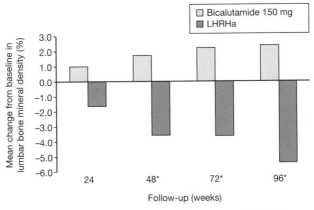

*Statistically significant difference between the two groups $P<0.0001$

Figure 11.3   Comparison of bicalutamide and luteinizing hormone-releasing hormone analogue (LHRHa) in their effects on bone mineral density with time [20].

In conclusion, whilst LHRHa remain the main hormonal therapy for all stages of prostate cancer, they carry an appreciable morbidity.

ANTIANDROGEN MONOTHERAPY

Antiandrogens (AAs) are compounds that block the effect of androgens. Two forms of AAs are available. Steroidal antiandrogens (CPA and megestrol acetate) block both androgen receptors of the prostate cells and central androgen receptors. Although CPA was the first AA and is widely used as first-line therapy in Europe, it has fallen from favour because of its high incidence of cardiovascular and respiratory side-effects. Non-steroidal AAs include flutamide, nilutamide and bicalutamide, with the last now standard in many countries.

In general, the therapeutic response of AAs as monotherapy is inferior to that of LHRHa. However, studies of bicalutamide 150 mg versus LHRHa have shown equivalence in survival terms for non-metastatic prostate cancer (Figure 11.4) [21]. For M1 disease there is a survival disadvantage for AA monotherapy.

The concerns about AA monotherapy, if therapeutically equivalent, are twofold. The long-term use of AAs may induce androgen receptor mutations and possible progression of hor-monally treated cancer. In addition, AAs have a different set of complications to LHRHa. In particular, diarrhoea and breast complications may result in treatment withdrawal. Between 60% and 75% of treated patients will suffer from breast enlargement or breast pain.

Bicalutamide 150 mg monotherapy has been extensively studied, and the EPC trials exam-ined its value either as an adjunct to standard therapy or as an alternative to watchful wait-ing. There appear to be significant advantages in terms of progression-free survival in locally advanced groups for bicalutamide 150 mg over placebo in patients treated primarily with radiation and as an alternative to watchful waiting. An overall survival advantage has been shown for men treated in the adjuvant setting after radiotherapy. Progression-free survival improved in the surgically treated patients. In the same study, patients in the watchful wait-ing arm with low-risk cancers in the bicalutamide arm showed a trend towards worse sur-vival than those on placebo. It appears, therefore, that in non-metastatic high-risk prostate cancer the therapeutic effect of bicalutamide 150 mg is beneficial and will improve disease control. The trend towards worsening survival in low-risk cancers precludes its use at earlier stages of disease progression.

MAXIMAL ANDROGEN BLOCKADE (COMBINED ANDROGEN BLOCKADE)

Maximal (combined) androgen blockade (MAB) combines removal of testicular androgens with blockade at cellular level of adrenal androgens (Figure 11.5). The rationale for MAB (Table 11.4) depends upon the belief that the small amounts of circulating androgens pro-duced by the adrenals (androstenedione and dihydroepiandrosterone) may play a role in prostate cancer growth at cellular level disproportionate to their circulating levels.

There are several theories to explain why MAB may increase the longevity of response of prostate cancers to hormonal therapy (see above). The addition of an antiandrogen will block the effect of adrenal androgens. Although adrenal androgens represent a small percentage of available circulating androgens, their effect on the androgen receptor (AR) may be dispro-

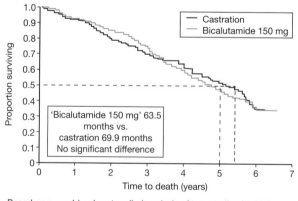

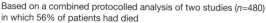

Figure 11.4   Comparison of survival with castration and bicalutamide in non-metastatic prostate cancer [21].

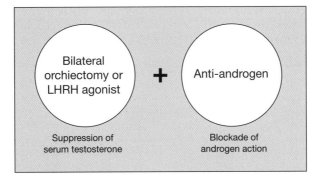

Figure 11.5   Combined androgen blockade describes suppression of serum testosterone levels in combination with androgen receptor blockade.

Table 11.4   Rationale for MAB

1   Inhibition of adrenal androgens
2   Tissue androgen level remains elevated despite castration levels of androgen in circulation
3   Prevention of androgen receptor (AR) amplification
4   Inhibition of ligand binding to AR
5   Direct effect on AR function inhibiting dissociation of heat shock protein
6   Inhibition of ligand-independent activation of AR
7   Alteration of coactivator and corepressor

portionate. Studies have shown that in hormone-refractory prostate cancer tissue androgen levels are similar to benign prostate tissue (Figure 11.6), thus presenting androgens to the AR in sufficient quantities to maintain cellular activity [22]. Antiandrogens may remove some of this additional androgen. It is probable that there is amplification both in number and sensitivity of AR following testosterone withdrawal; MAB may prevent amplification. There are several other points at which an antiandrogen may modify cellular response to androgens including affecting ligand binding, nuclear coactivator and corepressor activity and even ligand-independent AR activation.

MAB may be used in three ways: short term, long term and delayed or second line.

An antiandrogen may be added to a LHRHa to prevent flare response. This may last for 3–4 weeks and then the antiandrogen is discontinued whilst the LHRHa is continued.

MAB as a long-term strategy for improving hormonal control was first advocated by Labrie *et al.* [23]. He showed that a LHRHa plus flutamide increased the rate and duration of response. However, this series was non-randomized and his controls were historical. The first large randomized controlled trial was published by Crawford [24] when a survival advantage was reported for leuprolide plus flutamide compared with leuprolide alone (35.6 vs. 28.3 months) and this reached significance. It appeared that men with low-volume metastatic disease and good performance status fared better. Further studies seemed to validate Crawford's initial report but were later to be challenged by trials which failed to demonstrate any survival advantage for MAB.

In order to address the issue of whether MAB confers any clinical advantage, several meta-analyses have been published. The Prostate Cancer Trialists Collaborative Group (PCTCG) included data from 22 randomized controlled trials and more than 5000 patients [25]. Trends in favour of MAB were identified with a 5-year survival advantage of 3.4%; however, this did not reach statistical significance. A follow-up included five more studies

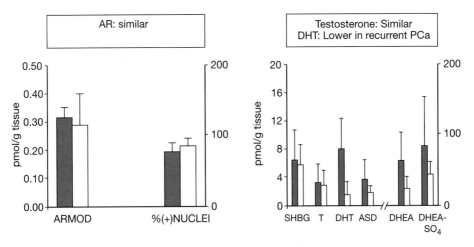

Closed bars: BPH (no treatment); Open bars: Recurrent PCa (after Hx)

Figure 11.6 Prostatic androgen receptor expression and tissue concentrations of androgen and SHBG levels in benign prostatic hyperplasia (BPH, closed bars) and recurrent hormone-refactory prostate cancer (PCa, open bars). ARMOD, androgen receptor mean optical density; %(+) nuclei, percentage nuclear staining; SHBG, sex-hormone-binding globulin; DHT, dihydrotestosterone; ASD, androstenedione; DHEAD, dehydroepiandrosterone; DHEAD-SO$_4$, dehydropiandrosterone sulphate [22]

with a total of 8275 patients [26]. Again, a non-significant survival advantage of 1.8% was demonstrated. Other studies appear to confirm only a small survival advantage for MAB over LHRHa monotherapy and this may well be outweighed by the added costs and withdrawals due to treatment toxicity.

Other authors, however, have interpreted the historical data on MAB in a different way. Klotz, in a review of the PCTCG meta-analyses, differentially explored the influence of AA type on response [27]. If the series are analysed according to whether the AA was steroidal (CPA) or non-steroidal (flutamide, nilutamide in these series), then the survival advantages for MAB become more significant. MAB with non-steroidal AA results in an overall 8% improvement in survival. The use of CPA for MAB confers a survival disadvantage of 13% over LHRHa monotherapy.

Klotz took this analysis further when comparing MAB with two different non-steroidal AAs, flutamide and bicalutamide. An indirect comparison of PCTCG and the Schellhammer trial produced a survival advantage for MAB with bicalutamide of 20% compared with LHRHa monotherapy.

In conclusion, MAB does show a small survival advantage for men with prostate cancer over LHRHa monotherapy. This is more marked when a non-steroidal AA is part of the regime.

INTERMITTENT HORMONAL THERAPY (IHT)

Hormonal therapy has traditionally been ongoing and lifelong. This was inevitable when surgical castration was the mainstay of such therapy. The advent of LHRHa and antiandrogens means there is scope for patients to have periods off therapy. There are theoretical and clinical reasons why intermittent therapy may be preferable to continuous treatment. The possibility that the pulsatile application of hormonal therapy may delay the development of hormonally independent prostate cancer growth has been suggested. This may be by cyclical reinduction of apoptotic potential by repeatedly withdrawing and reintroducing an LHRHa.

In addition, periods off therapy may be advantageous for patients by reducing treatment-associated morbidity. Several studies have looked at the use of IHT both as primary therapy for advanced disease and in patients with PSA relapse after radical therapy.

The Chiba study group [28] showed an improvement in quality of life measures in those treated by IHT.

The Canadian Prospective Trial of intermittent androgen suppression followed 109 men with failure after local radiation for 132 weeks [29]. In this series hormones were discontinued when PSA fell below 4 ng/l and recommenced after three consecutive rises above 4 ng/l. The median on-treatment period was 40 weeks with a non-treatment period of 46 weeks. The quality of life was markedly improved when off treatment.

The trials available exploring IHT show that patients may safely remain off therapy for between 50% and 70% of the time [29]. However, there are no good randomized controlled trials as yet mature to confirm an advantage or disadvantage in terms of survival for IHT over continuous therapy.

THE ROLE OF HORMONAL THERAPIES AS SECOND LINE AND BEYOND

If biochemical or other evidence of disease progression occurs in a patient being treated primarily with hormonal therapy the first question to be asked is whether there is still androgen dependence or is the prostate cancer now refractory to androgen withdrawal. There are several mechanisms by which further disease control can be achieved by manipulating the androgen control of the prostate cancer cell. These can be divided into stepping-up, stepping-down and alternatives.

STEP-UP THERAPY

If monotherapy is the primary modality then in a proportion of patients with disease progression stepping up from LHRHa to MAB or antiandrogen monotherapy to LHRHa or MAB will result in PSA response in up to 50%.

If primary antiandrogen monotherapy with bicalutamide 150 mg is used and consecutive PSA rises indicate disease progression, it is reasonable to add in a LHRHa in order to achieve MAB. There are no published series to inform as to the chance of response, its duration or any increase in survival.

If LHRHa was the prime therapy then second-line MAB may be achieved by adding an antiandrogen when the PSA rises. Bicalutamide, flutamide and CPA have all been utilized in this context. Response rates (a fall in PSA > 50%) have been reported in 20–50% with a mean duration of 3–6 months One trial [30] reported higher response rates with a mean duration of 14.5 months (Figure 11.7).

It is therefore reasonable practice in a patient treated with monotherapy to step up to MAB if there are three consecutive rises in PSA or other signs of progression [36].

STEP-DOWN THERAPY

In patients treated with either primary or secondary MAB progression, a rising PSA may occur and there may still be scope for hormonal manipulation. The use of an AA may result in AR mutations and these AR changes may allow the AA to become an agonist and stimulate prostate cell metabolism. Antiandrogen withdrawal may therefore theoretically produce a tumour response with a fall in PSA. PSA response rates of 15–50% have been reported for AA withdrawal, although there is no evidence that this translates into an improvement in survival [31–35]. Table 11.5 demonstrates that median survival is similar in patients with and without an antiandrogen withdrawal response [35].

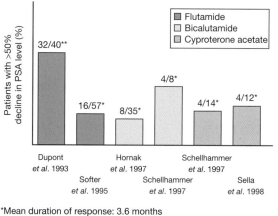

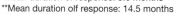

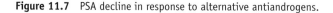

Figure 11.7   PSA decline in response to alternative antiandrogens.

Table 11.5   Relationship between prostate-specific antigen (PSA) response to antiandrogen withdrawal and survival [35]

A PSA response (50% reduction) to antiandrogen withdrawal does not translate into prolonged survival:
Median survival after PSA response to withdrawal = 13 months
Median survival in the absence of a PSA response = 12 months
$n = 82$

In men treated with MAB with evidence of disease progression the antiandrogen should be withdrawn before other interventions are considered.

OTHER OR ALTERNATIVE HORMONAL THERAPIES

When MAB has been fully explored and the antiandrogen withdrawn the scope for further hormonal manipulations may be limited. Antiandrogen switching may be considered. Miyake *et al.* reported 55 men on MAB with bicalutamide who were switched to flutamide at progression [36]. Forty-five per cent showed a decrease in PSA, with 22% classed as responders for a median period of 6 months.

Oestrogens have been employed following failure of primary therapy. The response to oestrogens is presumed to be in part mediated by inhibition of the feedback action of testosterone on pituitary luteinizing hormone production. They may also have a direct effect on the testes and a cytotoxic effect on prostate cancer cells. Oestrogens also increase circulating sex hormone-binding globulin thus reducing unbound testosterone. In androgen-independent prostate cancer, objective response rates of 5–19% have been reported for estramustine phosphate. Four trials of oestrogen second-line therapy reviewed by Oh [37] reported response rates of 20–65%.

Oh [37] (Figure 11.8) reviewed the reported series of second-line hormonal therapy. High-dose (150–200 mg) bicalutamide in three trials produced responses in approximately 20%. Corticosteroids produced similar response rates. The anti-fungal ketoconazole produced higher response rates. A 50% fall in PSA was reported in as many of 55% of cases; however, objective response was seen in only 2–20% (Table 11.6). PC SPES has also been shown in small series to produce response rates of up to 80%.

Table 11.6 Antiandrogen inhibition: ketoconazole [38, 39]

Antiandrogen withdrawal plus ketoconazole [38]
      55% of patients had >50% prostate-specific antigen (PSA) decrease
      Median response was 8.5 months
In patients undergoing flutamide withdrawal [39]
      Addition of ketoconazole raised PSA response from 11% to 27% (P = 0.0002)
      Objective response rate raised from 2% to 20% (P = 0.02)
      Deferred ketoconazole after antiandrogen withdrawal led to PSA and objective responses
      f 32% and 7% respectively

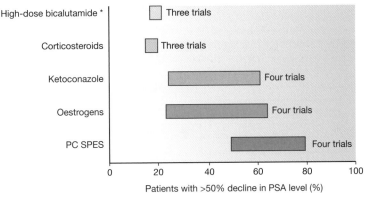

*150–200 mg/day

Figure 11.8 Response to alternative second-line hormone manipulations.

The problem with all these second-line therapies is a lack of data showing objective response. In almost all, series response is defined as a fall in PSA usually of more than 50% from baseline. In addition there are no randomized controlled trials to inform as to the proven value of any of these manoeuvres.

REFERENCES

1. Huggins C, Steven RE, Hodges CV. Studies on prostatic cancer. *Arch Surg* 1941; 43:209–23.
2. Blanchard EB, Young LD, Haynes MR, Scott RW Long term instructional control of heart rate without exteroceptive feedback. *J Gen Psychol* 1975; 92:291–2.
3. Glashan RW, Robinson MR. Cardiovascular complications in the treatment of prostatic carcinoma. *Br J Urol* 1981; 53:624–7.
4. MRC. Immediate versus deferred treatment for advanced prostatic cancer: initial results of the Medical Research Council Trial. The Medical Research Council Prostate Cancer Working Party Investigators Group. *Br J Urol* 1997; 79:235–46.
5. Studer UE, Hauri D, Hanselmann S et al. Immediate versus deferred hormonal treatment for patients with prostate cancer who are not suitable for curative local treatment: results of the randomized trial SAKK 08/88. *J Clin Oncol* 2004; 22:4109–18.
6. Schröder FH, Kurth KH, Fosså SD et al.; Members of the European Organisation for the Research and Treatment of Cancer Genito-urinary Group. Early versus delayed endocrine treatment of pN1–3 M0 prostate cancer without local treatment of the primary tumor: results of European Organisation for the Research and Treatment of Cancer 30846 – a phase III study. *J Urol* 2004; 172:923–7.
7. Bolla M. Adjuvant hormonal treatment with radiotherapy for locally advanced prostate cancer. *Eur Urol* 1998; 35(Suppl. S1):23–6.

8. Pilepich MV, Winter K, John MJ *et al.* Phase III radiation therapy oncology group (RTOG) trial 86-10 of androgen deprivation adjuvant to definitive radiotherapy in locally advanced carcinoma of the prostate. *Int J Radiat Oncol Biol Phys* 2001; 50:1243–52.
9. Pilepich MV, Winter K, Lawton CA *et al.* Androgen suppression adjuvant to definitive radiotherapy in prostate carcinoma – long-term results of phase III RTOG 85-31. *Int J Radiat Oncol Biol Phys* 2005; 61:1285–90.
10. Seay TM, Blute ML, Zincke H. Long-term outcome in patients with pTxN+ adenocarcinoma of prostate treated with radical prostatectomy and early androgen ablation. *J Urol* 1998; 159, 357–64.
11. Messing EM, Manola J, Sarosdy M *et al.* Immediate hormonal therapy compared with observation after radical prostatectomy and pelvic lymphadenectomy in men with node-positive prostate cancer. *N Engl J Med* 1999; 341:1781–8.
12. See WA, Wirth MP, McLeod DG *et al.* Bicalutamide as immediate therapy either alone or as adjuvant to standard care of patients with localized or locally advanced prostate cancer: first analysis of the early prostate cancer program. *J Urol* 2002; 168:429–35.
13. Freedland SJ, Humphreys EB, Mangold LA *et al.* Risk of prostate cancer-specific mortality following biochemical recurrence after radical prostatectomy. *JAMA* 2005; 294:433–9.
14. McLeod DG, Iversen P, See WA *et al.* Bicalutamide 150 mg plus standard care vs standard care alone for early prostate cancer. *BJU Int* 2006; 97:247–54.
15. Schally AV, Arimura A, Kastin AJ *et al.* Gonadotropin-releasing hormone: one polypeptide regulates secretion of luteinizing and follicle-stimulating hormones. *Science* 1971; 173:1036–8.
16. Siddall JK, Hetherington JW, Cooper EH, *et al.* Biochemical monitoring of carcinoma of prostate treated with an LH-RH analogue (Zoladex). *Br J Urol* 1986; 58:676–82.
17. Peeling WB, Griffiths GJ, Jones DR *et al.* The United Kingdom experience: clinical trials for carcinoma of the prostate monitored by ultrasound. *Prog Clin Biol Res* 1987; 237:161–76.
18. Kaisary AV, Tyrrell CJ, Peeling WB, Griffiths K. Comparison of LHRH analogue (Zoladex) with orchiectomy in patients with metastatic prostatic carcinoma. *Br J Urol* 1991; 67:502–8.
19. Aus G, Abbou CC, Bolla M *et al.* EAU guidelines on prostate cancer. *Eur Urol* 2005; 48:546–51.
20. Sieber PR, Keiller DL, Kahnoski RJ, Gallo J, McFadden S. Bicalutamide 150 mg maintains bone mineral density during monotherapy for localized or locally advanced prostate cancer. *J Urol* 2004; 171:2272–6, quiz 2435.
21. Iversen P, Tyrrell CJ, Kaisary AV *et al.* Bicalutamide monotherapy compared with castration in patients with nonmetastatic locally advanced prostate cancer: 6.3 years of followup. *J Urol* 2000; 164:1579–82.
22. Mohler JL, Gregory CW, Ford, OH, III, *et al.* The androgen axis in recurrent prostate cancer. *Clin Cancer Res,* 2004; 10:440–8.
23. Labrie F, Belanger A, Kelly PA, *et al.* Antifertility effects of luteinizing hormone-releasing hormone (LHRH) agonists. *Prog Clin Biol Res* 1981; 74:273–91.
24. Crawford ED Combined androgen blockade. *Eur Urol* 1996; 29(Suppl. 2):54–61.
25. Moul JW, Chodak G. Combination hormonal therapy: a reassessment within advanced prostate cancer. *Prostate Cancer Prostatic Dis* 2004; 7(Suppl. 1):S2–7.
26. Lukka H, Waldron T, Klotz L, Winquist E, Trachtenberg J. Maximal androgen blockade for the treatment of metastatic prostate cancer – a systematic review. *Curr Oncol* 2006;13:81–93.
27. Klotz L. Combined androgen blockade: an update. *Urol Clin North Am* 2006; 33:161–6, v–vi.
28. Sato N, Akakura K, Isaka S *et al.*; Chiba Prostate Study Group. Intermittent androgen suppression for locally advanced and metastatic prostate cancer: preliminary report of a prospective multicenter study. *Urology* 2004; 64:341–5.
29. Bruchovsky N, Klotz L, Crook J *et al.* Final results of the Canadian prospective phase II trial of intermittent androgen suppression for men in biochemical recurrence after radiotherapy for locally advanced prostate cancer: clinical parameters. *Cancer* 2006; 107:389–95.
30. Dupont A, Gomez JL, Cusan L, Koutsilieris M, Labrie F. Response to flutamide withdrawal in advanced prostate cancer in progression under combination therapy. *J Urol* 1993; 150:908–13.
31. Scher HI, Kelly WK. Flutamide withdrawal syndrome: its impact on clinical trials in hormone-refractory prostate cancer. *J Clin Oncol* 1993; 11:1566–72.
32. Hornak M, Bardos A, Goncalves F. [The antiandrogen withdrawal syndrome: decrease in prostate specific antigen serum levels after withdrawal of antiandrogens]. *Rozhl Chir* 1997; 76:435–7.
33. Schellhammer PF, Venner P, Haas GP *et al.* Prostate specific antigen decreases after withdrawal of antiandrogen therapy with bicalutamide or flutamide in patients receiving combined androgen blockade. *J Urol* 1997; 157:1731–5.

34. Sella A, Flex D, Sulkes A, Baniel J. Antiandrogen withdrawal syndrome with cyproterone acetate. *Urology* 1998; 52:1091–3.
35. Small EJ, Srinivas S. The antiandrogen withdrawal syndrome. Experience in a large cohort of unselected patients with advanced prostate cancer. *Cancer* 1995; 76:1428–34.
36. Miyake H, Hara I, Eto H. Clinical outcome of maximum androgen blockade using flutamide as second-line hormonal therapy for hormone-refractory prostate cancer. *BJU Int* 2005; 96:791–5.
37. Oh WK. Secondary hormonal therapies in the treatment of prostate cancer. *Urology* 2002; 60:87–92; discussion 93.
38. Small EJ, Baron AD, Fippin L, Apodaca D. Ketoconazole retains activity in advanced prostate cancer patients with progression despite flutamide withdrawal. *J Urol* 1997; 157:1204–7.
39. Small EJ, Halabi S, Dawson NA *et al.* Antiandrogen withdrawal alone or in combination with ketoconazole in androgen-independent prostate cancer patients: a phase III trial (CALGB 9583). *J Clin Oncol* 2004; 22:1025–33.

12

Chemotherapeutic strategies for treatment of advanced disease

Andrew J. Armstrong, Michael A. Carducci

INTRODUCTION

Hormone-refractory prostate cancer (HRPC) remains an incurable disease. However, therapeutic options have improved over the last several years, with the use of docetaxel-based chemotherapy, resulting in significant palliation of symptoms, objective and prostate-specific antigen (PSA)-based responses, improvements in pain and overall survival benefits [1–2]. A vast array of novel agents are currently in clinical trials using this docetaxel platform, as well as other novel combinations, with the goal of turning metastatic HRPC into a chronic symptom-free disease rather than an inevitably progressive one. New approaches to prognostic markers and resistance to hormonal and chemotherapeutic approaches have led to improved clinical stratification and identification of therapeutic targets. As chemotherapeutic options in earlier stage disease remain purely experimental at present, this chapter will focus on the clinical approach to treating men with metastatic HRPC, the current state of knowledge about the pathophysiology of hormone-refractory growth, and therapeutic strategies in the first-line setting and beyond.

DEFINITION OF HORMONE-REFRACTORY DISEASE

The most widely accepted criterion for the hormone-refractory state has been the demonstration of progressive, measurable or evaluable disease in the face of castrate levels of serum testosterone ($< 50\,ng/dl$) [3]. Biochemical progression after antiandrogen (bicalutamide, flutamide, nilutamide) withdrawal, as measured consecutively over a 4- to 6-week period, has been proposed for eligibility into clinical trials for HRPC. Patients are usually continued on gonadotrophin-releasing hormone agonists (GnRHa) during this time if tolerable. There is at this time no universally accepted definition of progression of hormone-refractory disease, however, and patients may have no measurable or evaluable disease with PSA-only progression and be termed hormone refractory or castration resistant [4]. These PSA-only hormone-refractory patients represent a heterogeneous group, and time to metastatic progression and death is highly variable, with a median of 1.5–3.5 years depending on PSA and PSA kinetic characteristics [5]. Survival in this common subgroup in the clinic is generally better than in patients with metastatic hormone-refractory disease but, as of 2006, chemotherapy remains unstudied in non-metastatic HRPC. In the TAX327 trial of docetaxel and prednisone com-

Andrew J. Armstrong, MD ScM, Duke Comprehensive Cancer Center, Department of Medicine, Division of Medical Oncology, Duke University Medical Center, Durham, North Carolina, USA
Michael A. Carducci, MD ScM, Associate Professor of Oncology and Urology, Sidney Kimmel Comprehensive Cancer Center, Johns Hopkins School of Medicine, Baltimore, Maryland, USA

pared with mitoxantrone and prednisone, 10% of patients had a rising PSA as the only indicator of progressive disease despite the presence of metastases [1]. In this subgroup, the median survival was approximately 21 months, compared with 16.8 months for those with progression defined by pain or radiologically measurable disease. This illustrates the need for randomization and stratification based on known prognostic factors in clinical trials of this heterogeneous patient population.

The demonstration of progressive disease in the face of continuous androgen suppression with GnRHa often leads to the introduction of combined androgen blockade with antiandrogens as second-line hormone manipulation. This can be followed by antiandrogen withdrawal and trials of third-line hormonal therapy, often with the androgen synthesis inhibitor ketoconazole and hydrocortisone or other antiandrogens. The response time to each of these manipulations is generally of the order of several months but some responses may be long or durable [6]. Eventually, prostate cancer growth becomes refractory to these manipulations. The indication for chemotherapy in practical terms has generally been metastatic progression despite the utilization of several hormonal options, manifested generally by clinically evident or radiographically measurable disease rather than biochemical (PSA) progression alone.

BIOLOGICAL BASIS FOR HORMONE-REFRACTORY GROWTH

Like many epithelial malignancies, prostate cancer represents a multistep cascade of events that contribute to the malignant phenotype, including evasion of apoptosis, growth factor independence, tissue invasion and metastasis, angiogenesis and immortality [7]. Many of these features are shared with tissue stem cells, and may be related to genomic instability and acquired somatic mutations, possibly as a result of increased susceptibility of prostate cancer cells to environmental toxins and oxidative damage. The methylation and subsequent loss of expression of glutathione s-transferase pi, a phase II detoxification enzyme probably involved in genomic protection from carcinogens, is one of the earliest changes seen during prostate cancer progression [8]. Loss of expression of the homeobox gene NKX3.1 may also increase the susceptibility to DNA damage early in prostate cancer pathogenesis [9]. Increased expression of multidrug resistance protein (MRP), myc, bcl-2, vascular endothelial growth factor (VEGF), cyclin-D1 and p53 have all been correlated with progression to the androgen-independent state, as have diminished levels of the tumour suppressors PTEN and p27-Kip1 [10, 11]. Bcl-2 is a unique antiapoptotic gene expressed in the basal regenerating compartment of the prostate that extends cell viability in the absence of cell proliferation [12]. While the cell of origin in prostate cancer remains unclear, these basal cells are typically androgen independent and may contain the putative prostate cancer stem cell responsible for relapse following androgen ablation. Destruction of the more differentiated compartment of luminal type cells that are androgen dependent would not be expected to eradicate these stem cells. Whether these regenerating cells are present from the beginning of prostate cancer development or acquired during progression remains to be determined. Efforts to identify phenotypic markers of these stem cells, such as telomerase, CD133, TMPRSS2–ETS fusion proteins and hedgehog signalling, are encouraging, and novel trial designs to test the hypothesis of the stem cell basis for prostatic malignancy are anticipated [13–17].

Resistance to cytotoxic therapy-induced programmed cell death may also be related to the relative inactivation of the phosphatase and tensin homologue deleted on chromosome 10 (PTEN) tumour-suppressor gene during the progression to the hormone-refractory state [18]. Loss of PTEN expression is seen in the majority of prostate metastases compared with 15% of early localized malignancies [19]. This tumour-suppressor gene restrains the activity of the Akt/PI3K survival pathway, which contributes to apoptotic resistance to cytotoxic agents, cell anchorage-independent growth, angiogenesis, nutrient driven proliferation and other stem-cell like phenotypes [20–22]. Inhibition of this pathway may thus be beneficial in advanced disease.

Resistance to cytotoxic therapy may be related to concurrent resistance to androgen deprivation and progression to HRPC. Up-regulation of the androgen receptor has been observed during progression to the androgen-refractory state [23]. Alterations in coactivators and corepressors of the androgen receptor may function as a biological signal amplification switch associated with increased androgen receptor expression, and may explain some of the lack of benefit and even paradoxical growth seen during treatment with antiandrogens [24]. Androgen receptor mutations, about 45% of which are activating mutations, have been observed in a minority of patients with HRPC and may lead to increased sensitivity to oestrogens, progestins and other non-androgen ligands [25, 26]. Increased sensitivity to local autocrine and paracrine stromal growth factors [i.e. epidermal growth factor (EGF), insulin-like growth factor-1 (IGF-1), interleukin 6 (IL-6)] that act either through traditional signalling pathways or cross-talk with androgen receptor signalling have been reported [27]. Transition to the hormone-refractory state may thus be accompanied by an amplification of or alteration in androgen receptor signalling, or a transition to dependence on growth factor kinase pathways [24]. PSA production may thus also become driven by non-androgen signals and may confound the use of PSA declines as a surrogate marker for investigational agents.

PROGNOSTIC MODELS

The predicted survival of men with HRPC is heterogeneous and depends on a number of factors, including performance status, baseline haemoglobin, baseline alkaline phosphatase and lactate dehydrogenase (LDH), baseline PSA, presence or absence of pain, disease sites (i.e. visceral metastases), disease kinetics, comorbidities and competing causes of death, and clinical state (type of progression) [28]. Currently, the median survival of men with asymptomatic non-metastatic HRPC is approximately 2–4 years, for asymptomatic metastatic HRPC approximately 20–24 months, and for symptomatic metastatic HRPC approximately 10–15 months [1, 5, 28]. Tables 12.1 and 12.2 illustrate those factors that contribute to the individu-

Table 12.1   Predicted median survival based on prostate cancer disease state

Disease state	Median overall survival
Rising PSA only HRPC	2–4 years
Asymptomatic Metastatic HRPC	20–24 months
Symptomatic HRPC	10–15 months
Metastatic HRPC relapsed after docetaxel	12 months

HRPC, hormone-refractory prostate cancer; PSA, prostate-specific antigen.

Table 12.2   Prognostic factors in metastatic HRPC

Performance status
Pain at baseline
Serum LDH (greater than normal)
Visceral metastases
Baseline haemoglobin
Baseline alkaline phosphatase
PSA kinetics (doubling time or velocity)
Gleason sum in primary tumour (>7)
Number of metastatic sites
Rising PSA only as progression type
Low albumin

LDH, lactate dehydrogenase; PSA, prostate-specific antigen.

alization of prognosis. PSA kinetics are emerging as an independent risk factor for mortality, including both PSA velocity and PSA doubling time (PSADT), and have been retrospectively evaluated in several relatively small studies [29–32]. Regardless of baseline PSA, PSA kinetics seems to be prognostic for mortality, and this marker has been validated now in a large independent data set (in press). The Halabi nomogram (Figure 12.1) for metastatic HRPC is a useful stratification tool for randomized trials in this population, with PSA kinetics, presence of pain and number of metastatic sites being likely additional measures of prognosis and stratification [28]. Given the multiple prognostic variables and heterogeneity of overall survival, randomized trials in this patient population are essential in the evaluation of novel therapies.

To date, a surrogate marker for overall survival in metastatic HRPC has yet to be validated. PSA response seems not to be a strong surrogate for overall survival in the large randomized trials, and recent reviews have shown a low association in other clinical trials [33]. Progression-free survival remains to be uniformly described in this disease state, and other candidate surrogates include change in PSA kinetics, PSA nadir, duration of response and pain response to chemotherapy [34].

HISTORICAL PERSPECTIVE

Controlled chemotherapy trials for HRPC began in the 1960s and 1970s with the United States National Prostatic Diseases Project and the systematic evaluation of chemotherapeutic agents, including 5-fluorouracil (5FU), cyclophosphamide and others. A full review of the background of chemotherapeutic agents is referenced, and Table 12.3 provides a comparison of selected single and combination chemotherapeutic agents in terms of response rates, survival and time to progression observed in phase II trials [35]. The results of the phase II trials of docetaxel and combination docetaxel and estramustine essentially led to the phase III

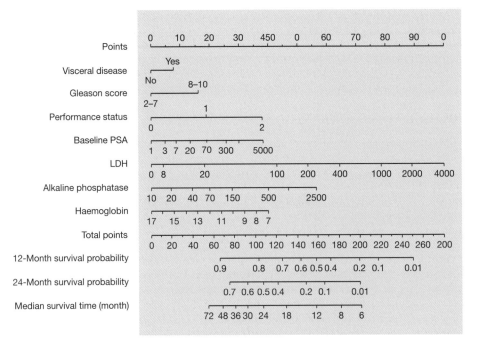

Figure 12.1 Nomogram for predicting survival in metastatic hormone-refractory prostate cancer. Reproduced with permission from the *Journal of Clinical Oncology*, all rights reserved [28].

Table 12.3   Selected chemotherapeutic agents with activity in hormone-refractory prostate cancer [35]

Agent	Number of patients	Survival (months)	Time to progression (months)	Measurable RR (%)	PSA RR (95% CI)
Docetaxel	810	9–18.9	4.6–5.1	12–28	38–48
Paclitaxel	126	9–13.5	NR	17	4–39
Mitoxantrone	255	12.3–23	3.7–8.1	13	33–48
Epirubicin	260	9–13	NR	31	24–32
Vinorelbine	154	10.2–17	2.9–7	7	4–28
Estramustine	113	NR	NR	40	21
Cyclophosphamide	53	8–12.7	NR	14	4
Doxorubicin	135	9–13	NR	22	NR
Gemcitabine	50	14.7	2.7	NR	NR
Cisplatin	29	NR	NR	10	NR
Paclitaxel, estra-mustine, etoposide, carboplatin (TEEC)	19	14.2	5.5	58	58
Docetaxel/estramustine	619	12–20	6–10	17–42	5–82
Ketoconazole, doxo-rubicin, vinblastine, estramustine (KAVE)	80	19–23.4	NR	61	56–67

NR, not reported; PSA, prostate-specific antigen; RR, response rate (defined for measurable disease by RECIST or WHO criteria, and for PSA as a 50% or greater decline from baseline).

studies discussed below based on the superior response rates as defined by declines in serum PSA greater than 50%, the tolerability of docetaxel and market pressures for agent development. However, mitoxantrone and prednisone remains an approved combination since 1996 for the palliation of symptoms in men with metastatic HRPC, and today is most commonly used in men who can not tolerate docetaxel-based therapy [36]. It is unclear what the role of mitoxantrone is as second-line therapy after docetaxel failure, given its low response rate in this setting and potential for cardiotoxicity [37]. Clearly, clinical trials remain an essential component of progress towards improved outcomes in this disease.

CHEMOTHERAPY FOR ADVANCED DISEASE, FIRST LINE

In 2004, docetaxel (Taxotere®) with prednisone was approved for use in the USA and Europe in metastatic HRPC based on the results of two large, phase III, randomized, multicentre, controlled trials: TAX327 and Southwest Oncology Group Protocol (SWOG) 9916 [1, 2]. The eligibility for these trials was similar and included progressive disease as defined by PSA progression or objective radiological progression in the face of castrate levels of testosterone. Despite this, there are some differences in baseline characteristics of the patients and conduct of each trial, shown in Table 12.4. Notably, SWOG 9916 subjects had lower PSA values at baseline, were less heavily pretreated, had less pain and visceral metastases at baseline, and slightly better performance status compared with TAX327 subjects, making cross-trial comparisons difficult. In addition, the chemotherapy doses and schedules were different in these two trials. In TAX327, patients were randomized to one of three arms: docetaxel 75 mg/m^2 every 3 weeks, docetaxel 30 mg/m^2 weekly for 5 of 6 weeks, and mitoxantrone 12 mg/m^2 every 3 weeks up to 10 cycles or 30 weeks of therapy in total. In SWOG 9916, patients were randomized into two groups: docetaxel 60 mg/m^2 every 3 weeks on day 2, with estramustine 280 mg daily for days 1–5 versus mitoxantrone 12 mg/m^2 every 3 weeks with treatment continuing until disease progression, adverse events or 12 cycles of docetaxel or 144 mg/m^2

Table 12.4 Comparison of baseline and response characteristics in the TAX327 and SWOG 9916 trials [1, 2]

Trial	TAX327 (D3P, D1P, MP) (n = 1006)	SWOG 9916 (D+E+P vs. MP) (n = 674)
Baseline characteristics		
Baseline PSA, median	108–123	84–90
Prior estramustine	18–20%	None
Age, median (years)	68–69	70
Caucasian (%)	>90	82–86
PS (% poor)	12–14	10–12
PSA-only progression (%)	10	18–19
Visceral metastases	22–24	18–19
Pain at baseline	45	36
Prior hormonal manipulations (per cent over 2)	21–25	NR
Outcomes (per arm)	D3, D1, MP	DE, MP
PSA response rate (%)	45, 48, 32	50, 27
Tumour response rate (%)	12, 8, 7	17, 11
Pain response (%)	35, 31, 22	NR
Median survival (months)	18.9, 17.4, 16.5	17.5, 15.6
Time to progression (months)	Not defined, reported	6.3, 3.2
Follow-up time (months)	21	32

NR, not reported; PS, performance status; PSA, prostate-specific antigen.

of mitoxantrone. Finally, the doses of steroids were very different in each arm of the trials, making it difficult to separate the true antitumour effects of docetaxel. For example, while all patients received 5 mg of prednisone twice daily, the every-3-weeks docetaxel arms in both trials received 8 mg dexamethasone for three doses prior to chemotherapy while only one dose was given in the weekly docetaxel arm, and mitoxantrone arms did not receive supplemental steroids. Thus, some of the efficacy seen in these trials may be due to some of the known antitumour effects of high doses of steroids on an intermittent basis [38].

The major results of the TAX327 and SWOG trials are shown in Table 12.4 and Figure 12.2 [1, 2]. In summary, overall survival in TAX327 was improved by 2.5 months with 3-weekly docetaxel (18.9 vs. 16.5 months, HR 0.76) but not statistically significantly prolonged in the weekly docetaxel arm (17.4 months). The trial was not designed for a formal comparison of the docetaxel schedules, and the confidence intervals around the median survival estimates for these groups clearly overlap. However, based on this result, docetaxel received regulatory approval in the USA and Europe. Surprisingly, PSA response rates were higher for weekly docetaxel, as were duration of pain and PSA responses, despite the lack of survival advantage.

Toxicity in the every-3-weeks versus weekly docetaxel arms was notable for more haematological toxicity in the every-3-week arm (3% vs. 0% neutropenic fever), but slightly lower rates of nausea and vomiting, fatigue, nail changes, hyperlacrimation and diarrhoea [1]. Neuropathy, alopecia and peripheral oedema were slightly more common in the every-3-week arm. Quality of life as measured by the Functional Assessment of Cancer Therapy–Prostate (FACT–P) scoring system did not differ significantly among the docetaxel schedules but was more favourable than the mitoxantrone arm [34]. In extrapolating the use of docetaxel to large populations of men with HRPC, it is also important to point out significant reports of interstitial pneumonitis, extravasation injuries, colitis, excess tearing and maculopapular rash that may occur with docetaxel but were not seen in TAX327 [39].

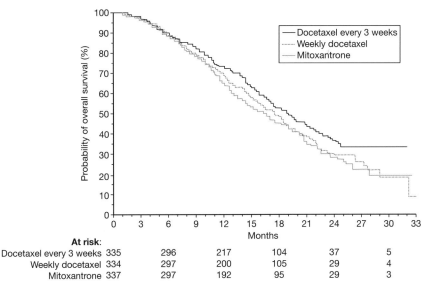

Figure 12.2   Survival estimates for every-3-weeks docetaxel, weekly docetaxel and every-3-weeks mitoxantrone in the TAX327 trial [1]. Copyright 2004, Massachusetts Medical Society. All rights reserved.

While a similar survival advantage was seen in SWOG 9916 with docetaxel and estramustine, this came at a cost of increased cardiovascular, gastrointestinal and thromboembolic toxicity, despite the use of low-dose anticoagulant prophylaxis (2 mg coumadin and 325 mg aspirin) [2]. These rates may be attributable to the oestrogenic properties of estramustine, leading to an approximately 7–15% incidence of thromboembolic disorders [40]. Despite a 50% PSA response rate, enthusiasm for estramustine has significantly diminished as a result of roughly similar overall survivals across these two trials for docetaxel-based chemotherapy.

COMBINATIONS WITH MOLECULARLY TARGETED AGENTS

While a comprehensive discussion of novel therapies for metastatic HRPC is discussed in subsequent chapters, a brief mention of therapeutic strategies and ongoing clinical trials is warranted here. Table 12.5 lists some of the agents currently in phase II–III development in metastatic HRPC.

ANTIANGIOGENIC AGENTS

Prostate cancer is known to overexpress VEGF and its receptors, and VEGF levels correlate with disease stage and perhaps survival in the metastatic setting, with levels falling after surgical resection of primary tumours [41, 42]. The mechanism of abnormal VEGF production in prostate cancer may be related to aberrant hypoxia-induced signalling (HIF1α) but essentially remains unclear, as does the mechanism of action of anti-VEGF therapies in other solid tumours. Potential mechanisms include a normalization of vasculature for facilitated delivery of chemotherapy, a decrease in oncotic interstitial pressure from leaky capillary membranes, improved recruitment of mature dendritic cells and immunostimulation, and true anti-neovascularization effects [43–47]. A multicentre phase III study, CALGB 90401, is currently randomizing patients to docetaxel or docetaxel and bevacizumab, including prednisone in each arm, and is now open with a goal accrual of 1020 patients over 3 years. This

Table 12.5 Selected novel agents in phase II–III development in metastatic hormone-refractory prostate cancer

Target	Agent, Sponsor	Phase	Brief eligibility overview
VEGF	Bevacizumab (Avastin), CALGB 90401	III	Docetaxel±bevacizumab in metastatic HRPC, first line
Vitamin D receptor	Calcitriol (DN101), Novacea	III	ASCENT II: docetaxel±DN101 in metastatic HRPC
Endothelin axis	Atrasentan, SWOG	III	SWOG S0421: docetaxel±Atrasentan in metastatic HRPC
Vaccine strategies	Prostate GVAX, Cell Genesys Provenge, Dendreon TRICOM, NCI, ECOG	III	GVAX (VITAL-1) and Provenge (D9902B), first-line metastatic, asymptomatic HRPC VITAL-2: docetaxel±GVAX in symptomatic HRPC
EGFR (HER2/HER3)	Lapatinib, ECOG	II	Rising PSA setting only (non-metastatic)
Immunomodulation	Lenalidomide, DOD Prostate Cancer Clinical Trial Consortium	II	Rising PSA population or metastatic HRPC after local therapy
PTEN/Akt and mTOR pathway	Temsirolimus, Wyeth Everolimus, Novartis Rapamycin, DOD/Johns Hopkins AP23573, Ariad	I-II	Preoperative pharmacodynamic and dose-finding studies; combination with docetaxel in metastatic HRPC: Dana Farber and MSKCC, RAD001 with gefitinib (MSKCC)

DOD, Department of Defense; ECOG, Eastern Cooperative Oncology Group; EGFR, epidermal growth factor receptor; HER human epidermal growth factor receptor; HRPC hormone-refractory prostate cancer; MSKCC, Memorial Sloan Kettering Cancer Center; NCI, National Cancer Institute; SWOG, Southwest Oncology Group Protocol; VEGF, vascular endothelial growth factor.

follows the results of a phase II study that demonstrated the safety and PSA response efficacy of docetaxel, estramustine and bevacizumab in HRPC [48].

Additional agents with antiangiogenic properties include thalidomide and its analogues, such as lenalidomide, as well as small molecule inhibitors of the VEGF receptor tyrosine kinase such as sorafenib and sutent [49, 50]. These agents are in phase II development in HRPC. Thalidomide analogues probably have multiple mechanisms of action, including inhibition of VEGF, improved T cell costimulatory function, tumour necrosis factor (TNF) alpha inhibition and a decrease in interleukin6 (IL-6) levels [50]. A phase II randomized study of thalidomide and docetaxel in HRPC demonstrated an impressive 53% PSA response rate (> 50% decrease in PSA), and improved time to progression and overall survival; however, this study was underpowered and complicated by a high rate of thrombosis, sedation and neuropathy in the experimental arm, necessitating the introduction of therapeutic low molecular weight heparin prophylaxis [51]. Novel thalidomide analogues are in phase II development in prostate cancer, and are expected to have a lower incidence of vascular and neurotoxic adverse events [52]. The high potency of these agents in terms of T-cell stimulation, antiangiogenic properties and oral availability make them attractive as therapeutic agents.

GROWTH FACTOR PATHWAYS

In metastatic hormone-refractory prostate cancer, several classes of agents that modify growth factor signalling pathways hold some promise and are in early-phase trials. These include rapamycin analogues that target the Akt/PI3 kinase/mTOR pathway, heat shock protein 90 (HSP90) inhibitors, and inhibitors of upstream growth factor receptors in prostate cancer such as human epidermal growth factor receptor (HER)-2/3, IGF-R, IL-6R and platelet-derived growth factor receptor (PDGFR). Akt activation and/or PTEN loss have been linked to hormonal resistance, chemotherapeutic insensitivity, biologically aggressive behaviour, advanced Gleason score and relapse after local therapy [18, 21]. Mouse models of PTEN loss or Akt activation have demonstrated growth inhibition, restoration of chemosensitivity and improved time-to-progression with inhibitors of this pathway, including rapamycin analogues [53–57]. Mechanistic dose-finding pre-prostatectomy studies are in progress in prostate cancer with three rapamycin analogues: temsirolimus, everolimus and rapamycin itself [57–60]. The development of these agents will be dependent on the establishment of surrogate markers of biological effect, the identification of subgroups of responders, and drug characteristics such as dose, pharmacokinetic variability and tolerability. All agents in this class have a well-described pattern of toxicity, including stomatitis, acneform rash, glucose intolerance, nausea, fatigue, mild thrombocytopenia, arthralgias, electrolyte abnormalities and possibly increased risks of infection [61]. Their long-term immunosuppressive safety in prostate cancer patients has yet to be tested, but has been evaluated favourably in renal cell carcinoma and other tumour types [62, 63]. The use of these agents in combination with docetaxel is under investigation and requires careful monitoring due to metabolic and myelosuppressive interactions. As these agents are primarily cytostatic in prostate cancer, combination therapy with other biological agents may be necessary.

Epidermal growth factor receptor (EGFR) tyrosine kinase inhibitors such as gefitinib and trastuzumab have not been successful in metastatic prostate cancer; and it is possible that EGFR and HER2 may not carry the same importance in the majority of prostate cancer cases as they do in some lung cancer or breast cancer cases [64, 65]. Indeed, HER2 amplification in prostate cancer is rare, unlike the case in subsets of breast cancer [66]. Recent findings suggest that HER-2/HER-3 dimerization and activation led to optimization of androgen receptor (AR) signalling in the setting of androgen depletion, pointing to a potential novel therapeutic target [67]. The HER1/HER2 intracellular kinase inhibitor lapatinib is the subject of a recently completed Eastern Cooperative Oncology Group (ECOG) phase II study in men with a rising PSA after local therapy.

The endothelin axis may be an important mediator of the bone–prostate cancer interface and a paracrine signalling target. Endothelin receptors are overexpressed in metastatic HRPC and higher levels of endothelin correlate with progressive disease [68]. While endothelin is a potent vasoconstrictive agent, it may also regulate cellular mitogenic pathways in prostate cancer and osteoblasts, and play a role in the mediation of bone-related pain from metastatic prostate cancer. Atrasentan has been developed as a highly selective endothelin (ET)-A receptor antagonist and is the most clinically developed agent of this class in prostate cancer [69]. In the phase III trial, 809 patients with metastatic HRPC were randomized to placebo or 10 mg of oral atrasentan, with the primary clinical endpoint being time to progression (TTP) [70]. Although TTP was not found to be statistically significantly different from placebo in the intent-to-treat analysis, several secondary endpoints indicated clinical activity, including improvements in quality of life scores, pain scores and reductions in the rise of laboratory markers including alkaline phosphatase and PSA. While atrasentan was not approvable based on these data and out of concerns for cardiovascular toxicity, these results clearly point to biological activity of the endothelin axis in modulating osteoblastic metastases, and emphasize the importance of trial design in this population. Further development of this agent in combination with docetaxel is under way in SWOG 0421 or in select bone-only subgroups of patients. Phase III trial results in non-metastatic prostate cancer are due to be reported in late 2006. Another ET-A receptor antagonist, ZD4054, is also in phase II development at this time [71].

Prostate cancer cells express high levels of PDGFR, and this signalling pathway utilizes the PI3 kinase/Akt pathway which has been implicated in prostate cancer progression [72]. While single agent activity of imatinib, an oral PDGFR tyrosine kinase inhibitor, has been modest, the combination of imatinib 600 mg and docetaxel 30 mg/m^2 weekly for 4 out of 6 weeks demonstrated a > 50% PSA reduction in 8 out of 21 patients (38%), with several durable (> 18 month) responses [72]. A second-line randomized trial of this combination sponsored by the NCI Prostate Cancer SPORE clinical consortium is under way, with preliminary results demonstrating little if any benefit over docetaxel alone [73].

IMMUNOLOGICAL APPROACHES

As the prostate is a non-vital organ, induction of anti-prostate auto- or alloimmunity may be clinically beneficial without undue organ toxicity. Several vaccination strategies have progressed into phase III testing in prostate cancer, including Provenge, a prostate acid phosphatase (PAP)-activated dendritic cell-based vaccine, and Prostate GVAX, a whole-cell allogeneic vaccine [74]. Both of these agents are under evaluation in the phase III setting. Provenge [Sipuleucel-T] is a proprietary process of antigen-delivery to activated antigen presenting cells, collected from patients through leukapheresis, stimulated with fusion PAP-granulocyte-macrophage colony-stimulating factor (PAP-GMCSF) protein, and reinjected intravenously every 2–4 weeks [75]. Initial results from small phase II–III studies (D9901 and D9902A) involving a total of 225 patients with asymptomatic metastatic HRPC did not significantly demonstrate improved time to disease or pain progression, the primary endpoints [76]. While not originally powered to detect a survival benefit, overall survival was improved by an average of 4 months in each study. Analyses based on chance imbalances in prognostic factors and use of chemotherapy after vaccination did not reduce this survival finding. A confirmatory phase III study of Provenge in minimally symptomatic men with HRPC is ongoing and powered to detect a difference in survival.

Prostate GVAX® is a form of active immunotherapy using whole cell allogeneic prostate cell lines (PC-3 and LnCaP) virally transduced to express an immune adjuvant granulocyte–macrophage colony-stimulating factor (GMCSF), lethally irradiated and injected intradermally [77]. Given that GMCSF probably facilitates the maturation and activation of dendritic cells, initial work extrapolated early melanoma studies to mouse models of prostate cancer with results showing prolonged survival and tumour regression [77, 78]. A phase II study of prostate GVAX was conducted in 34 patients with metastatic HRPC and demonstrated a median survival of 26 months in select, asymptomatic patients [79]. A further evaluation of 80 patients with metastatic HRPC treated at higher doses demonstrated one partial PSA response and improvement in markers of bone turnover, with survival analysis still ongoing [80]. A phase III trial of GVAX® versus docetaxel (VITAL-1) in 600 men with minimally symptomatic metastatic HRPC is currently accruing patients, and a second phase III study examining docetaxel and prednisone with or without GVAX has been initiated (VITAL-2).

Finally, several other vaccine approaches are in phase II–III testing and include the recombinant vaccinia-fowlpox PSA vaccine (TRICOM) and the BLP25 MUC1 liposomal vaccine MUC-1 [74, 81]. The use of vaccines alone or in combination with chemotherapy or biological agents, such as cytotoxic T lymphocyte-associated protein 4 (CTLA4) blocking antibodies, may improve immune responses and overcome tumour tolerance, potentially at the expense of autoimmunity [82, 83].

DIFFERENTIATING AGENTS

In prostate cancer, epidemiological data suggest that the vitamin D receptor is a potential therapeutic target, given the link of vitamin D deficiency with prostate cancer incidence [84]. *In vitro*, calcitriol may have growth inhibitory, proapoptotic, and differentiating properties in prostate cancer, thus leading to a rationale for clinical trials [85]. Based on favourable phase II results of calcitriol and docetaxel in combination, Beer *et al.* recently reported interim results from a phase II randomized trial [AIPC (androgen-independent prostate cancer) Study of Calcitriol Enhancing Taxotere (ASCENT)] of docetaxel and prednisone with or without DN101 , a proprietary oral calcitriol analogue [86]. In this randomized multi-institutional study of 250 men with progressive metastatic HRPC treated with weekly docetaxel with or without DN101, the primary endpoint was PSA response rate, a typical phase II endpoint. With a median follow-up of 18.3 months, neither PSA nor clinical response endpoints were met (6-month PSA response 58% vs. 49%, $P = 0.07$, and measurable disease response rate of 29% vs. 24%, $P = 0.58$ in the placebo vs. treated subjects respectively). However, despite being underpowered to detect a difference in survival, the estimated median survival was non-significantly prolonged with DN-101, from 16.4 to 23.5 months (HR 0.70, 95% CI 0.48–1.03, $P = 0.07$), and better tolerated than docetaxel alone [87]. This difference became significant with a prespecified multivariate adjustment based on chance imbalances in this small sample size. A larger study with typical phase III survival endpoints is under way (ASCENT II) to confirm these findings.

Other strategies that may induce terminal differentiation of prostate cancer cells include inhibitors of histone deacetylase and DNA methyltransferase, enzymes responsible for the epigenetic silencing of gene expression. Histones maintain DNA in a closed, coiled configuration, and this activity is mediated by a reversible acetylation process, in which acetylation of lysine residues on select histone tails favours transcription. Aberrant hypermethylation and gene silencing of specific promoter regions in prostate cancer has been described, such as the antioxidant enzyme GST-pi and the tumour suppressor p21 [88]. The rationale behind agents that target histone deacetylase or DNA methyltransferase is their ability to induce broad gene re-expression in preclinical models of prostate cancer which may induce apoptosis, up-regulate p21 signalling and arrest growth [89, 90]. Histone deacetylase (HDAC) subtypes may be critical to the tailoring of these agents to disease states. Further confounding mechanistic assumptions are the effects on protein signalling independent of their epigenomic effects [91]. Phase II studies using suberoylanilide hydroxamic acid (SAHA), an orally bioavailable HDAC inhibitor, in metastatic HRPC are ongoing, and a phase II study is planned of the HDAC inhibitor MS-275 in combination with cis-retinoic acid based on promising preclinical and phase I results [92, 93].

As the antiapoptotic Bcl-2 protein is overexpressed in metastatic HRPC, and resistance to cell death seems to be dominant over proliferation in these tumours, proapoptotic strategies are attractive therapeutically [94]. The mechanism of Bcl-2 overexpression is unclear, however, and could be related to PTEN loss and/or Akt pathway activation, thus providing a common mechanism for the observed joint occurrences with tumour progression [95]. Agents that target bcl-2 have been tested and current results have demonstrated feasibility and safety but unclear efficacy or target validation in prostate cancer, and newer compounds are anticipated to explore this strategy [96].

CHEMOTHERAPY FOR ADVANCED DISEASE, SECOND LINE

Given that disease-free survival after initiation of docetaxel-based chemotherapy is of the order of 4–6 months, many patients will be eligible for second- or third-line agents, with a median expected survival in this subgroup of approximately 12 months [37]. As of 2006, there are no approved second-line agents for metastatic HRPC, and the options include watchful waiting, radiation to symptomatic sites, clinical trials, or off-protocol chemotherapy such as mitoxantrone and prednisone for palliation of symptoms. Select patients do derive response benefit from docetaxel retreatment and many patients have undertaken intermittent chemotherapy, with prolonged treatment-free intervals [97]. There is some preliminary and preclinical evidence that low-dose metronomic chemotherapy with taxanes or cyclophosphamide may have some clinical benefit in prostate cancer [98, 99].

The dose limitations of docetaxel therapy in metastatic HRPC are predominantly those of peripheral neurotoxicity and myelotoxicity, and the search for well-tolerated novel cytotoxic compounds continues, both in the front line and in the second-line setting. One agent in development for second-line therapy is satraplatin, a novel oral platinum analogue that may fulfil a niche in second-line therapy if it is well tolerated and has been shown to improve survival over corticosteroids in the maturing SPARC (Satraplatin and Prednisolone Against Refractory Cancer) phase III trial [100].

The epothilones are a class of microtubule-targeting cytotoxic agents in development for second-line and relapsed HRPC. While sharing a common mechanism of action with the taxanes, they are not generally susceptible to P-glycoprotein induced drug efflux [101]. The epothilone-B analogue BMS-247550 (Ixabepilone) has been studied in a first-line phase II

Table 12.6 Agents in phase II–III trials for use in second-line therapy after docetaxel failure in metastatic hormone-refractory prostate cancer

Agent	Phase	Trial, Sponsor
Satraplatin	III	SPARC Trial (Spectrum Pharmaceuticals): prednisone ± satraplatin
Epothilone B Analogue BMS-247550 (Ixabepilone)	II	ECOG: BMS vs. mitoxantrone and prednisone
Targeted cytotoxics and radiopharmaceuticals: MLN2704 ^{177}Lu ^{90}Y J591	II	MLN2704: MSKCC, Millenium Pharmaceuticals J591: Cornell University
PDGFR: Imatinib(Gleevec)	II	ECOG, MD Anderson and Prostate Cancer Foundation with docetaxel
Sunitinib	II	Phase II, Massachusetts General Hospital
SAHA	II	Phase II, DOD Prostate Cancer Clinical Trials Consortium

DOD, Department of Defense; ECOG, Eastern Cooperative Oncology Group; MSKCC, Memorial Sloan Kettering Cancer Center; PDGFR, platelet-derived growth factor receptor; SAHA, suberoylanilide hydroxamic acid.

trial of men with HRPC [102]. Initial results demonstrated comparable PSA declines and progression-free survival to that seen with docetaxel-based therapy. Use of these drugs may be limited by dose-limiting neurotoxicity similar to that seen with the taxanes, and other agents that may target microtubules with reduced neurotoxicity are under evaluation, such as E7389, an analogue of the marine compound halichondrin B [103]. The use of BMS 247550 in taxane-resistant HRPC is being investigated currently in the second-line setting compared with mitoxantrone and prednisone and has shown similar PSA declines of about 20% [37].

Finally, monoclonal antibodies targeted to prostate cancer cells with tagged cytotoxic agents represent a novel approach to therapy. One agent, MLN2704 is a prostate-specific membrane antigen (PSMA) conjugated maytansinoid agent and is in phase I/II trials currently in HRPC [104]. Radioimmunotherapy with bound radioactive agents to monoclonal antibodies has also shown some promise and is also in phase II trials [105–108]. Table 12.6 provides an overview of second-line clinical trials that are ongoing in metastatic HRPC.

CONCLUSIONS

Today, we are fortunate to have a number of clinical trial options for men with advanced metastatic hormone-refractory prostate cancer, including combination approaches with antiangiogenic compounds, active immunotherapy and anti-tolerance approaches, novel growth factor pathway inhibitors, and differentiation and proapoptotic agents. The rational development of these agents against therapeutic targets in prostate cancer is essential, and thus continued progress in the understanding of the molecular biology of prostate cancer progression and hormone-refractory growth is essential. Novel hormonal agents, prostate cancer stem cell-specific therapies and disease-specific mutation selective agents are all in early stage development, and appropriately powered clinical trials are encouraged in all settings as the principal therapeutic strategy in this unfortunately common and incurable disease.

DISCLOSURES

Funding for some of the studies described in this chapter was provided by Aventis and Abbott Laboratories. Dr Carducci is a paid consultant and on the Speakers Bureau for Aventis and Abbott Laboratories. He has participated as an investigator in studies described in this chapter. The terms of this arrangement are being managed by the Johns Hopkins University in accordance with its conflict of interest policies.

REFERENCES

1. Tannock IF, de Wit R, Berry WR *et al.* Docetaxel plus prednisone or mitoxantrone plus prednisone for advanced prostate cancer. *N Engl J Med* 2004; 351:1502–1512.
2. Petrylak DP, Tangen CM, Hussain MHA *et al.* Docetaxel and estramustine compared with mitoxantrone and prednisone for advanced refractory prostate cancer. *N Engl J Med* 2004; 351:1513–1520.
3. Bubley GJ, Carducci MA, Dahut W *et al.* Eligibility and response guidelines for phase II clinical trials in androgen-independent prostate cancer: recommendations from the Prostate-Specific Antigen Working Group. *J Clin Oncol* 1999; 17:3461–3467.
4. Scher HI, Eisenberger M, D'Amico AV *et al.* Eligibility and outcomes reporting guidelines for clinical trials for patients in the state of a rising prostate specific antigen: recommendations from the Prostate-Specific Antigen Working Group. *J Clin Oncol* 2004; 22:537–556.
5. Smith MR, Kabbinavar F, Saad F *et al.* Natural history of rising serum prostate-specific antigen in men with castrate nonmetastatic prostate cancer. *J Clin Oncol* 2005; 23:2918–2925.
6. Small EJ, Halabi S, Dawson NA *et al.* Antiandrogen withdrawal alone or in combination with ketoconazole in androgen-independent prostate cancer patients: a Phase III trial (CALGB 9583). *J Clin Oncol* 2004; 22:1025–1033.
7. Hanahan D, Weinberg RA. The hallmarks of cancer. *Cell* 2000; 100:57–70.

8. Lee WH, Morton RA, Epstein JI *et al.* Cytidine methylation of regulatory sequences near the p-class glutathione-s-transferase gene accompanies human prostate cancer carcinogenesis. *Proc Natl Acad Sci USA* 1994; 91:11733–11737.

9. Ouyang X, DeWeese TI, Nelson WG *et al.* Loss–of-function of Nkx3.1 promotes increased oxidative damage in prostate carcinogenesis. *Cancer Res* 2005; 65:6773–6779.

10. Isaacs JT. The biology of hormone refractory prostate cancer: why does it develop? *Urol Clin NA* 1999; 26:263–273.

11. Nelson WG, De Marzo AM, Isaacs WB. Mechanisms of disease: prostate cancer. *N Engl J Med* 2003; 349: 366–381.

12. McDonnell TJ, Troncoso P, Brisbay SM *et al.* Expression of the protooncogene bcl-2 in the prostate and its association with emergence of androgen-independent prostate cancer. *Cancer Res* 1992; 52:6940–6944.

13. Karhadkar SS, Bova GS, Abdallah N *et al.* Hedgehog signaling in prostate regeneration, neoplasia, and metastasis. *Nature* 2004; 431:707–712.

14. Biroccio A and Leonetti C. Telomerase as a new target for the treatment of hormone-refractory prostate cancer. *Endo Rel Cancer* 2004; 11:407–421.

15. Richardson GD, Robson CN, Lang SH *et al.* CD133, a novel marker for human prostatic epithelial stem cells. *J Cell Sci* 2004; 117:3539–3545.

16. Tomlins SA, Rhodes DR, Perner S *et al.* Recurrent fusion of TMPRSS2 and ETS transcription factor genes in prostate cancer. *Science* 2005; 310:644–648.

17. Polyak K, Hahn WC. Roots and stems: stem cells in cancer. *Nat Med* 2005; 11:296–299.

18. McMenamin ME, Soung P, Perera S *et al.* Loss of PTEN expression in paraffin-embedded primary prostate cancer correlates with high Gleason score and advanced stage. *Cancer Res* 1999; 59:4291–4296.

19. Whang YE, Wu X, Suzuki H *et al.* Inactivation of the tumor suppressor PTEN/MMAC1 in advanced human prostate cancer through loss of expression. *Proc Natl Acad Sci USA* 1998; 95:5246–5250.

20. Cantley LC, Neel BG. New insights into tumor suppression: PTEN suppresses tumor formation by restraining the phosphoinositide 3-kinase/AKT pathway. *Proc Natl Acad Sci USA* 1999; 96:4240–4245.

21. Ayala G, Thompson T, Yang G *et al.* High levels of phosphorylated form of akt-1 in prostate cancer and non-neoplastic prostate tissues are strong predictors of biochemical recurrence. *Clin Cancer Res* 2004; 10:6572–6578.

22. Vivanco I, Sawyers CL. The phosphatidylinositol 3-kinase-akt pathway in human cancer. *Nat Rev Cancer* 2002; 2:489–501.

23. Chen CD, Welsbie DS, Tran C *et al.* Molecular determinants of resistance to antiandrogen therapy. *Nature Medicine* 2004; 10:33–38.

24. Scher HI, Sawyers CL. Biology of progressive, castration-resistant prostate cancer: directed therapies targeting the androgen-receptor signaling axis. *J Clin Oncol* 2005; 23:8253–8261.

25. Tilley WD, Buchanan G, Hickey TE *et al.* Mutations in the androgen receptor gene are associated with progression of human prostate cancer to androgen independence. *Cancer Res* 1996; 2:277–285.

26. Marcelli M, Ittman M, Mariani S *et al.* Androgen receptor mutations in prostate cancer. *Cancer Res* 2000; 60:944–949.

27. Culig Z, Hobisch A, Cronauer MV *et al.* Androgen receptor activation in prostatic tumor cell lines by insulin-like growth factor-I, keratinocyte growth factor, and epidermal growth factor. *Cancer Res* 1994; 54:5474–5478.

28. Halabi S, Small EJ, Katoff PW *et al.* Prognostic model for predicting survival in men with hormone-refractory metastatic prostate cancer. *J Clin Oncol* 2003; 21:1232–1237.

29. Rozhansky F, Chen MH, Cox MC *et al.* Prostate-specific antigen velocity and survival for patients with hormone-refractory metastatic prostate carcinoma. *Cancer* 2006; 106:63–67.

30. Scotte F, Banu E, Oudard S *et al.* Prostate-specific antigen doubling time (PSADT) before the onset of chemotherapy as survival predictor for hormone refractory prostate cancer patients. *J Clin Oncol* 2005; 23(16S):4551 (abstract).

31. Srinivas S, Balu V, King C. Utility of prostate specific antigen doubling time in patients with androgen independent prostate cancer. *J Clin Oncol* 2005; 23(16S): 4631 (abstract).

32. Semeniuk RC, Venner PM, Hanson SA. A retrospective review of prostate specific antigen doubling time in men with hormone refractory prostate cancer. *J Clin Oncol* 2005; 23(16S):4666 (abstract).

33. Roessner M, de Wit R, Tannock IF *et al.* Prostate-specific antigen (PSA) response as a surrogate endpoint for overall survival: analysis of the TAX327 study comparing docetaxel plus prednisone with mitoxantrone plus prednisone in advanced prostate cancer. *J Clin Oncol* 2005; 23(16S):4554 (abstract).

34. Berthold DR, Pond G, De Wit R *et al.* Association of pain and quality of life response with PSA response and survival of patients with metastatic hormone refractory prostate cancer treated with docetaxel or mitoxantrone in the TAX327 study. *Proc Am Soc Clin Oncol* 2006; 24(18S):4516 (abstract).

35. Armstrong AJ, Carducci MA. Chemotherapy for advanced prostate cancer. In: Kirby R, Partin AW, Feneley M, Parsons JK eds. *Prostate Cancer Principles and Practice.* Taylor and Francis, London, 2006, pp. 989–1004.

36. Tannock IF, Osoba D, Stocklet MR. Chemotherapy with mitoxantrone plus prednisone or prednisone alone for symptomatic hormone-resistant prostate cancer: a Canadian randomized trial with palliative endpoints. *J Clin Oncol* 1996; 14:1756–1764.

37. Lin AM, Rosenberg JE, Weinberg VK *et al.* Clinical outcome of taxane-resistant hormone-refractory prostate cancer patients treated with subsequent chemotherapy (ixabepilone or mitoxantrone/prednisone. *J Clin Oncol* 2006; 24(18S):4558 (abstract).

38. Nishimura K, Nonomura N, Satoh E *et al.* Potential mechanism for the effects of dexamethasone on growth of androgen-independent prostate cancer. *J Natl Cancer Inst* 2001; 93:1739–1746.

39. Khan MA, Carducci MA, Partin AW. The evolving role of docetaxel in the management of androgen independent prostate cancer. *J Urol* 2003; 170:1709–1716.

40. Lubiniecki GM, Berlin JA, Weinstein RB *et al.* Thromboembolic events with estramustine phosphate-based chemotherapy in patients with hormone-refractory prostate carcinoma: results of a meta-analysis. *Cancer* 2004; 101:2755–2759.

41. George DJ, Halabi S, Shepard TF *et al.* Prognostic significance of plasma vascular endothelial growth factor levels in patients with hormone-refractory prostate cancer treated on Cancer and Leukemia Group B 9480. *Clin Cancer Res* 2001; 7:1932–1936.

42. Duque JL, Loughlin KR, Adam RM, Kantoff PW, Zurakowski D, Freeman MR. Plasma levels of vascular endothelial growth factor are increased in patients with metastatic prostate cancer. *Urology* 1999; 54: 523–527.

43. Gabrilovich DI, Ishida T, Nadaf S *et al.* Antibodies to vascular endothelial growth factor enhance the efficacy of cancer immunotherapy by improving endogenous dendritic cell function. *Clin Cancer Res* 1999; 5:2963–2970.

44. Ferrara N, Gerber H, LeCouter J. The biology of VEGF and its receptors. *Nature Med* 2003; 9:669–676.

45. Willett CG, Boucher Y, di Tomaso E *et al.* Direct evidence that the VEGF-specific antibody bevacizumab has antivascular effects in human rectal cancer. *Nature Med* 2004; 10:145–147.

46. Fox WD, Higgins B, Maiese KM *et al.* Antibody to vascular endothelial growth factor slows growth of an androgen-independent xenograft model of prostate cancer. *Clin Cancer Res* 2002; 8:3226–3231.

47. Jain RK. Normalization of tumor vasculature: an emerging concept in antiangiogenic therapy. *Science* 2005; 307:58–62.

48. Picus J, Halabi S, Rini B *et al.* The use of bevacizumab (B) with docetaxel (D) and estramustine (E) in hormone refractory prostate cancer (HRPC): Initial results of CALGB 90006. *J Clin Oncol* 2003; 22:1578 (abstract).

49. Bartlett JB, Dredge K, Dalgleish AG. The evolution of thalidomide and its ImiD derivatives as anticancer agents. *Nature Rev Cancer* 2004; 4:314–322.

50. Zakarija A and Soff G. Update on angiogenesis inhibitors. *Curr Opin Oncol* 2005; 17:578–583.

51. Figg WD, Dahut W, Duray P *et al.* A randomized phase II trial of thalidomide, an angiogenesis inhibitor, in androgen-independent prostate cancer. *Clin Cancer Res* 2001; 7:1888–1893.

52. Capitosti SM, Hansen TP, Brown ML. Thalidomide analogues demonstrate dual inhibition of both angiogenesis and prostate cancer. *Bioorg Med Chem* 2004; 12:327–336.

53. Majumder PK, Febbo PG, Bikoff R *et al.* MTOR inhibition reverses Akt-dependent prostate intraepithelial neoplasia through regulation of apoptotic and HIF-1-dependent pathways. *Nat Med* 2004; 10:594–601.

54. Neshat MS, Mellinghoff IK, Tran C *et al.* Enhanced sensitivity of PTEN-deficient tumors to inhibition of FRAP-mTOR. *Proc Natl Acad Sci* 2001; 98:10314–10319.

55. Podsypanina K, Lee RT, Politis C *et al.* An inhibitor of mTOR reduces neoplasia and normalizes p70/s6 kinase activity in PTEN +/- mice. *Proc Natl Acad Sci* 2001; 98:10320–10325.

56. Grunwald V, DeGraffenried L, Russel D *et al.* Inhibitors of mTOR reverse doxorubicin resistance conferred by PTEN status in prostate cancer cells. *Cancer Res* 2002; 62:6141–6145.

57. Gera JF, Mellinghoff IK, Shi Y *et al.* Akt activity determines sensitivity to mammalian target of rapamycin (mTOR) inhibitors by regulating cyclin D1 and c-myc expression. *J Biol Chem* 2004; 279:2737–2746.

58. Tabernero J, Rojo F, Burris H *et al.* A phase I study with tumor pharmacodynamic evaluation of dose and schedule of the oral mTOR inhibitor Rapamycin (RAD001) in patients with advanced solid tumors. *J Clin Oncol* 2005; 23(16S):3007 (abstract).

59. Thomas G, Speicher L, Reiter R *et al.* Demonstration that temsirolimus preferentially inhibits the mTOR pathway in the tumors of prostate cancer patients with PTEN deficiencies. *AACR-NCI-EORTC International Conference on Molecular Targets and Cancer Therapeutics*, Philadelphia, PA 2005; C131 (abstract).

60. Hidalgo M, Rowinsky EK. The rapamycin-sensitive signal transduction pathway as a target for cancer therapy. *Oncogene* 2000; 19:6680–6686.

61. Raymond E, Alexandre J, Faivre S *et al.* Safety and pharmacokinetics of escalated doses of weekly intravenous infusion of CCI-779, a novel mTOR inhibitor, in patients with cancer. *J Clin Oncol* 2004; 22:2336–2347.

62. Atkins MB, Hidalgo M, Stadler WM *et al.* Randomized phase II study of multiple dose levels of CCI-779, a novel mammalian target of rapamycin kinase inhibitor, in patients with advanced refractory renal cell carcinoma. *J Clin Oncol* 2004; 22:909–918.

63. Hudes F, Carducci M, Tomczak P *et al.* A phase 3, randomized, 3-arm study of temsirolimus or interferon-alpha or the combination of TEMSR+IFN in the treatment of first-line, poor-risk patients with advanced renal cell carcinoma. *J Clin Oncol* 2006; 24(18S):LBA4 (abstract).

64. Schröder FH, Wildhagen MF. ZD1839 (gefitinib) and hormone resistant (HR) prostate cancer – final results of a double blind randomized placebo-controlled phase II study. *J Clin Oncol* 2004; 22(14S):4698 (abstract).

65. Canil CM, Moore MJ, Winquist E *et al.* Randomized phase II study of two doses of gefitinib in hormone-refractory prostate cancer: a trial of the National Cancer Institute of Canada-Clinical Trials Group. *J Clin Oncol* 2005; 23:455–460.

66. Ziada A, Barqawi A, Glode LM *et al.* The use of trastuzumab in the treatment of hormone refractory prostate cancer: phase II trial. *Prostate* 2004; 60:332–337.

67. Mellinghoff, IK, Vivanco I, Kwon A *et al.* Her2/neu kinase-dependent modulation of androgen receptor function through effects on DNA binding and stability. *Cancer Cell* 2004; 6:517–527.

68. Nelson J, Bagnato A, Battistini B *et al.* The endothelin axis: emerging role in cancer. *Nat Rev Cancer* 2003; 3:110–116.

69. Yin JJ, Mohammad KS, Kakonen SM *et al.* A causal role for endothelin-1 in the pathogenesis of osteoblastic bone metastases. *Proc Natl Acad Sci USA* 2003; 100:10954–10959.

70. Carducci M, Nelson JB, Saad F *et al.* Effects of atrasentan on disease progression and biological markers in men with metastatic hormone-refractory prostate cancer: Phase 3 study. *J Clin Oncol* 2004; 22(14S): 4508 (abstract).

71. Lassiter LK and Carducci MA. Endothelin receptor antagonists in the treatment of prostate cancer. *Sem Oncol* 2003; 30:678–688.

72. Mathew P, Thall PF, Jones D *et al.* Platelet-derived growth factor receptor inhibitor imatinib mesylate and docetaxel: a modular phase I trial in androgen-independent prostate cancer. *J Clin Oncol* 2004; 22:3323–3329.

73. Mathew P, Thall PF, Johnson MM *et al.* Preliminary results of a randomized placebo controlled double-blind trial of weekly docetaxel combined with imatinib in men with androgen independent metastatic prostate cancer and bone metastases. *J Clin Oncol* 24; 18S:4562 (abstract).

74. Webster WS, Small EJ, Rini BI, and Kwon ED. Prostate cancer immunology: biology, therapeutics, and challenges. *J Clin Oncol* 2005; 23:8262–8269.

75. Burch PA, Croghan GA, Gastineau DA *et al.* Immunotherapy (APC8015, Provenge®) targeting prostatic acid phosphatase can induce durable remission of metastatic androgen-independent prostate cancer: a phase 2 trial. *Prostate* 2004; 60:197–204.

76. Small EJ, Schellhammer PF, Higano CS *et al.* Results of a placebo-controlled phase III trial of immuno-therapy with APC8015 for patients with hormone refractory prostate cancer. *J Clin Oncol* 2005; 23(16S): 4500 (abstract).

77. Dranoff G, Jaffee E, Lazenby A *et al.* Vaccination with irradiated tumor cells engineered to secrete murine granulocyte-macrophage colony-stimulating factor stimulates potent, specific, and long-lasting immunity. *Proc Natl Acad Sci USA* 1993; 90:3539–3543.

78. Vieweg J, Rosenthal FM, Bannerji R *et al.* Immunotherapy of prostate cancer in the Dunning rat model: use of cytokine gene modified tumor vaccines. *Cancer Res* 1994; 54:1760–1765.

79. Simons J, Higano C, Corman J *et al.* A phase I/II trial of high dose allogeneic GMCSF gene-transduced prostate cancer cell line vaccine in patients with metastatic hormone-refractory prostate cancer. *J Clin Oncol* 2003; 22:667 (abstract).

80. Small E, Higano C, Smith D *et al.* A phase 2 study of an allogeneic GMCSF gene-transduced prostate cancer cell line vaccine in patients with metastatic hormone-refractory prostate cancer (HRPC). *J Clin Oncol* 2004; 22(14S):4565 (abstract).

81. Kaufman HL, Wang W, Manola J *et al.* Phase II randomized study of vaccine treatment of advanced prostate cancer (E7897): a trial of the Easter Cooperative Oncology Group. *J Clin Oncol* 2004; 22:2122–2132.

82. Richman CM, Denardo SJ, O'Donnell RT *et al.* Combined modality radioimmunotherapy in metastatic prostate cancer and breast cancer using paclitaxel and a MUC-1 monoclonal antibody, m170, linked to yttrium-90: a phase I trial. *J Clin Oncol* 2004; 22:2554 (abstract).

83. Hurwitz AA, Foster BA, Kwon ED *et al.* Combination immunotherapy of primary prostate cancer in a transgenic mouse model using CTLA-4 blockade. *Cancer Res* 2000; 60:2444–2448.

84. Vijayakumar S, Mehta RR, and Boerner PS. Clinical trials involving vitamin D analogues in prostate cancer. *Cancer J* 2005; 11:362–373.

85. Peehl DM, Skowronski RJ, Leung GK *et al.* Antiproliferative effects of 1,25-dihydroxyvitamin D3 on primary cultures of human prostatic cells. *Cancer Res* 1994; 54:805–810.

86. Beer TM, Eilers KM, Garzotto M *et al.* Weekly high-dose calcitriol and docetaxel in metastatic androgen-independent prostate cancer. *J Clin Oncol* 2003; 21:123–128.

87. Beer TM, Ryan CW, Venner PM *et al.* Interim results from ASCENT: a double-blinded randomized study of DN-101 (high dose calcitriol) plus docetaxel in androgen-independent prostate cancer. *J Clin Oncol* 2005; 23(16S):4516 (abstract).

88. Kopelovich L, Crowell JA, Fay JR. The epigenome as a target for cancer chemoprevention. *J Natl Cancer Inst* 2003; 95:1747–1757.

89. Gilbert J, Gore SD, Herman JG *et al.* The clinical application of targeting cancer through histone acetylation and hypomethylation. *Clin Cancer Res* 2004; 10:4589–4596.

90. Carducci MA, Gilbert J, Bowling MK *et al.* A phase I clinical and pharmacologic evaluation of sodium phenylbutyrate in patients with refractory solid tumor malignancies. *Clin Cancer Res* 2001; 7:3047–3055.

91. Kristeleit R, Fong P, Aherne GW, de Bono J. Histone deacetylase inhibitors: emerging anticancer therapeutic targets? *Clin Lung Cancer* 2005; 7 (Suppl 1):S19–30.

92. Kelly WK, O'Connor OA, Krug LM *et al.* Phase I study of an oral histone deacetylase inhibitor suberoylanilide hydroxamic acid, in patients with advanced cancer. *J Clin Oncol* 2005; 23:3923–3931.

93. Pili R, Rudek M, Altiok S *et al.* Phase I study pharmacokinetic and pharmacodynamic study of the histone deacetylase inhibitor MS-275 in combination with 13-cis retinoic acid in patients with advanced solid tumors. *J Clin Oncol* 24; 18S:3055 (abstract).

94. Mita M, Tolcher AW. Novel apoptosis inducing agents in cancer therapy. *Curr Probl Cancer* 2005; 29:8–32.

95. Huang H, Cheville JC, Pan Y *et al.* PTEN induces chemosensitivity in PTEN-mutated prostate cancer cells by suppression of bcl-2. *J Biol Chem* 2001; 276:38830–38836.

96. Tolcher AW, Chi K, Kuhn J *et al.* A phase II, pharmacokinetic, and biological correlative study of oblimersen sodium and docetaxel in patients with hormone-refractory prostate cancer. *Clin Cancer Res* 2005; 11:3854–3861.

97. Beer TM, Ryan CW, Venner PM *et al.* Intermittent chemotherapy in metastatic androgen-independent prostate cancer: initial results from ASCENT. *J Clin Oncol* 2006; 24(18S):4518 (abstract).

98. Glode LM, Barqawi A, Crighton F *et al.* Metronomic therapy with cyclophosphamide and dexamethasone for prostate carcinoma. *Cancer* 2003; 98:1643–1648.

99. Kerbel RS, Kamen BA. The antiangiogenic basis of metronomic chemotherapy. *Nat Rev Cancer* 2004; 4:423–436.

100. Sternberg CN, Hetherington J, Paluchowska PHTJ *et al.* Randomized phase III trial of a new oral platinum, Satraplatin (JM-216) plus prednisone or prednisone alone in patients with hormone refractory prostate cancer. *J Clin Oncol* 2003; 22:1586 (abstract).

101. Goodin S, Kane MP, Rubin EH. Epothilones: mechanism of action and biologic activity. *J Clin Oncol* 2004; 22:2105–2125.

102. Hussain M, Faulkner J, Vaishampayan U *et al.* Epothilone B analogueue BMS-247550 administered every 21 days in patients with hormone refractory prostate cancer. A Southwest Oncology Group Study (S0111). *J Clin Oncol* 2004; 22(14S):4510 (abstract).

103. Synold TW, Morgan RJ, Newman EM *et al.* A phase I pharmacokinetic and target validation study of the novel anti-tubulin agent E7389: a California Cancer Consortium trial. *J Clin Oncol* 2005; 23(16S): 3036 (abstract).
104. Henry MD, Wen S, Silva MD *et al.* A prostate-specific membrane antigen-targeted monoclonal antibody-chemotherapy conjugate designed for the treatment of prostate cancer. *Cancer Res* 2004; 64:7995–8001.
105. Bander NH, Nanus DM, Milowsky MI *et al.* Targeted systemic therapy of prostate cancer with a monoclonal antibody to prostate-specific membrane antigen. *Semin Oncol* 2003; 30:667–677.
106. Milowsky MI, Nanus DM, Kostakoglu L *et al.* Phase I trial of yttrium-90–labeled anti–prostate specific membrane antigen monoclonal antibody J591 for androgen-independent prostate cancer. *J Clin Oncol* 2004; 22:1–10.
107. Henry MD, Wen S, Silva MD *et al.* A prostate-specific membrane antigen-targeted monoclonal antibody-chemotherapeutic conjugate designed for the treatment of prostate cancer. *Cancer Res* 2004; 64:7995–8001.
108. Scott, AM. Radioimmunotherapy of prostate cancer: does tumor size matter? *J Clin Oncol* 2005; 23:4567–4569.

13

Molecular strategies and clinical trial design in the treatment of advanced prostate cancer

Don Newling

INTRODUCTION

With a heightening awareness of the molecular signalling pathways responsible for the development and progression of prostate cancer has come a paradigm shift in the identification of targets for new therapeutic endeavours. The use of targeted therapies at different stages of the disease is leading to new concepts in how the activity of these agents may be measured in terms of the design of clinical trials and the progression of the use of new molecules from the laboratory setting to the clinic.

In recent years the pivotal role of the androgen receptor in prostate cancer progression has been confirmed [1] (Figure 13.1). In the hormone-sensitive disease stages the receptor is stimulated by androgens and possibly also by oestrogens and other steroid molecules, whereas in the more advanced disease, particularly in the so-called hormone-refractory state, the androgen receptor at very low levels of androgen is stimulated by a series of growth factors and cytokines.

The hope for the future is the identification of specific targets at different stages of the disease and in individual patients, which will lead to tailored therapy for prostate cancer, an

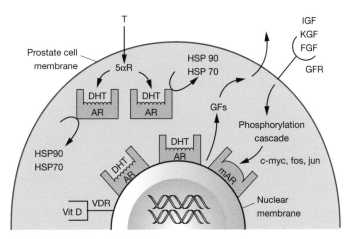

Figure 13.1 The role of the androgen receptor (AR).

Don Newling, MBBChir. FRCS, Medical Director (Urology), AstraZeneca, Alderley Park, Macclesfield, UK

important step on the way to truly personalized medicine [2]. In order to establish the value of an individual therapy it is important to be certain that at a given clinical stage of prostate cancer or even in a particular cancer that the target for that new therapy is present, that the expression of that target is a reflection of the disease process and that therefore a proof of principle and proof of concept will undoubtedly be followed by a specific and beneficial therapeutic effect for a given treatment [3].

Prostate cancer is a heterogeneous tumour and, because of this, it is likely that identification of a single target and therapeutic inhibition of that target will not result in complete ablation of a tumour. Rather, targeted therapies will be used in conjunction with other more established therapeutic options in combination therapy, a more multidisciplinary approach to the management of this disease.

UNDERSTANDING THE BIOLOGY OF PROSTATE CANCER

As the prostate gland is a secondary sexual organ, rather like the breast, proliferating epithelium is largely under the control of hormones produced by the primary sex organ, the testicle. In addition, androgenic hormones are produced by the adrenal gland and converted in the periphery to testosterone. The androgens arrive on the prostate cell in the bloodstream bound to sex hormone-binding globulin. On reaching the prostate epithelium, testosterone diffuses passively into the cytoplasm of the cell where it is converted to dihydrotestosterone by 5-alpha-reductase. This more active androgen attaches to the androgen receptor and, by a process of dimerization, sheds heat shock proteins and binds to the nucleosome and via activation of the androgen response element the process of proliferation starts. At the same time, in the stroma of the prostate, the arrival of testosterone stimulates the production of peptide growth factors, which diffuse out of stromal cells and alight on their own specific receptors on the epithelial cell. By this completely independent pathway in every prostate cancer there is an element of a hormone-unresponsive, i.e. hormone-refractory, cell line. After androgen withdrawal as a therapeutic option by surgical or medical castration, the androgen receptor becomes sensitive to the same growth factors as well as to other agents, such as cytokines, in order for the proliferation of the epithelial cell to be maintained. A number of cofactors, proteins, need to be available and their presence seems to be necessary both in the hormone-sensitive and hormone-refractory state [4].

Many growth factors have been identified as being of significance in the development of prostate cancer. Amongst these are vascular endothelial growth factor (VEGF), platelet-derived growth factor (PDGF), insulin-like growth factor (IGF) and the endothelin growth factor. Even when the appropriate growth factor pathway is inhibited, there are what are described as survival pathways within the prostate epithelial cells involving a number of kinases and the PTEN, Akt and mTOR pathways; so even when the hormones are removed, the androgen receptor is blocked and the growth factor receptors are inhibited in one way or another, there is still a mechanism for prostate cancer cells to survive. There is increasing evidence that the cells make use of the *myc* oncogene pathway and the hedgehog transcription pathway [5].

TARGETING THE ANDROGEN RECEPTOR

Since the end of the nineteenth century, castration has been used as a treatment for the management of an enlarged prostate gland. Here, although the androgen receptor remains intact, with the source of androgens removed, it is less active. The androgens from the adrenal gland can also be surgically removed by carrying out an adrenalectomy or even hypophysectomy [6].

Since the late 1970s, androgen receptor antagonists have been available that inhibit the activation of the receptor and, therefore, proliferation of the epithelium by blocking the receptor at the cellular level. The androgen receptor is active in almost all tissues of the body and by blocking it, the action of the androgens elsewhere is also inhibited. Because testosterone levels are not diminished by androgen receptor antagonists, the changes associated with castration such as loss of body strength, of cognitive facility and of bone mineral density do not occur. Unfortunately, because testosterone tends to rise with the use of an androgen receptor antagonist, there is a conversion peripherally to oestrogens which gives rise to the important side effect of non-steroidal antiandrogen treatment of gynaecomastia [7].

The effects of these traditional methods of androgen suppression leave the androgen receptor intact and available for stimulation by non-hormonal sources such as growth factors and cytokines. Recent studies have shown that, contrary to what was formerly believed, progression after androgen ablation is accompanied by up-regulation and increased expression of the androgen receptor, which makes it more sensitive to stimulation by very small amounts of androgens as well as non-androgens as described above. In addition to the androgenic ligand or non-androgenic ligand, the androgen receptor requires the presence of a number of cofactors such as cofactors A and R and heat shock proteins to activate the transcription pathways leading to proliferation, apoptosis inhibition and secretion of proteins such as prostate-specific antigen (PSA).

Comparative microarray analyses have shown an increased expression of enzymes involved in steroid precursor synthesis pathways in castration-resistant tumours in comparison with castration-sensitive tumours. The genes involved in fatty acid and steroid metabolism are also up-regulated. These findings suggest sources of steroids, albeit small compared with the combined production of the testes and adrenals but which, in the presence of an up-regulated androgen receptor, may well be adequate to maintain ligand-dependent stimulation of prostate cancer after castration therapy. Furthermore, mechanisms involving the sequestration of androgen molecules by the production of steroid hormone-binding globulin by prostate epithelial and stromal cells will further support the continued ligand-bound androgen receptor stimulation [8].

The ideal inhibition of the activities of the androgen receptor would be its destruction or complete down-regulation. Compounds causing oestrogen receptor down-regulation are now in widespread clinical use and work is still ongoing to develop a selective androgen receptor down-regulator (SARD). Such a targeted therapy would remove the androgen receptor not only from the influence of androgens but also in the so-called hormone-refractory state from the influence of growth factors and cytokines [9].

Recent work by Bhattacharyya *et al.* [10] has shown that the oestrogen receptor down-regulator fulverstrant down-regulates androgen receptor expression and diminishes androgenic responses in human prostate cancer cell lines. This may indicate that the androgen receptor has mutated in such a way that the oestrogenic moiety in fulverstrant can bind to it or that, fortuitously, this molecule has found an alternative binding site to the ligand-binding domain on the androgen receptor from where it is able to bring about down-regulation. Inhibition of the activities of cofactors with antisense oligonucleotides and the antibiotic geldanamycin, which suppresses the functional maturation of heat shock protein substrates, are other approaches under investigation for the reduction of androgen receptor expression [11].

INHIBITING THE GROWTH FACTOR PATHWAYS

Growth factor inhibition may be achieved by producing monoclonal antibodies to the growth factor itself and thereby binding it in the blood before it reaches its own receptor, the development of antibodies to the receptor itself or by blocking the transcription process, the beginning of the phosphorylation cascade following arrival of the growth factor on its receptor. Identification of the transcription processes distal to the receptor activation has led to the identification of other agents that can block a particular pathway at a more distal level (Figures 13.2 and 13.3). The growth factors particularly involved in hormone-refractory prostate cancer (HRPC) proliferation are VEGF, PDGF and the IGF pathway (Table 13.1).

In addition, the endothelin axis seems to be particularly important in prostate cancer. The two receptors for endothelin 1 are strongly expressed in prostate cancer. Overall, inhibition of these receptors gives rise to inhibition of proliferation of the cells and a proapoptotic pathway activation leading to accelerated programmed cell death. In addition, inhibition of endothelin receptor A prevents osteoblastosis, a process that occurs in prostate cancer secondary deposits in bone. It also has a positive and beneficial effect on the appreciation of pain

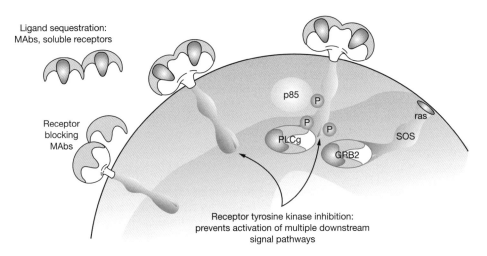

Figure 13.2

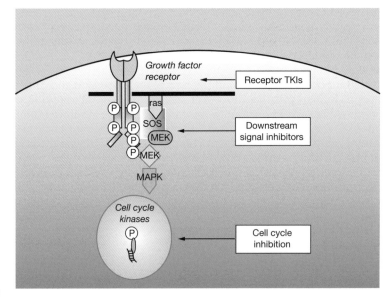

Figure 13.3

Figure 13.2 and **Figure 13.3**   Different approaches to inhibition of growth factor signalling and the downstream transcription processes including cell cycle inhibition.

Table 13.1   Major growth factors in prostate cancer proliferation

Family	Members
IGF	IGF I, II and insulin
PDGF	PDGF AA, AB and BB
EGF	EGF, TGF alpha, pox virus growth factor and amphiregulin
TGF	TGF beta 1–5, BMP 2–6, inhibin A and B
FGF	FGFa, FGFb, FGF5 and 6, and KGF
VEGF	VEGF1, VEGF2 and VEGF3
Endothelins	E1, E2 and E3

BMP, bone morphogenic protein; EGF, epidermal growth factor; FGF, fibroblast growth factor; IGF, insulin-like growth factor; KGF, keratinocyte growth factor; PDGF, platelet-derived growth factor; TGF, transforming growth factor; VEGF vascular endothelial growth factor.

due to bony metastases. Stimulation of the endothelin receptor B, on the other hand, causes apoptosis and also reduces pain by increasing the production of endorphins. Considerable work is in progress to develop a specific, selective endothelin receptor A antagonist that has no effect on the endothelin B axis and would, therefore, have marked beneficial results at all stages of prostate cancer (Figure 13.4) [12].

CELL CYCLE INHIBITION

In the past, classical chemotherapy and radiotherapy have been the means of inhibiting normal progression of cell cycling and proliferation. Both applications are effective but cause widespread damage to normal tissues, adjacent to the irradiated area in the case of radiotherapy and to regions of necessary high cell turnover, such as the gut and bone marrow, in the case of chemotherapy. A deeper knowledge of the different steps in the cell cycle and more precise detailing of the mechanics of mitosis have led to the development of more accurate targeting of stages in the cell cycle that can be identified in malignant cells but that occur less frequently in normal cells. The formation of the mitotic spindle is just such a process that occurs at increased frequency in rapidly dividing cells and can be inhibited by cytotoxic compounds like the taxanes or estramustine. Both these treatment options have found

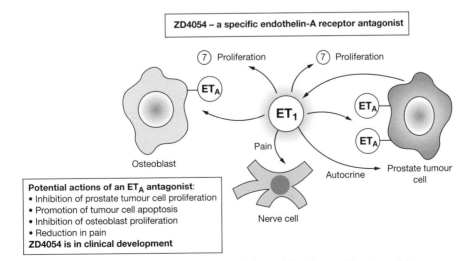

Figure 13.4   The endothelin axis in prostate cancer and the activity of a specific antagonist.

a place in the management of advanced prostate cancer, but both compounds do affect normally dividing cells, giving rise to less frequent, but similar, side-effects as traditional chemotherapy. Recently, more selective cell cycle inhibitors have been identified that inhibit the cell cycle kinases responsible for the build-up of DNA and protein synthesis. More selective than spindle formation inhibitors and traditional chemotherapeutics, these compounds have not yet the specificity necessary to only attack the malignant phenotype. The identification of another group of nuclear enzymes that play a highly significant role in mitosis and are dramatically overexpressed in malignant cells holds promise for more specific cell cycle inhibition. The aurora kinases are responsible for the activation of kinetochores – nuclear inclusions that direct the pattern of DNA distribution along the mitotic spindle. Inhibition of this process leads to overproduction of DNA molecules, which leads to cytostasis and cell death, but almost exclusively in malignant cells [13].

DNA instability is a hallmark of the malignant phenotype. Grossly abnormal nuclear aberrations are not compatible with cell survival. Less severe aberrations activate various DNA repair mechanisms within the cell that allow cell survival, but frequently with a propensity for uncontrolled proliferation. Inhibition of the enzymes responsible for these repair processes such as chK kinases and the PARP enzymes will interrupt the survival pathway and the abnormal cells will die [14].

THE VITAMIN D AXIS

In addition to the androgens and other steroid molecules and their receptors, the secosteroid 1,25-dihydroxyvitamin D3 and its receptors play a role in the growth and function of the normal and neoplastic prostate. Initial studies were of an epidemiological nature, linking observations of the high incidence of prostate cancer with low levels of vitamin D in the elderly, in Afro–Caribbeans, in Scandinavians and in migrant Asians who adopt a Western diet [15]. Vitamin D appears to exert its antiproliferative effects through a membrane-associated receptor and a nuclear receptor. The membrane-associated receptor may be linked to the IGF pathway. In the absence of the vitamin D ligand, the nuclear receptor dimerizes with a retinoic acid receptor to stimulate proliferation [16]. A number of polymorphisms in the gene coding for the nuclear receptor have been associated with varying levels of prostate cancer risk [17]. Experimentally, vitamin D has been shown to reduce the invasive potential of DU-145 cells in matrigel cultures as well as to reduce the metastatic potential of *in vivo* cultures [18]. Vitamin D analogues are now being developed that will inhibit the vitamin D receptor-stimulated proliferation of prostate epithelial cells, while not giving rise to the hypercalcaemia that occurred with earlier derivatives. It is presumed that management of prostate cancer with vitamin D analogues will probably be most beneficial in early disease and they may even be used in the prophylaxis of clinical cancer [19]. At the present time, however, the initial search for efficacy is directed against hormone-refractory disease, alongside taxotere combination therapy.

THE PREVENTION OF METASTASES

If DNA instability and uncontrolled cellular proliferation is one hallmark of malignancy, then invasion and metastatic potential is another. For this potential to be optimized, there needs to be alterations both within the malignant cell and in its normal relationships with neighbouring cells in the tissue. The normal epithelial cell has a well-defined cytoskeleton that maintains its rigidity and its close relation and adherence to surrounding structures, such as other epithelial cells and the basement membrane of the tissue. These cellular interfaces are preserved by the cadherin/catenin axis along with a group of molecules called integrins. During the development of the malignant phenotype, the cytoskeleton fails to be established, which increases the mobility and fluidity of the cells and disrupts the normal cell-to-cell and cell-to-basement membrane adherence. This allows the now malleable cell to break away from its surrounding structures and to invade through tissue planes. The next step in the metastatic process is entry into the surrounding neovasculature which, under the influence of VEGF and other growth factors, is leaky and allows invasion of the malignant cells through the endothelium and into the vessel lumen. The process is aided and abetted by the matrix metalloproteinases which, in turn, are up-regulated via the endothelin axis along with VEGF.

The establishment of the cytoskeleton and the maintenance of the integrity of cell/cell and cell/basement membrane relationships are under the control of a number of enzymatic pathways. Among the most important of these is the Src/Abl kinase pathway. Inhibitors of these non-membrane-bound tyrosine kinases are now entering phase II/III trials [20].

IMMUNOTHERAPY AND GENE THERAPY

The fact that malignant cells with their aberrant behaviour produce peptides and proteins not found in normal cells has long been recognized. Why such proteins do not give rise to a significant immune response in all cases has long puzzled oncologists. The explanation is probably complex and almost certainly varies from tumour to tumour. In some cases, the steadily increasing trickle of antigens into the bloodstream may cause immune paralysis, such as is seen in certain infectious situations. Alternatively, there may be a shift in the balance of cytokines as a result of the presence of the malignancy or a masking of the major histocompatibility complex molecules that thwarts the antigen presenting cells. However, spontaneous remissions of certain tumours do occur and, over the years, it has been repeatedly observed that when this happens there is often a significant infiltration of the primary tumour with tumour-infiltrating lymphocytes (TILs), suggesting a significant type II immune response.

Early attempts at immunotherapy in prostate cancer using antibodies to PSA and prostate-specific membrane antigen (PSMA), even with the addition of cytokine soups, rarely got further than small phase II studies and responses were anecdotal rather than of statistical significance. Presenting tumour-associated antigens with adjuvants such as BCG with or without TILs and cytokines, was only marginally more successful as the 'foreign' proteins gave rise to such a brisk type I immune response that the antigens did not stay around long enough for a type II response to be mounted [21].

Two vaccine therapies that show much more promising results have recently almost completed phase III studies. The first is an autologous vaccine against prostate acid phosphatase (PAP) produced in a recombinant form and administered as an infusion three times over a 4-week period. In patients with HRPC, there appear to be survival benefits compared to placebo. The other compound is an allogeneic vaccine produced from two prostate cancer cell lines, HP3 and LNCaP, that have been engineered to produce granulocyte–macrophage colony-stimulating factor (GMCSF). This vaccine is being compared with standard chemotherapy, and in combination with chemotherapy against chemotherapy alone [22].

The lack of consistency of abnormal gene expression and the heterogeneity of the majority of clinical prostate cancers has complicated the search for an effective gene therapy for this disease. Initial efforts at replacing mutated tumour-suppressor genes, such as p53, Rb and p21, with transfected wild types were hampered by immune responses to the viral vectors and low percentages of successful subsequent expression. The introduction of oncolytic viruses have, thus far, resulted in their attachment to normal tissues and unacceptable side-effects. Antisense gene therapy using a transfect with a viral or non-viral vector of genes that is highly expressed in aggressive cancers, e.g. transforming growth factor (TGF) beta or bcl-2, is an exciting possibility which is being explored in a variety of phase I studies at the present time. The above techniques require high rates of efficient transfection to be successful and, thus far, this has proved difficult [23]. An alternative methodology has been developed involving the so-called suicide genes which may circumvent these difficulties. The underlying principle of this technique is the conversion of a prodrug to a cytotoxic agent after transfection of the cancer cell with a transgene. Destruction of the transfected cell is accompanied by a significant bystander effect, which means that not all cells have to be transfected. The herpes simplex virus thymidine kinase gene is one such gene that phosphorylates the prodrug ganciclovir converting it to a false-base and inhibiting DNA polymerase. Other genes are under investigation together with PSA promoters and enhancer sequences. The majority of these gene therapies require direct injection into the prostate tumour and, as yet, remain in phase I or early phase II development [24].

CLINICAL TRIALS – NEW APPROACHES

As was mentioned in the introduction, the new targeted therapies inhibiting growth factor pathways and transcription pathways are going to become part of a more holistic approach to prostate cancer. Once the molecular identification of an individual tumour has been carried out by scrupulous histological examination and immunohistocytochemical evaluation of possible targets, then a cocktail of treatments will be necessary. These may be given sequentially or simultaneously, depending on the necessity of urgent therapy. As with all approaches to malignancies, the smaller the target the better chance there is that it will be eliminated. In localized prostate cancer surgical extirpation of the prostate gland or even of the tumour itself will result in cure in a very high proportion of cases. In more advanced cases, we know that the combination of radiotherapy and early hormonal therapy can result in cure; where cure is not necessarily the complete removal of all vestiges of the tumour but may simply be control of the tumour for long enough for the patient to have a normal lifespan and die of unrelated causes. Here, cure is synonymous with control of the tumour. When tumour presents at a more advanced stage, it may still be beneficial to try and ablate the primary tumour in order to debulk the tumour mass and make the residual tumour more amenable to simple therapies, i.e. novel targeted therapy.

The use of therapeutic manoeuvres in early stage disease is bedevilled in prostate cancer by the fact that the majority of patients will have multiple therapies during the life cycle of the disease and, therefore, the influence of a given therapy administered early is unlikely to impact on overall survival and unlikely to give rise to a registerable option in early stage disease.

PSA is a correlate of prostate cancer activity but not a true surrogate. However, in early stage disease after prostatectomy, delay of the reappearance of PSA in comparison with placebo therapy would be an indication of tumour treatment efficacy. In more advanced disease, PSA doubling time (PSADT) is an indication of tumour activity; again, not so far accepted as a registerable endpoint but nevertheless an important clinical endpoint, that determines therapeutic options for the clinician. In more advanced disease, the evaluation of compounds is still limited by conflicting comorbidities in this elderly population. Progression-free survival, an important clinical endpoint, is now used as an indication of treatment efficacy although, once more, it remains a non-registerable endpoint as far the regulatory authorities are concerned. One very important clinical step on the road to prostate cancer mortality is the appearance of metastases. This is an important determinate of changes in clinical activity such as a change of therapy but, because it is not a true surrogate for survival, is not accepted as a registerable endpoint.

With acceptance of the feasibility of using intermittent hormone ablation in the management of advanced disease, there comes the option of introducing novel therapies in the interval between cycles of hormone treatment; compared with placebo this would also be an indication of efficacy of a compound by postponing the subsequent reintroduction of hormone therapy and the rise in PSA that precedes it [25].

CONCLUSIONS

The 'holy grail' of management of prostate cancer will be the personalization of treatment options based on histological, cytological and biochemical evaluation of primary tumours, metastases and the patient as a whole. Such a patient evaluation will enable individual therapy programmes to be designed, which will be maximally effective and minimally intrusive, protecting the patient's quality of life while, hopefully, increasing its length.

There needs to be a radical rethink of the design and performance of clinical trials in this disease if we are going to optimize the progress that has been made in our understanding of its molecular biology.

REFERENCES

1. Scher Hi, Buchanan G, Gerald W *et al.* Targeting the androgen receptor: improving outcomes for castrate resistant prostate cancer. *Endocrine Related Cancer* 2004; 11:459–476.
2. Eaton CL, Davies P, Phillips ME. Growth factor involvement and oncogene expression in prostatic tumours. *J Steroid Biochem* 1988; 30:341–345.
3. Koutsilieris M, Dimopoulos MA, Doillon C *et al.* The molecular concept of prostate cancer. *Cancer* 1996; 9:89–94.
4. Griffiths K, Morton MS, Aspects of the cell biology of prostate cancer. In: Kaisary AV, Murphy GP, Denis L, Griffiths K eds. *Text Book of Prostate Cancer Pathology, Diagnosis and Treatment.* Martin Dunitz, London, 1999, pp. 51–75.
5. Bissonnette RP, Echeverri F, Mahboubi A *et al.* Apoptotic cell death induced by c-myc is inhibited by bcl-2. *Nature* 1992; 359:552–554.
6. Newling D, Fossa SD, Andersson L *et al.* Assessment of hormone refractory prostate cancer. *Urology* 1997; 49:46–53.
7. Iversen P, Tyrell CJ, Kaisary AV *et al.* Casodex (bicalutamide) 150-mg monotherapy compared with castration in patients with previously untreated nonmetastatic prostate cancer: results from two multicenter randomized trials at a median follow-up of 4 years. *Urology* 1998; 51:389–396.
8. Gregory CW, Hamil KG, Kim D *et al.* Androgen receptor expression in androgen-independent prostate cancer is associated with increased expression of androgen-regulated genes. *Cancer Res* 1998; 58: 5718–5724.
9. Culig Z, Hobisch A, Cronauer MV *et al.* Regulation of prostatic growth and function by peptide growth factors. *Prostate* 1996; 28:392–405.
10. Bhattacharyya RS. Krishnan AV , Swami S, Feldman D. Fulvestrant (ICI 182, 780) down-regulates androgen receptor expression and diminishes androgenic responses in LNCaP human prostate cancer cells. *Mol Cancer Ther* 2006; 5:1539-1549.
11. Grenert JP, Sullivan WP, Fadden P *et al.* The amino-terminal domain of heatshock protein 90(hsp90) that binds geldanamycin is an ATP/ADP switch domain that regulates hsp90 confirmation. *J Biol Chem* 1997; 272: 23843–23850.
12. Nelson JB, Chan-Tack K, Hedican SP *et al.* Endothelin-1 production and decreased enothelin B receptor expression in advanced prostate cancer. *Cancer Res* 1996; 56:663–668.
13. Rieder CL, Khodjakov A. Mitosis through the microscope: advances in seeing inside live dividing cells. *Science* 2003; 300(5616):91–96.
14. Zhou BB, Bartek J. Targeting the checkpoint kinases: chemosensitization versus chemoprotection. *Nat Rev Cancer* 2004; 4:216–225.
15. Schwartz GG, Hulka BS. Is vitamin D deficiency a risk factor for prostate carcinoma (hypothesis). *Anticancer Res* 1990; 10(5A):1307–1311.
16. Strugnell SA, Deluca HF. The vitamin D receptor-structure and transcriptional activation. *Pro Soc Exp Biol Med* 1997; 215:223–228.
17. Hustmyer FG , Deluca HF, Peacock M. ApaI, BsmI, EcoRV and TaqI polymorphisms at the human vitamin D receptor gene locus in Caucasians, Blacks and Asians. *Hum Mol Genet* 1993; 2:487.
18. Schwarta GG, Lokeshwar BL, Selzer M *et al.* 1,25-dihydroxyvitamin D and EB1089 inhibit prostate cancer metastasis in vivo. In: *Vitamin D: Chemistry, Biology and Clinical Applications of the Steroid Hormone.* University of California Press, Riverside, 1997, pp. 489–490.

19. Blumenfield AJ, Fleshner N. Casselman B *et al.* Nutritional aspects of prostate cancer: a review. *Can J Urol* 2000; 7:927–935; discussion 936.

20. Hennequin, LF, Allen J, Costello GF *et al.* The discovery of AZD0530: a novel oral highly selective and dual-specific inhibitor of the Src and Abl family kinases. *Proceedings of the American Association for Cancer Research*, Anaheim, CA 2005; 2537 (abstract).

21. Patel B, Belldegrun A. Gene and immune-based therapy for prostate cancer. In: *New Perspective in Prostate Cancer*. Belldegrun A, Kirby RS, Newling DWW eds. ISIS Medical, Oxford 2000, pp. 273–285.

22. Corman JM, Small E, Smith D *et al.* Immunotherapy with GVAX Vaccine for prostate cancer improves predicted survival in metastatic hormone refractory prostate cancer: results from two phase 2 studies. *J Urol* 2006; 175:976 (abstract).

23. Sanda MG. Biological principles and clinical development of prostate cancer gene therapy. *Semin Urol Oncol* 1997; 15:43.

24. Hall SJ, Mutchnik SE, Chan Sh *et al.* Adenovirus-mediated herpes simplex virus thymidine kinase gene and ganciclovir therapy leads to systemic activity against spontaneous and induced metastasis in an orthotopic mouse model of prostate cancer. *Int J Cancer* 1997; 70:183–187.

25. De Reijke THM, Collette L. EORTC prostate cancer trials: what have we learnt? *Crit Rev Oncol Hematol* 2002; 43:159–165.

14

Therapeutic strategies of palliative care and quality of life for advanced prostate cancer

Christopher Farnham, Omar Al-Salihi, Faye Lim

INTRODUCTION

Managing patients with advanced prostate cancer is a challenge to all members of the multidisciplinary team. These patients often have numerous problems – physical, social and psychological. It is all too easy to lose sight of the bigger picture – that of improving the patient's quality of life and treating symptoms without increasing the patient's morbidity.

WHY PALLIATIVE CARE?

Palliative care has traditionally been the active total care of patients whose disease is not being treated with a curative intent [1]. However, this can now be applied as an approach at all stages of the patient's journey. This approach has been recognized in the UK by National Institute for Clinical Excellence (NICE) guidance [2] in urological cancers and in the publication of *Improving Outcomes in Urological Cancers Manual* and *Improving Supportive and Palliative Care for Adults with Cancer Manual*.

Palliative care as an approach looks at the individual and uses a multidisciplinary approach to providing care either in the person's home, in hospital or in the hospice. It focuses on quality of life as well as symptom control.

This chapter is written from the perspectives of both the oncologist and palliative care physician and hopes to put the message across that symptom control should be part of the patient's journey from the point of diagnosis to death. Symptom control should be the responsibility of all members of the multidisciplinary team and primary care team. Where the treatment occurs should be determined by patient choice.

We aim to give an overview of the treatment strategies available to treat the common symptoms of advanced prostate cancer. It is important that they are used appropriately and at the right time as the window of opportunity may be narrow.

Carcinoma of the prostate is now the second most common cause of cancer death in the UK for men [3], and it is anticipated that this will increase with an aging population. In this group, 60% will have advanced disease when they are first seen [4] and this translates into symptoms. As with many cancers the disease can take on a chronic pattern with good hormonal control but, because of patient age, there are often a multitude of other medical problems that also need to be treated actively.

Christopher Farnham, MB BS BSc FRCP, Consultant in Palliative Care, St John's Hospice, Hospital of St John and St Elizabeth, London, UK
Omar Al-Salihi, BSc MBBS MRcP FRCR, Consultant Oncologist, University College London Hospital, London, UK
Faye Lim, MBBS BSc MRCP, Specialist Registrar in Oncology, University College London Hospital, London, UK

Treatments are changing for prostate carcinoma, but they remain essentially palliative in nature and they often cause a raft of side-effects that need to be palliated themselves. Data looking at prostate cancer deaths showed that 61% of patients needed palliative interventions (radiation, urological intervention) before death and that, on average, they spent 5 weeks in hospital [6]. This shows that the use of acute services is high for this group. However, separate data shows that the same group are the third most common being referred to hospital-based palliative care services, have the third longest survival and the oldest age of death. In addition they have the third highest use of inpatient palliative services. Clearly this significant use of health resources should be considered in the planning of healthcare strategies [7].

Palliative care has been shown to be effective in this patient group for both continuity and cost-effectiveness [8].

PALLIATION FROM DIAGNOSIS TO DEATH

As stated earlier, the treatment of symptoms should start at the point of diagnosis. We have roughly divided the symptoms experienced by patients into three categories – generic, prostate-/treatment-specific and end of life symptoms. As physicians, it is important to monitor the changes in symptoms with cancer progression and adapt our treatments accordingly.

GENERIC SYMPTOMS

The patient with cancer of the prostate can experience a wide range of symptoms.

GENERAL PAIN

Pain is a common symptom in all patients with cancer [9] and men with prostatic cancer are no different. An approach to pain that divides it up into four domains is helpful. These are:

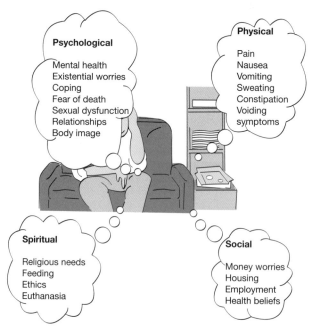

Figure 14.1 The four domains of pain [10].

physical, psychological, social and spiritual [10] (Figure 14.1). These constitute a concept of 'total pain', where considering one element alone leads to inadequate pain treatment.

An example of this was a man dying of prostate cancer with metastatic back pain that was poorly controlled with oral opioids. However, having made his will and seen his newly born grandson, his pain scores significantly reduced on the same analgesic regime.

When approaching the management of cancer pain it is important to assess the cause of the pain and treat this, if appropriate. Treatment may include radiotherapy, bisphospho-nates or renal stenting.

The aim of pain relief should be as follows:

1   Take a detailed pain history.
2   Identify what is the cause of the pain.
3   Identify if this is a somatic or a neuropathic pain.
4   Identify if this is likely to be an opioid-responsive pain.

Then apply the WHO analgesic ladder [10] to decide the best analgesic regime (Figure 14.2).

PAIN DUE TO BONE METASTASIS

The Role of Radiotherapy

Radiotherapy plays an important role in the palliation of bone pain secondary to bone metas-tasis [11–13]; it is especially useful in controlling incident pain [11, 12]. Up to 65% of patients with bone disease suffer from pain and the average survival after the appearance of bone metastases is between 2 and 4 years. The spine, pelvis, proximal thigh and upper arm bone tend to be frequently affected [12].

Both retrospective and prospective studies have shown that palliative radiotherapy to single sites is very effective in producing partial and total pain relief and reduction in stiff-ness in up to 80–90% of cases [11]. The use of a single fraction of radiation has been shown to provide good pain relief. Sze *et al.* carried out a systematic review of randomized studies investigating the effectiveness of a single fraction versus multiple fractions [11] and found no difference between the two fractionations with regards to pain response. For spinal bone metastases, often a single 8-Gy fraction treated to depth is used. Pelvic, hip and shoulder metastases are treated using a parallel-opposed pair and again a single 8-Gy fraction is used. All use megavoltage X-rays.

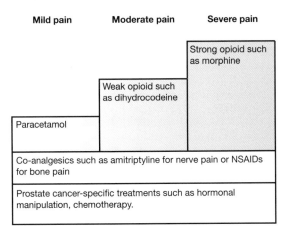

Figure 14.2   The WHO analgesic ladder.

Many patients also develop metastases of the ribs. These are often very painful and debilitating. These areas can be treated using superficial X-rays (220 kv or 225 kv). This is more appropriate due to the preferential bone absorption as a result of the photoelectric process. Complete or partial pain relief is achieved in 30–60% and 70–80% of patients. Pain relief occurs from a few days to weeks and lasts up to 6 months.

In individuals with multiple painful bone metastases, hemi-body radiotherapy is sometimes undertaken [14, 15]. Usually one half of the body is irradiated with a single 6- or 8-Gy fraction [13]. Patients should be given an anti-emetic before and 5 days after treatment of the lower body due to irradiation of large parts of the bowel. After the treatment, the blood counts must be closely watched as patients may become pancytopaenic due to toxicity of the bone marrow. If both halves of the body are to be treated, there should be a gap of 6 weeks to allow recovery of the bone marrow. This treatment is not suitable for individuals who have been heavily treated with chemotherapy. Most patients report a response at 48–96 h post radiotherapy that lasts around 4 months [14, 15].

Retreatment with Radiotherapy

Often, patients re-present to the clinician with pain in the same area that was previously treated with radiation. In most cases this does not pose too much of a problem, the exception being if the area is the spinal cord. Rades *et al.* investigated the feasibility and effectiveness of re-irradiation after primary radiotherapy to the spinal cord with a single 8-Gy fraction or five fractions each of 4 Gy. The median follow-up was 8 months. The study showed that spinal re-irradiation appears safe and effective provided the cumulative effective dose was not greater than a biological effective dose (BED) of 100 Gy. (In simple terms, BED is a measure of the effect of a course of fractionated or continuous irradiation.) Beyond this dose, there is an increased risk of radiation myelopathy. Retreatment occurs more frequently in patients who have previously been treated with a single fraction compared with those who have received multiple fractions [16, 17]. It is also important to take into account the time interval between treatments as this has an impact on the extent of normal tissue repair and the risk of tissue toxicity.

The Role of Radioisotopes in the Palliation of Bone Metastases

Focal radiotherapy is less helpful in individuals who have diffuse metastatic bone disease. Hemi-body radiotherapy in some cases may not be appropriate and the systemic administration of radioisotopes may be a viable alternative. Strontium-89 and samarium-153 are radioisotopes that are licensed for use in the treatment of metastatic bone cancer. They are both beta-emitters, which preferentially accumulate in bones with high osteoblastic activity. Radioactive dose tends to be high in metastases but low in the bone marrow hence this is a safe treatment to give to previously irradiated patients. Rhenium-186 and rhenium-188 are currently under investigation. Strontium-89 is given as a single intravenous injection of 150 MBq (4 mCi) of strontium-89 chloride. The documented response rates range from 40% to 95% and usually start 1–4 weeks after the infusion. Pain relief usually lasts up to 18 months and there is associated decrease in analgesia use [18, 19]. The most common side-effect seen is marrow suppression; in particular thrombocytopenia and neutropenia.

Bauman *et al.* carried out a systemic review of the use of radiopharmaceuticals in palliating bone pain. Six randomized phase III trials, two randomized phase II and one randomized crossover trial were reviewed. They concluded that the use of single agent radioisotopes should be considered as a possible option for palliating patients with multiple sites of bone pain [18].

The Role of Chemotherapy

Palliative chemotherapy in prostate cancer may have a beneficial effect at reducing pain. Studies report response rates ranging from 40 to 50% of treated patients [20]. Rapidly growing tumours may compress nerves and organs leading to pain. In this situation, palliative chemotherapy may decrease the tumour volume. This, however, is probably an oversimplification of the pain relief mechanism, especially where chemotherapy is also effective in patients with stable disease. There is an anti-inflammatory effect of chemotherapy that may alleviate metastatic bone pain; possible mechanisms include modulation of local production of prostaglandins and cytokines by the tumour.

It is important to make sure that the side-effects are tolerable. Current chemotherapy agents include docetaxel, mitoxantrone, vinorelbine and oral cyclophosphamide.

The Role of Bisphosphonates

Bisphosphonates are composed of a phosphorus–carbon–phosphorus backbone. Their pharmacological properties are determined by the R1 and R2 carbon side chains. They have a high affinity to calcium phosphate because of a hydroxyl group at the R1 position. The R2 side chain determines the antiresorptive potency.

Of all the bisphosphonates tested zoledronic acid is the most potent, having activity that is 100 times that of either pamidronate or clodronate and more than 1000 times that of etidronate [21].

Bisphosphonates act by inhibiting both normal and pathological osteoclast-mediated bone resorption. Bisphosphonates affect the attachment, differentiation and survival of osteoclasts and hence this affects their activity. They also affect osteoclastic activity via effects on osteoblasts.

There have been three randomized trials assessing the effect of bisphosphonates in men with androgen-independent prostate cancer and bone metastases (Table 14.1). These are the Zometa 039 trial, the Protocol 032/INT 05 trial and the NCIC Pr06 trial [22]. The Zometa 039 trial looked at the efficacy of zoledronic acid over 15 months. The primary endpoint was the proportion of men that experienced one or more skeletal-related events [23]. Protocol 032/INT 05 investigated the effect of pamidronate on pain, analgesic use and the proportion of patients who developed a skeletal-related event [24]. The NCIC Pr06 study looked at the efficacy of clodronate in men with symptomatic prostate cancer. Patients were asked to complete a pain index and quality of life questionnaire, as well as document their analgesic use. The primary endpoint in this study was a two-point decrease in the pain index or a 50% reduction in analgesic use [25]. The results from the three studies indicated that zoledronic acid but not the other bisphosphonates decreased the risk of skeletal complications in men diagnosed with both prostate cancer that was androgen independent, and bone metastases.

Zoledronic acid is usually given at a dose of 4 mg as a 15-min infusion into a peripheral vein. This is repeated every 3–4 weeks. The side-effects related to treatment include a transient flu-like syndrome comprising fever, arthralgia and myalgia starting within 24 h of treatment. Asymptomatic hypocalcaemia and renal toxicity are the other common side-effects. There is also an increased risk of osteonecrosis of the jaw but mainly in patients with poor oral hygiene or existing dental problems.

Table 14.1 Summary of trials and the effect on skeletal complications in androgen-independent prostate cancer patients

Trial	Bisphosphonate used	Risk of skeletal complications
Zometa 039	Zoledronic acid	Decreased
Protocol 032/INT05	Pamidronate	No effect
NCIC Pr06	Sodium clodronate	No effect

Currently, there is an ongoing trial (CALGB/CTSU 90202) defining the role of zoledronic acid in hormone-sensitive metastatic prostate cancer. This will provide information about the long-term effects and the optimal timing of bisphosphonate usage in patients with bone metastasis.

In summary, there is evidence to support the use of zoledronic acid in men with androgen-independent metastatic prostate cancer. There is improvement in pain and a reduction in skeletal complications. There are, however, limited data on the optimal duration of therapy. Current practice guidelines suggest it is continued till the occurrence of either treatment-related adverse events or a substantial decline in performance status.

SPINAL CORD COMPRESSION

Radiation and Spinal Cord Compression
Unfortunately, a great number of patients still present to clinicians or hospital with symptoms and signs of cord compression. In individuals whose spine is riddled with metastases or who have a single metastases but are considered to be medically unsuitable for an operation, or have a lifespan that is less than 3 months, radiation may be used [13, 26]. Often the fractionation used is determined by the prognosis and the general medical state of the individual.

A longer survival is associated with a higher risk of spinal cord compression recurrence [16]. Patients with advanced disease that progresses at a slow rate are treated with longer fractionation courses. By using longer fractionation courses of radiotherapy (5×4 Gy, 10×3 Gy, 15×2.5 Gy), better local control is obtained. This is explained by the higher total radiation dose given. There is also a trend towards better survival [16].

A short course of radiation or a single 8-Gy fraction is given to patients with poor prognosis (< 6 months survival or poor chance of neurological recovery). These patients are identified by their unfavourable histology, neurological dysfunction and poor performance status. For neurological dysfunction, these tend to be cases where paraplegia has been present for more than 48 h; treatment in established paraplegia will rarely improve neurological function and is given more for pain relief. Patients who are unwell are distressed by the daily visits to the oncology department and the set-up required prior to treatment.

Surgery and Radiotherapy
In selected patients presenting with spinal cord compression, it is appropriate to use a combined modality treatment – surgery and radiotherapy [13, 27]. These patients tend to be those who have a good performance status and are either ambulant or have presented with a short history (< 24 h) of immobility. These patients should be treated within 24 h of diagnosis.

After laminectomy or anterior fixation, radiotherapy is given. There has been one randomized controlled trial by Patchell et al. that compared surgery and post-operative radiotherapy to radiotherapy alone in a selected group of good performance patients with a single site of cord compression [27]. Their primary endpoint was the ability to walk, while the secondary endpoint was urinary continence, muscle strength and functional status, the need for corticosteroids and opioid analgesics and survival time. The trial showed that patients treated with the combined modality retained the ability to walk for a longer period, those who were unable to walk were more likely to regain the ability to do so, and there was a decreased need for corticosteroids and opioid analgesics. Hence, combined treatment was far more superior. The radiation fractionation used in the trial was 30 Gy in 10 fractions. This has not been compared with other dose fractionation regimes and so the current UK practice is to deliver 30 Gy in 10 fractions or 20 Gy in five fractions [13].

FATIGUE AND ANAEMIA

Often patients with advanced prostate cancer are anaemic, the pathophysiology of which is unclear. This leads to fatigue and patients may require regular transfusions.

Johansson *et al.* carried out a multicentred study investigating the efficacy of epoetin-beta on haemoglobin and quality of life in men with hormone-refractory prostate cancer. The study showed that a higher dose of epoetin resulted in a larger rise in the haemoglobin, and an improvement in the quality of life and fatigue levels [28]. The drug was very well tolerated. This was further confirmed by Bogdanos *et al.* [29]. These improvements increase incrementally up to a haemoglobin level of 12 g/dl.

Epoetin is a recombinant form of the hormone erythropoietin. It binds to and activates the erythroid progenitor cells stimulating formation of mature erythrocytes. Epoetin causes an increase in the reticulocyte count, haemoglobin concentration and the haematocrit in a dose-proportional manner. Individuals who are likely to benefit are those who have adequate bone marrow reserve (neutrophils $> 1.5 \times 10^9/l$ and platelets $> 100 \times 10^9/l$) and ferritin stores.

HYPERCALCAEMIA

Patients with hypercalcaemia may present with non-specific symptoms such as fatigue, anorexia, polyuria, nausea, weakness, constipation, lethargy and confusion. With rising levels of calcium neurological symptoms may develop such as fits, altered behaviour and coma, and impaired renal function may also develop. There is a direct correlation between the symptom severity and the level of ionized calcium.

Treatment of hypercalcemia is aimed at improving the renal function, quality of life and the mental status. Any calcium, vitamin D supplements and thiazide diuretics should be stopped. The patient should receive isotonic saline infusion to encourage renal excretion of calcium as well as bisphosphonates.

Pamidronate restores normocalcemia in 60–100% of patients and is often the bisphosphonate of choice. It is usually given at a dose of 60–90 mg as an infusion over 2–4 h. Zoledronic acid, which is the most potent bisphosphonate, can also be given and is highly effective. The fall in calcium is very rapid and is maintained for several weeks.

Other measures that could be used include calcitonin, which opposes the physiological effects of parathyroid hormone (PTH) on bone and calcium resorption at the renal tubules. The initial dose given is 5 IU/kg body weight given either subcutaneously or intramuscularly every 12 h. This may be dose-escalated to a maximum of 10 IU/kg body weight every 6 h according to response. Tachyphylaxis is a common side-effect; otherwise it is well tolerated. Because calcitonin is derived from salmon, 40–70% of patients develop antibodies against it, which may rarely result in hypersensitivity reactions.

Dialysis is rarely indicated except in the patient who develops hypercalcemia that is complicated by renal failure.

FRACTURES AND NEAR FRACTURES

Pain can be an indicator of a pathological or impending pathological fracture. When deciding on the appropriate management, one should take into consideration the life expectancy of the patient, whether the fracture is displaced and whether it affects weight-bearing bones.

For impending fractures, there should be early diagnosis and intervention to decrease pain and prevent disability. Radiological signs that may prompt prophylactic surgical intervention include more than 50% cortical bone destruction, a lytic lesion greater than 2.5 cm and a pathological avulsion fracture.

Radiotherapy should then be considered following surgical fixation of pathological fracture to provide pain relief, promote bone healing and halt local tumour progression.

PROSTATE-SPECIFIC/TREATMENT-RELATED SYMPTOMS

UROLOGICAL PROBLEMS

Urinary Tract Infections

Urinary tract infection is a very common problem. Foreign bodies in the urinary tract are a frequent cause. These include urinary catheters, nephrostomy tubes and ureteric stents. Intermittent self-catheterization can also lead to urinary tract infections. Permanent catheters cause disruption of the normal defence barriers and the normal flora of adjacent skin. Bacteria often coat the mucosal and catheter surfaces with a biofilm that protects them from the mechanical effects of urine flow, as well as the immune system and antibiotics.

Patients with urinary tract infection present with temperature, suprapubic pain and offensive urine. Infection may ascend the urinary tract and cause pyelonephritis – fever, flank pain, raised inflammatory markers and positive blood cultures. This can contribute to decreased in quality of life as well as increased morbidity and mortality.

By far the most common pathogen is *Escherichia coli* (*E. coli*); it is responsible for up to 75% of infections. Antibiotic treatment should be according to local clinical guidelines, should be as specific as possible and given for the shortest period necessary to eradicate the infection.

Haematuria

Haematuria is another common symptom that can be very distressing for the patient. Haematuria can occur after radiotherapy or as a result of local disease progression. It may be associated with urinary tract infection or with a catheter or other foreign material in the urinary tract.

Radiation to the pelvis can cause telangiectasia of the bladder, which can rupture and cause haemorrhage. Often haematuria is self-limiting and requires little intervention provided the patient is voiding satisfactorily. Haematuria should be investigated fully to rule out other sinister pathology.

Bleeding due to progressing local disease can be difficult to manage. Palliative radiotherapy may be considered provided the maximum tolerance limit has not been reached with previous radiation treatment to the pelvis. Other interventions would include laser coagulation to the bleeding prostate, which provides good palliation, as well as the use of intravesical tranexamic acid in combination with etamsylate [30]. Etamsylate is a haemostatic agent that is thought to increase the capillary vascular wall resistance and platelet adhesiveness in the presences of a vascular lesion via inhibition of the biosynthesis and actions of prostaglandins [31].

Urinary Obstruction

Bladder outflow or ureteric obstruction can be caused by progressing prostate cancer, or gross pelvic lymphadenopathy, or stricture formation in the urethra. Patients often present with an insidious rise in the urea and creatinine, and a decrease in the urine output. Often pain is absent unless there is acute obstruction. If not diagnosed, patients may present in acute renal failure with life-threatening hyperkalaemia.

Management depends on the cause and site of obstruction. If the prostate is the cause of obstruction, urethral catheterization may relieve the problem. In bilateral ureteric obstruction it may be necessary to insert ureteric stents. If the ureters cannot be cannulated cystoscopically, unilateral or bilateral nephrostomy tube(s) may be placed percutaneously, with the option for antegrade placement of ureteric stent(s) to restore internal urinary drainage. Ureteric stents and nephrostomy tubes need to be replaced every 3–6 months in view of the risks of encrustation and obstruction. Particularly in the patient with a poor prognosis, management must consider the quality of life and wishes of the individual.

SEXUAL AND ERECTILE DYSFUNCTION

A large portion of men with prostate cancer do not regain normal sexual function after treatment [32]. Men are as troubled by the loss of sexual desire as they are about erectile dysfunction. Schover *et al.* carried out a survey to identify factors that were associated with a good sexual outcome [32]. The positive factors included younger age, patients with much younger partners, and the importance they place on preserving sexual function.

As the prostate cancer progresses, the sexual function is often not considered by the clinician. At this stressful time, patients require support and close emotional contact from their spouses and this may include intercourse [33]. Again there is very little documentation of the importance of impotence and the effect on intimate relationships between couples, however we should consider this and approach it with sensitivity. Many patients and clinicians are too embarrassed to bring up the topic and may be grateful if it is discussed.

Provided there are no overriding contraindications, management options should be offered. These include oral medications such as sildenafil, inflatable penile prosthesis, penile injections and vacuum devices. It should be noted that the most successful treatments tend to be the most invasive: penile prosthesis and injections have a response rate of 50–75%, compared with 39% for oral medications [34, 35].

HOT FLUSHES

Eight per cent of men on gonadotrophin-releasing hormone agonists will experience hot flushes, and a survey carried out by Karling *et al.* revealed that 27% of men found this side-effect to be the most bothersome. The treatments available include progestins, these have been shown to decrease hot flushes by 85%, and venlaflaxine. A pilot study done at the Mayo clinic showed a decrease in the number and severity of hot flushes [36]. This effect is not specific to venlaflaxine but seems to be one that is shared by all selective serotonin reuptake inhibitors (SSRIs). Care needs to be taken when prescribing the drug to patients with epilepsy, ischaemic heart disease or those who are on cytochrome P450 inhibitor drugs. Clinicians should also look out for the uncommon but life-threatening long QT syndrome that can sometimes occur.

Acupuncture, soya products and vitamin E have also shown some success in decreasing the hot flushes. Acupuncture seems to have the highest response rate at 70% [37]. These interventions should be offered to men with advanced prostate cancer as they are likely to continue with hormone suppression therapy indefinitely.

END OF LIFE SYMPTOMS

PSYCHOLOGICAL SYMPTOMS

Much has been written about depression in cancer patients [38] and it is important to screen for this. Various burdensome tools have been used, but simply asking the patient 'Do you think that you could be depressed?' is often adequate. Other simple tools such as the 'Distress thermometer' [38] have been used in the oncology outpatient setting. NICE guidance recognizes the need for all staff to have the ability to support the psychological needs of patients, but it is also important to be able to refer early on to psychological medicine and psychiatry when needed.

Throughout treatment it is important to help the patient and their supporters to deal with the uncertainty that the disease brings, and to help the patient retain the feeling of being a part of the decision-making process [39]. As death approaches it is vital to allow opportunity to explore the patient's fears about the future and to allow for preparation. This might involve alerting family abroad, drawing up a will, decisions about refusing treatment or making spiritual preparations.

Prior to death, 85% of patients with cancer will develop symptoms of delirium [40]. This often encompasses 'terminal agitation', but can be due to opioid analgesia, renal deterioration, antimuscarinic drugs, metabolic abnormalities, dehydration or psychoactive drugs [41, 42]. Simple reversible measures such as choosing a different drug or a trial of subcutaneous fluid might be helpful.

CONTINUING CARE

The patient rarely seeks medical attention alone, and carers also need consideration. Work done specifically with caregivers looking after patients with prostate cancer has shown that the burden of caring adversely affects their quality of life [43]. Other work compared caregivers looking after patients with breast or prostate cancer. This has highlighted the levels of anxiety experienced as well as an increased level of depression in female caregivers [43].

As death approaches there is good evidence that excellent care is far from 'the norm' in hospitals [44]. It is all too common for medical entries to dry up in the notes, and most doctors have witnessed deaths that leave them feeling at best frustrated and at worst woefully inadequate. Diagnosing dying is difficult at the best of times but the stigma of death and the feeling of having failed the patient still lingers [45]. The palliative care approach to caring for patients in hospice, hospital and community settings has been shared through clinical pathways such as the Liverpool Integrated Care Pathway for the Dying [46]. This pathway has helped clinicians deliver care at a difficult time for all, and provides guidance about care both for the dying patient and their family. Importantly, it also recognizes the need for good bereavement support and practical advice such as 'parking permits, canteen opening hours for relatives, and where and how to register a death'.

The importance of palliative care and the deficiencies in its provision are often underestimated. A recent study in the USA evaluated guidelines for life-limiting illnesses and found only 10% had a significant palliative care content and 64% had minimal content [47]. In the UK, the NHS Cancer Plan 2000 states that 'the care of all dying patients must improve to the level of the best' [48], but it is only with increasing awareness of the palliative resources available and using them appropriately that we will be able to serve the needs of our patients well.

REFERENCES

1. World Health Organization. 2006.
2. National Institute for Clinical Excellence. *Improving Outcomes in Urological Cancers Manual*. NICE, UK, 2002.
3. Office for National Statistics. *Mortality Statistics-Cause, England and Wales,1999*. Stationery Office, London, 2000.
4. Newling DW. The palliative therapy of advanced prostate cancer, with particular reference to the results of recent European clinical trials. *Br J Urol* 1997; 79(Suppl 1): 72–81.
5. Aus G. Need for hospital care and palliative treatment for prostate cancer treated with non-curative intent. *J Urol* 1995; 154 (no.2Pt1): 466–469.
6. Green JS. An investigation into the use of palliative care services by patients with prostate cancer. *Am J Hosp Palliat Care* 2002; 19:259–262.
7. Esper P. A new concept in cancer care: the supportive care program. *Am J Hosp Palliat Care* 1999; 16: 13–22.
8. Twycross R, Wilcock A. *Symptom Management in Advanced Cancer, 3rd edn*. Radcliff Medical Press, Oxford, 2001, 18 pp.
9. George R, Farnham C. *Palliative Care and Pain Control in HIV and AIDS. ABC of AIDS*, 3rd edn. BMJ Publishing Group, London, 2005
10. World Health Organization. *Cancer Pain Relief*. WHO, Geneva, 1986.
11. Sze WM, Shelley MD, Held I *et al*. Palliation of metastatic bone pain: single fraction versus multifraction radiotherapy – a systematic review of randomised trials. *Clin Onc* 2003; 15: 345–352.

12. Saarto T, Janes R, Tenhunen M *et al.* Palliative radiotherapy in the treatment of skeletal metastases. *Eur J Pain* 2002; 6:323–330.

13. The Royal College of Radiologists. *Board of the Faculty of Clinical Oncology. Radiotherapy Dose-Fractionation.* June 2006.

14. Kuban DA, Schellhammer PF, el-Mahadi AM. Hemibody irradiation in advanced prostatic carcinoma. *Urol Clin North Am* 1991; 18:131–137.

15. Nseyo UO, Fontanesi J, Naftulin BN. Palliative hemibody irradiation in hormonally refractory metastatic prostate cancer. *Urology* 1989; 34:76–79.

16. Rades D, Fehlauer F, Schulte R *et al.* Prognostic factors for local control and survival after radiotherapy of metastatic spinal cord compression. *J Clin Oncol* 2006; 24:3388–3393.

17. Rades D, Stalpers LJ, Veniga T *et al.* Spinal irradiation after short-course RT for metastatic spinal cord compression. *Int J Radiat Oncol Biol Phys* 2005; 63:872–875.

18. Bauman G, Charette M, Reid R *et al.* Radiopharmaceuticals for the palliation of painful bone metastasis – a systemic review. *Radiother Oncol* 2005; 75:258–270.

19. Finlay IG, Mason MD, Shelley M. Radioisotopes for the palliation of metastatic bone cancer: a systematic review. *Lancet Oncol* 2005; 6:392–400.

20. Berthold DR, Sternberg CN, Tannock IF. Management of advanced prostate cancer after first-line chemotherapy. *J Clin Oncol* 2005; 23:8247–8252.

21. Michaelson MD, Smith MR. Bisphosphonates for treatment and prevention of bone metastases. *J Clin Onc* 2005; 23:8219–8224.

22. Dearnaley DP, Sydes MR, Mason MD *et al.* A double-blind, placebo-controlled, randomised trial of oral sodium clodronate for metastatic prostate cancer (MRC PR05 Trial). *J Natl Cancer Inst* 2003; 95:1300–1311.

23. Saad F, Gleason DM, Murray R *et al.* A randomised, placebo-controlled trial of zoledronic acid in patients with hormone-refractory metastatic prostate cancer. *J Natl Cancer Inst* 2002; 94:1458–1468.

24. Small EJ, Smith MR, Seamon JJ *et al.* Combined analysis of two multi center, randomised, placebo-controlled studies of pamidronate disodium for the palliation of bone pain in men with metastatic prostate cancer. *J Clin Oncol* 2003; 21:4277–4284.

25. Ernst D, Tannock I, Venner P *et al.* Randomised placebo controlled trial of mitoxantrone /prednisone and clodronate versus mitoxantrone /prednisone alone in patients with hormone refractory prostate cancer (HRPC) and pain: National Cancer Institute of Canada Clinical Trials Group study. *J Clin Oncol* 2002 ; Suppl abstr. 705.

26. Maranzano E, Latini P. Effectiveness of radiation therapy without surgery in metastatic spinal cord compression: final results from a prospective trial. *Int J Radiat Oncol Biol Phys* 1995; 32:959 –967.

27. Patchell RA, Tibbs PA, Regine WF *et al.* Direct decompressive surgical resection in the treatment of spinal cord compression caused by metastatic cancer: a randomised trial. Lancet 2005; 366(9486):643–648.

28. Johansson JE, Wersall P, Brandberg Y *et al.* Efficacy of epoetin beta on hemoglobin, quality of life, and transfusion needs in patients with anemia due to hormone-refractory prostate cancer – a randomised study. *Scand J Urol Nephrol* 2001; 35:288–294.

29. Bogdanos J, Karamanolakis D, Milathianakis K *et al.* Epoetin beta (NeoRecomon) corrects anaemia in patients with hormone-refractory prostate cancer and bone metastases. *Anticancer Res* 2004; 24(3b):1957–1961.

30. Dean A, Tuffin P. Fibrinolytic inhibitors for cancer-associated bleeding problems. *J Pain Symptom Management* 1997; 13:20–24.

31. Garay RP, Chiavaroli C, Hannaert P. Therapeutic efficacy and mechanism of action of ethamsylate, a long-standing hemostatic agent. *Am J Ther* 2006; 13:236–247.

32. Schover LR, Fouladi RT, Warneke CL *et al.* Defining sexual outcomes after treatment for localized prostate carcinoma. *Cancer* 2002; 95:1773–1785.

33. Soloway CT, Soloway MS, Kim SS *et al.* Sexual, psychological and dyadic qualities of the prostate cancer 'couple'. *BJU Int* 2005; 95:780–785.

34. Miller DC, Wei JT, Dunn RL *et al.* Use of medications or devices for erectile dysfunction among long term prostate cancer treatment survivors: potential influence of sexual motivation and /or indifference. *Urology* 2006; 68:166–171.

35. Schover LR, Fouladi RT, Warneke CL *et al.* The use of treatments for erectile dysfunction among survivors of prostate carcinoma. *Cancer* 2002; 95:2397–2407.

36. Quella SK, Loprinzi CL, Sloan J *et al.* Pilot evaluation of venlafaxine for the treatment of hot flushes in men undergoing androgen ablation therapy for prostate cancer. *J Urol* 1999; 162:98–102.

37. Holzbeierlein JM, McLaughlin MD, Thrasher JB. Complications of androgen deprivation therapy for prostate cancer. *Curr Opin Urol* 2004; 14:177–183.

38. Roth A. Rapid screening for psychologic distress in men with prostate carcinoma. A pilot study. *Cancer* 1998; 82:1904–1908.

39. de Haas H, Koedoot N. Patient centred decision making in palliative cancer treatment: a world of paradoxes. *Patient Educ Couns* 2003; 50:43–49.

40. Periera J, Hanson J, Bruera E. The frequency and clinical course of cognitive impairment in patients with terminal cancer. *Cancer* 1997; 79:835–842.

41. Lundstrom SH, Furst CJ. The use of corticosteroids in Swedish palliative care. *Acta Oncol* 2006; 45:430–437.

42. Strang P. The effect of megestrol acetate on anorexia, weight loss and cachexia in cancer and AIDS patients (review). *Anticancer Res* 1997; 17:657–662.

43. Grov EK, Dahl AA. Anxiety, depression, and quality of life in caregivers of patients with cancer in late palliative phase. *Ann Oncol* 2005; 16:1185–1191.

44. Ellershaw J *et al.* Care of the dying: setting standards for symptom control in the last 48 hours of life. *JPSM* 2001; 21:12–17.

45. Ellershaw J, Ward C. Care of the dying patient: the last hours or days of life. *BMJ* 2003; 326:30–34.

46. Ellershaw J, Wilkinson S. The Marie Curie Liverpool Integrated Care Pathway for the Dying Patient. *Care of the Dying: a Pathway to Excellence.* Oxford University Press, Oxford, 2003.

47. Mast K, Salama M. End of life content in treatment guidelines for life limiting diseases. *J Palliat Med* 2004; 7:754–773.

48. National Health Service. *NHS Cancer Plan.* Department of Health, London, 2000.

Section IV

Management of complications

15

Treatment strategies for spinal cord compression and fractures

Alistair J. Stirling, Adrian C. Gardner, Roger M. Tilman

INTRODUCTION

The spine is the commonest site of pain due to instability skeletal metastasis [1] and prostate cancer is one of the most common tumours to metastasize to bone. Spinal metastasis causes a spectrum of clinical presentations from pain due to instability and fracture to neurological compromise [epidural and spinal cord compression (ESCC)]. In prostate cancer, ESCC is much more common than pathological fracture. ESCC is in itself not fatal; nevertheless, incapacitating pain and subsequent neurological compromise, such as paraplegia and loss of sphincter control have major social and clinical implications. Complete loss of neurological function is irretrievable and, therefore, prevention of ESCC is desirable whenever possible. Although the average survival for prostate cancer patients after a diagnosis of metastatic spinal cord compression is only 5 months [2], the morbidity of metastatic spinal disease is such that an aggressive approach to management is justified. The aims of this chapter are to review the current management of metastatic prostate cancer to the spine.

TREATMENT STRATEGIES FOR SPINAL CORD COMPRESSION

PATHOANATOMY

At post mortem the incidence of prostate carcinoma histologically is 24–46% in men over 50 years of age. Metastatsis most commonly occurs to lymph nodes but bone is the second commonest site [3] and is seen in up to 84% of cases at post-mortem [4–7]. The spine is the most commonly involved site for bone metastasis. Within the spine the commonest site is the vertebral bodies of the thoracic and lumbar regions, which reflects the greater volume of bone in the vertebral bodies, their anatomical relationship to the prostate and Batson's valveless vertebral venous plexus, which drains directly from the pelvis to the spine. The commonest site of symptomatic neural compression is the thoracic region (67%), with 27% in the lumbar spine and 6% in the cervical spine [8, 9], in part reflecting the narrower volume of the spinal canal in the thoracic spine.

Ninety per cent of prostatic spinal metastases are osteoblastic [10]. Spinal deformity is therefore unusual, although epidural compression is not uncommon, being the initial sign of malignancy in 36% of patients with epidural metastasis [11]. By contrast, the majority of

Alistair J. Stirling, MBChB FRCS, Consultant Spinal Surgeon, Royal Orthopaedic Hospital NHS Trust, Birmingham, UK
Adrian C. Gardner, FRCS, Specialist Registrar in Orthopaedics and Trauma, Royal Orthopaedic Hospital NHS Trust, Birmingham, UK
Roger M. Tilman, FRCS, Consultant Orthopaedic Oncologist, Royal Orthopaedic Hospital NHS Trust, Birmingham, UK

spinal metastases from other primary tumours are osteolytic. Osteolytic metastases weaken bone resulting in pathological fracture with the potential for neurological compromise as a result of bony compression rather than tumour compression. Understanding this fundamental difference between the modes of presentation for prostate cancer and metastasis from other primaries is vital for the recognition of why epidural and spinal cord compression is significantly more common in prostate cancer than spinal instability at presentation.

CLINICAL FEATURES

The Patient

The problems of spinal metastases and, in particular, imminent neural compromise in patients with prostatic carcinoma should not override an overall appreciation of the individual's social, family and general medical circumstances, as well as previous treatment. An informed and realistic discussion between the doctor and the patient and his family regarding the potential benefits, risks and limitations is required before embarking on a treatment programme that may impinge significantly upon the time they have available.

An appreciation of biological rather than chronological age as well as appreciation of important comorbidity is mandatory before deciding upon the scale of justifiable surgical intervention.

The Disease

Definition of the patient's prognosis in terms of the stage of disease, previous treatment and responsiveness to adjuvant modalities is a prerequisite to surgical planning. For example, the difference in life expectancy between newly diagnosed hormone-naive prostate cancer and hormone resistant disease with visceral involvement would often alter the surgical strategy and technique employed.

Presentation

Patients may present to the spinal surgical team by a variety of different routes: as an acute admission, as a referral from a clinic with unexplained musculoskeletal pain or as an existing patient referred by an oncologist or member of the prostate care team [12]. Osborn et al. [13] investigated symptoms at presentation in a retrospective study of four large series of spinal metastases from prostate cancer. It was concluded that patients at risk of, or with established, ESCC present with four main initial symptoms: back pain, weakness, autonomic and sensory loss (Table 15.1).

Back Pain

The most frequent symptom reported in up to 100% of adult ESCC patients is back pain resulting mainly from the involvement of bone by metastatic tumour [14–17]. The type of pain and the relieving and aggravating factors reflect the underlying local pathological process. At first, pain may be local in origin due to the periosteum stretching as the metastasis enlarges, and this is sometimes accompanied by somatic referred pain. Radicular pain may also develop if root compression occurs [13]. Prostate cancer patients suffer pain for a median duration of 12 months before the onset of ESCC [18]. Localized pain may be relentless and exacerbated by anything that raises cerebrospinal fluid pressure such as straining, coughing or sneezing [13, 19]. With increasing occlusion of the spinal canal, pain may be aggravated by lying down, in contrast to degenerative spinal disease which is often relieved on lying down, leading to the red flag symptom of night pain.

Pain aggravated by standing, and more particularly with spinal movement, is usually termed mechanical. In the setting of osteoblastic metastasis this is thought to represent 'creaking' of dense but not necessarily strong metastatic bone (Figure 15.1). Alternatively,

Table 15.1 Presenting complaints

Back pain
Sensory dysfunction
Weakness
Autonomic dysfunction

in the unusual circumstance of osteolytic prostatic metastasis, this may be due to imminent fracture.

Patients often recognize the pain from cancer metastases as different to any previous, longstanding, mechanical, low back pain of degenerative origin and it is felt higher up the spine. There may be spinal tenderness on examination of the back [20]. Care should be taken when attributing pain to degenerative spinal disease in patients with a history of prostate cancer who should be carefully evaluated for spinal metastases [19, 21]. Symptomatic neurological compromise in the form of sensory loss, weakness and autonomic dysfunction, typically develop after pain, often but not always in this sequence.

The neurological presentation differs with the level of neural compression and the direction of its impingement on the spinal cord. Cord compression above T12 typically results in an upper motor neurone (UMN) picture, whilst at the conus and below, a lower motor neurone (LMN) picture is seen. If compression is initially anterior, weakness, loss of pain and temperature sensation may precede compromise of light touch and proprioception (dissociated sensory loss) due to the anterior position in the spinal cord of the spinothalamic tract (pain and temperature sensation) and corticospinal tract (motor) versus the posterior position of the dorsal columns (fine touch and proprioception). Conversely, if compression is initially posterior, the reverse may apply.

Weakness

Weakness is usually bilateral and frequently involves the muscle groups below the lesion [13]. The degree of weakness and ambulatory ability at diagnosis are important clinical predictors of outcome [14, 20]. In ESCC complete loss of motor power is usually irreversible even after treatment, whereas in 93% of ambulatory patients and 83% of paraparetic patients walking ability was maintained after appropriate therapy [16]. Once weakness is present, progression to ESCC in prostate cancer patients is relatively swift.

Autonomic and Sensory Dysfunction

Autonomic dysfunction in a cancer patient with ESCC is thought to be an unfavourable prognostic sign [14]. Symptoms of bowel and bladder problems, such as incontinence and urinary retention are frequent in these patients at diagnosis (57%) depending on the level of

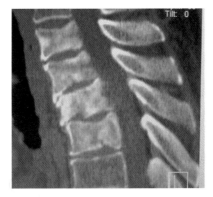

Figure 15.1 Dense weak bone with end plate fractures.

the compression [19]. It has been reported that over half of patients (51%) report symptoms of numbness and paraesthesiae, whilst on examination a sensory loss is found in 78% [19].

CLINICAL ASSESSMENT

A complete history and examination with particular attention to neurological status is necessary in a patient presenting with any combination of these symptoms [12].

Examination
In addition to a routine general examination with particular attention to excluding visceral metastasis, neurological examination should assess mental status, cranial nerves, motor and sensory examination, reflexes and cerebellar function [21]. Posture, stance and gait allow a rapid functional assessment of this and, thus, it is important to ask the patient to walk if possible. This then allows an assessment of the ability to tiptoe walk, heel walk and single knee dip, and this will often reveal latent weakness or proprioceptive loss not apparent on bed assessment. If there is a significant history of mechanical spinal pain, plain radiographs of the painful area to exclude incipient spinal collapse should be obtained prior to standing and walking assessment.

OBSERVATION AND PREOPERATIVE MANAGEMENT

Clear and definitive instruction to nursing and junior medical staff is mandatory in patients with potential or actual ESCC. This should include the type and frequency of neurological observation and action to be taken if deterioration occurs. If instability is suspected, suitable measures to minimize spinal movement and loading should be instituted such as the provision of a collar for the cervical spine, or bed rest for the thoracolumbar spine.

IMAGING AND DIAGNOSIS (TABLE 15.2)

Magnetic Resonance Imaging
Magnetic resonance imaging (MRI) is considered the gold standard diagnostic test for imaging vertebral and spinal metastases with a risk of ESCC (Figure 15.2) [13]. MRI is non-invasive, gives excellent anatomical detail of the spinal cord and is able to image the desired spinal segments irrespective of a cord compression preventing the flow of myelographic contrast (Figure 15.3). Several studies [22–24] have demonstrated that spinal MRI is as sensitive as other modalities for detecting spinal epidural metastases. It should be routine practice to image the entire spine as there is the potential to miss asymptomatic non-contiguous lesions. In line with other guidelines [12], it is recommended that all patients should receive an urgent MRI of the entire spine.

Radiography
Prior to the availability of MRI, definitive diagnosis of ESCC required myelography, a highly invasive test for patients who are already in pain. Consequently, routine investigations such as conventional radiography were used to determine those patients at low risk of ESCC in

Table 15.2 Investigations required

Full neurological examination
Full general examination
Plain radiographs of the entire spine
Urgent MRI of the entire spine
Chest radiograph
CT of chest and abdomen
Bone scan

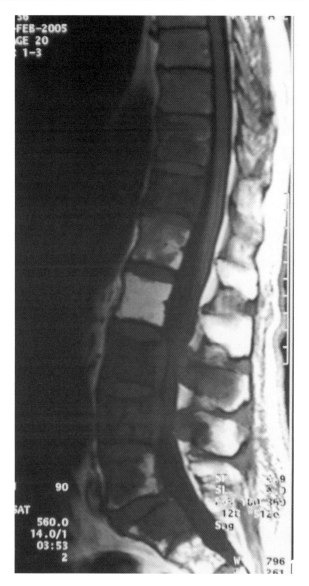

Figure 15.2 MRI scan showing sclerotic bone.

whom myelography would not be required. Conventional radiography has the ability to demonstrate vertebral abnormalities in up to 85% of patients with ESCC from both osteoblastic and osteolytic lesions or vertebral collapse [14, 18]. Portenoy *et al.* [25] studied the probability of epidural metastatic disease based on the presence of symptoms and radiographical or bone scan changes. (The study was not controlled with MRI.) Where there was a localized sign and the radiograph was abnormal, the probability of epidural disease was 0.9; however, where the radiograph was normal it was only 0.1. The risk was increased to 0.95 if both the radiograph and bone scan were abnormal, and reduced to 0.02 if the radiograph and bone scan were normal.

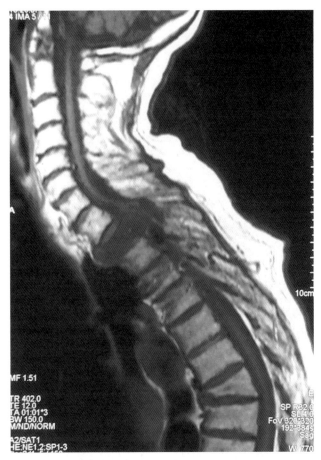

Figure 15.3 MRI scan showing cord compression.

For osteolytic metastases, lesions need to be >1 cm and over 50% of the bone has to be destroyed before these are necessarily evident using conventional radiography. In advanced hormone resistant cancers, the multiplicity of bony metastases and the fact that the majority are osteoblastic rather than osteolytic means that a high number of false-negatives result. It is therefore unlikely that radiographs alone have enough predictive value to warrant their routine use in predicting prostate cancer patients at risk from ESCC (Figure 15.4).

Myelography
Although MRI has largely replaced myelography there are still some circumstances in which myelography is useful. MRI is contraindicated in those with pacemakers, some intracranial vascular clips and with intraocular metallic foreign bodies. In addition, MRI images of the spine are usually grossly distorted by the presence of ferrous implants from previous spinal surgery. For this reason, the majority of implants are now titanium. If a second episode of ESCC has developed despite prior surgery with implants, myelography combined with computed tomography (CT) will usually provide sufficient information on which to base management decisions.

Radionuclide Bone Scans
Radionuclide bone scans are a useful single test for staging prostate cancer and are more sensitive than radiographs at detecting vertebral metastases (Figure 15.5) [26, 27]. They do

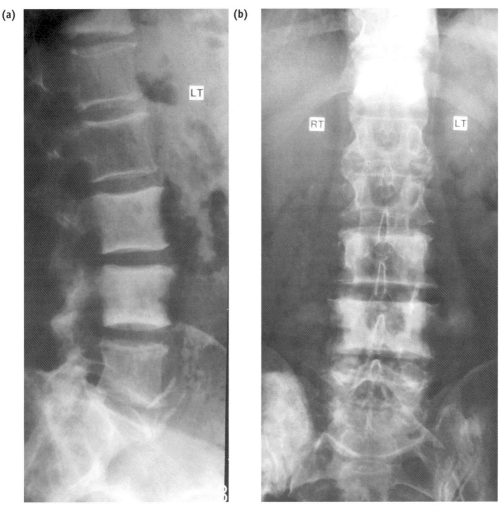

Figure 15.4 Prostatic infiltration of the spine showing sclerosis of the L3 and L4 vertebral bodies: (a) a lateral radiograph, (b) an anteroposterior radiograph.

not, however, provide sufficient detail to be of value for surgical planning as discriminating which of the often multiple vertebral site(s) is responsible for neural compression and the direction of that compression is not possible. In the context of spinal metastatic disease in practice, isotope bone scans are used only to define extraspinal osseous disease and its extent, and this can usually be delayed until after spinal surgery, if necessary. Beware the 'Super Scan' where there is uptake across the entire skeleton due to widespread disease and the lack of uptake differentiation can lead to the scan being reported as normal. In the presence of deteriorating neurology, appropriate surgical intervention should not be delayed.

Computed Tomography
MRI has for practical purposes superseded CT where available. This is on the basis of the higher sensitivity of MRI and lack of ionizing radiation. However, there are circumstances in which MRI is contraindicated or the presence of ferrous implants may render it useless as mentioned above.

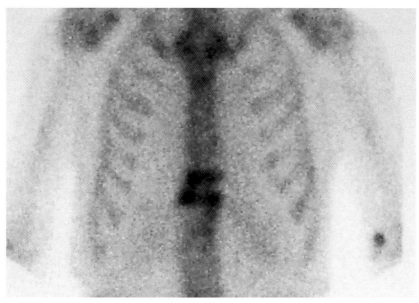

Figure 15.5   Radionucleotide scan showing increased uptake in the thoracolumbar spine.

Spinal CT can be a useful test to define a high risk of ESCC if MRI cannot be used and it has been shown that cortical disruption at multiple vertebral levels indicates a high chance (> 90%) of epidural tumour (Figure 15.6) [28]. It may also assess bony and anatomical details prior to surgery, for example bony dimensions for instrumentation or the course of the vertebral artery.

BIOPSY OF SPINAL LESIONS

A spinal biopsy is recommended if the lesion is a solitary bony lesion and there is doubt as to the underlying pathology. In these cases imaging with a bone scan, an MRI of the lesion and spine and percutaneous bone biopsy need to be performed before surgery to prevent inappropriate procedures [12]. Experienced surgeons should generally perform percutaneous biopsies, under X-ray control [12] to prevent a biopsy compromising future surgical margins should the mass prove to be a primary tumour. CT-guided biopsy by specialist radiologists may be an alternative option. A trephine biopsy is usually required and specialist bone pathologists should examine the histology for an accurate interpretation of the sample.

TREATMENT SELECTION

SCORING SYSTEMS

Various prognostic scoring systems for spinal metastases have been developed, to aid selection of surgical candidates and surgical techniques [29, 30]. Whilst these have been validated for spinal metastases in general, there are no published data specific to prostatic spinal metastatic disease. Given the structural difference from other osteolytic metastases, the applicability of such scoring systems to metastatic prostate cancer in the spine remains undefined.

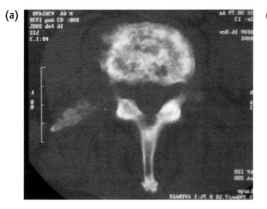
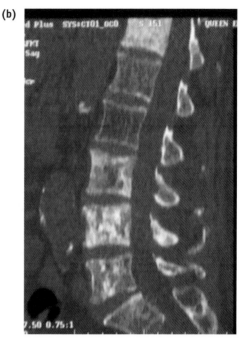

Figure 15.6 CT images of prostatic infiltration of the spine: (a) axial; (b) sagittal.

TREATMENT OPTIONS

RADIOTHERAPY (TABLE 15.3)

The response of epidural metastases to radiotherapy is well documented [31, 32]. Radiotherapy has been shown to produce significant pain relief in more than 90% of patients, and in two-thirds of patients a significant or complete improvement in neurology is achieved [25]. However, in the presence of paraplegia, the success of radiotherapy in combination with both steroids and androgen deprivation has proved to be substantially less than in patients who were paraparetic [33]. Whether radiotherapy is better in terms of outcome, both in the short and long term, when compared to surgery and radiotherapy has recently been addressed in a randomized controlled trial by Patchell *et al.* [34]. This study showed conclusively that the ability to walk was maintained for longer with surgery followed by radiotherapy, compared with radiotherapy alone. This significant benefit was demonstrated for both those patients who were walking and those who were unable to walk prior to intervention. The requirements for post-intervention analgesia and corticosteroids were also reduced in the surgical group. This study analysed all causes of metastatic epidural spinal cord compression, not just that secondary to prostate cancer, and concluded that surgery and radiotherapy

Table 15.3 Indications for radiotherapy [12]

No spinal instability
Radiosensitive tumour
Stable or slow neurological progression
Multi-level disease
Surgery precluded by general condition
Poor prognosis
Postoperative adjuvant treatment

was better than radiotherapy alone, and that, if possible, surgery should be the first choice for management [34]. The Radiation Therapy Oncology Group (RTOG) evaluated different dose-fractionation irradiation schedules in a randomized controlled trial [35] to determine their palliative effectiveness in patients with osseous metastases. The frequency, promptness and duration of pain relief were used to indicate the degree of response. Ninety per cent of patients experienced some relief of pain and 54% achieved eventual complete pain relief. However, the optimal dose-fractionation scheme for treating ESCC is still unknown. Most radiation oncologists adhere to standard schedules of 25–36 Gy with an average of 20 Gy over five fractions being chosen because it is considered to be a relatively well-tolerated dose for the spinal cord. There may be no optimal plan for every metastatic prostate cancer patient because each plan constructed will represent a compromise between delivery of the highest dose possible to control progression of the local tumour and palliate pain effectively, whilst limiting the effect on the spinal cord.

Radiotherapy is efficacious in terms of preventing further local tumour growth and ameliorating pain with minimal side-effects. The neurological outcome of radiotherapy depends on a number of factors. Firstly, the degree of functional limitation at initiation of radiotherapy will alter the outcome of therapy. This is important because it has been reported that radiotherapy may preserve the ability to walk in 80–100% of patients who start treatment when still able to walk [14, 32, 36]. Secondly, the extent of subarachnoid impingement will also affect the outcome of treatment. Epidural metastases that produce a minor impression on the thecal sac will have a better outcome than a large mass that completely obliterates the subarachnoid space. This has been confirmed in clinical studies, but is of weak value [37, 38].

In the era of MRI, the response of spinal metastases to radiotherapy has not been thoroughly investigated. The average life expectancy for patients undergoing radiotherapy for ESCC is between 3 and 6 months. Survival rates are higher in patients who were walking when treatment was initiated and in radiosensitive tumours, such as prostate with a single metastasis. The risk of recurrence increases with the length of survival and 50% of 2-year survivors will develop recurrence [14].

HORMONE DEPRIVATION THERAPY

Hormonal manipulation has been successfully employed in hormone-naive patients with ESCC from prostate cancer and there is a definite relationship between neurological deficit at presentation and response to hormone therapy. However, in patients who have complete paraplegia at the time of presentation hormone therapy is of little benefit [39].

SURGERY (TABLE 15.4)

A variety of surgical strategies can be employed for neoplastic spinal disease. Appropriate selection is dependent upon the individual case and requires tailoring accordingly. The objectives from a patient perspective (Table 15.5) are to minimize pain and to maximize or maintain neurological function with the minimum procedure adequate to the predicted life expectancy. As a rough rule of thumb, surgery and the associated recovery time should not involve more than 50% of the predicted remaining life expectancy, a minimum of 3 months. From a spinal perspective the objectives are to ensure adequate decompression, to ensure

Table 15.4 Indications for surgery

Spinal instability
Clinically significant neurological compression, in particular by bone

Table 15.5   Objectives of surgery

Maintenance or restoration of spinal cord function
Correction of spinal instability
Preservation of as many normal motion segments as possible

the maintenance, or restoration, of spinal cord or nerve root function, and to eliminate actual or potential spinal instability with preservation of as many normal motion segments as possible [12].

From a tumour perspective, given that metastatic prostatic carcinoma is almost always present at multiple sites by the time ESCC develops, the technical complexity of extralesional excision appropriate to primary spinal tumours is not applicable. Similarly, aggressive attempts at radical intralesional procedures are also inappropriate.

In the majority of patients with ESCC from prostatic metastases, the clinical problem is local tumour-related pain with accompanying root or cord compression syndromes rather than spinal instability. In the absence of symptoms or imaging evidence of instability and posterior compression, neural compression symptoms *may* be adequately managed by decompression alone, often in the form of laminectomy with, as necessary, specific root decompression in isolation.

If osteolytic metastases are present or if there is significant instability pain and/or there is other imaging evidence of potential or actual progressive deformity, techniques of stabilization may be required. They may also be necessary if adequate decompression in itself results in iatrogenic destabilization. For example, distal to T10, posterior decompression that removes one or both facet joints requires stabilization. Above this in the thoracic spine, the presence of the rib cage anteriorly may well provide enough support for surgical stabilization to be unnecessary.

Surgery may also be indicated if the tumour is found to be radioresistant or is progressing despite adequate radiotherapy [40]. A variety of surgical strategies and techniques are available for treatment of metastatic disease of the spine. Metastatic and hormone-refractory prostate cancer (HRPC) patients may benefit from specific techniques of surgical decompression and stabilization dependent upon the location of their metastases.

TECHNIQUES OF SPINAL SURGICAL RECONSTRUCTION AND STABILIZATION

Advances in spinal surgical techniques now permit excision and/or stabilization of any area of the spine (provided there are not multiple adjacent levels involved). It is, however, important to stress that the scale of the procedure should be proportionate to the prognosis and take into account the potential consequences of surgery in relation to other comorbidities. For example, in the cervical spine, decompression and reconstruction may often be undertaken more satisfactorily and over fewer segments from the front of the neck. In the thoracolumbar spine, although the same may apply in a fit patient with a prognosis sufficient to justify spinal reconstruction through an approach which opens the chest, many patients may not be medically fit to undergo this sort of extensive surgery. Indeed, given the prognosis for most patients the benefits of decompression with stabilization from the back of the spine will usually outlive the patient.

Posterior stabilization techniques now usually include pedicle screw fixation above and below the areas involved together with interconnecting rods with a bony fusion if appropriate (Figure 15.7). Anterior techniques usually include corpectomy (removal of the vertebral body) with titanium cage or cement reconstruction and an anterior plate fixed to the levels above and below for stability. Combined anterior and posterior reconstruction, except in

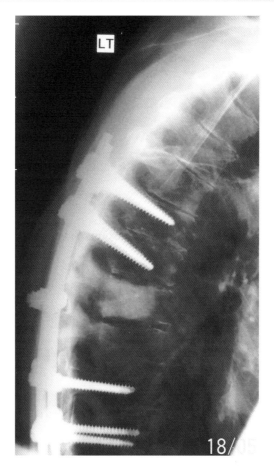

Figure 15.7   Posterior pedicle screw construct with sclerotic vertebra.

very unusual circumstances, remains difficult to justify. It should, however, be stressed that evidence-based comparison is not available in matching cases comparing these approaches.

A paucity of studies evaluating the surgical management of prostatic metastases to the spine means that interpretation of results must be measured. Most studies are retrospective and non-randomized in nature, and patient selection in these cohorts becomes a significant issue. The heterogeneous nature of the patient cohorts between studies, as well as confounding factors such as inconsistent application of adjuvant radiotherapy and varying radiotherapy regimes, additionally reinforces this point. However, the literature does justify a surgical approach to metastatic prostate cancer to the spine [40]. It must be noted though that, similar to radiotherapy, the results of surgery are superior in the absence of neurological compromise, especially paraplegia. The recent study by Flynn *et al.* [8] is worthy of note as it demonstrated that surgery and radiotherapy has a better outcome than radiotherapy alone especially in the paraparetic patient.

This concurs with the experience from our own unit, where 36 patients with metastatic prostate cancer to the spine were managed between 1993 and 2000. Interestingly, metastatic disease to the spine was the first indication of the disease in four patients. Most of the patients underwent a posterior procedure and most had a course of radiotherapy.

Our results compare favourably with the literature but also highlight the disadvantages of surgical management with one case of deep infection. The results of surgery can also be compromised by the development of ESCC or vertebral collapse at a site outside the previous surgery.

It should be noted that surgery after a course of radiotherapy is associated with a higher rate of wound breakdown and infection and a window of at least 6 weeks should ideally be left between the end of the radiotherapy and subsequent surgery to allow full recovery of the soft tissues covering the spine [41].

SUPPORTIVE MEASURES

ANALGESIA

A systematic approach to regular assessment, review and treatment needs to be adopted. It is important to elicit the type, nature and intensity of pain together with the impact on the patient and quality of life. Treatment should be in line with the World Health Organization (WHO) guidance, with medication given regularly (to prevent pain) and selected by the 'ladder', a stepwise progression from non-opioids to 'weak' opioids to strong opioids with appropriate adjuncts [33].

STEROID TREATMENT

Corticosteroids are an integral part of the therapy of ESCC [13]. Steroids initiated immediately after diagnosis may benefit the prostate cancer patient by relieving pain and improving neurological function. Corticosteroids such as dexamethasone perform a principal role in supportive treatment and have also been demonstrated to improve outcomes. A randomized trial of dexamethasone in patients undergoing radiotherapy for ESCC from solid tumours found that a significantly higher percentage were ambulatory on dexamethasone at long-term follow-up [42]. Dexamethasone is the most frequently used agent in the clinical environment; however, no prospective studies have investigated the optimal dose and schedule for patients with ESCC and this remains an area for debate. Supportive evidence of daily doses ranging from 16 to 96 mg is available [32, 43]. In the absence of data, an initial dose within this range is justifiable; however, regardless of the dose used, dexamethasone should be tapered as tolerated, since complications can arise rapidly.

EXTERNAL BRACING

A reduction in pain and an improvement in ambulation may be seen with the application of an external brace even in patients who have not shown evidence of spinal instability [21]. Modern braces are more lightweight and less cumbersome than traditional braces allowing for enhanced comfort.

CONCLUSIONS

The treatment of metastatic prostate cancer to the spine is uniquely different to that of other spinal metastases and in many cases there is no 'one size fits all' answer as to the optimal management of these patients. It is imperative to involve spinal surgeons with the knowledge, interest and capability to evaluate neural compromise and potential or actual spinal instability before deciding on the appropriateness or otherwise of surgical intervention and the techniques involved.

An individual approach based on knowledge and understanding of the current treatment options available and the patient's unique situation and presentation is the best approach to this complex clinical problem.

TREATMENT STRATEGIES FOR FRACTURES

The management of a metastatic lesion in a long bone follows a very similar path to that already outlined for a spinal metastasis and guidelines for this are well established [12, 44]. An isotope bone scan is the ideal 'skeletal survey' for looking for lesions throughout the skeleton. Plain radiographs can be very misleading about the extent of a lesion and CT scanning will give a greater understanding of the osseous anatomy and any skeletal deficiencies. MRI may be useful to assess the presence of any associated soft tissue mass.

The treatment of bone pain is multifactorial including hormonal therapy, radiotherapy and chemotherapy. The length of radiotherapy course required for the palliation of bone pain from metastasis is not yet clear and research in this field continues [45]. There may be a role for hemi-body irradiation or systemic isotope therapy [46]. Bisphosphonates have been used to reduce bone pain from prostate metastasis with mixed results [47].

Biomechanically, the effect of an osteolytic metastasis on bone strength depends on whether the metastasis acts as a stress riser acting to reduce torsional rigidity by approximately 60% or as an open section defect decreasing torsional rigidity by almost 90%. The effects of osteoblastic metastasis on bone strength are not as well known but are thought to reduce bone stiffness rather than strength [47, 48].

Second to the vertebral bodies other common areas of metastasis for prostate cancer are the sternum, pelvis, ribs and femurs. The presentation of appendicular skeletal metastasis is with pain, with or without associated fracture. As previously mentioned, prostate metastases tend to be osteoblastic rather than osteolytic and so pathological fractures in the long bones are uncommon [48]. An osteolytic metastasis represents progression of disease and an increased potential to fracture. However, these fractures have a high potential for union after fixation [48].

Bone pain from metastatic disease is thought to be mediated via stimulation of endosteal nerve endings by chemical agents released from destroyed bone such as prostaglandins and substance P, stretching of the periosteum due to increasing size of the tumour and inflammation of the soft tissues around the tumour [47].

The operative management of appendicular metastasis is dependent on the location of the lesion, the presence of a fracture or an assessment of a future pathological fracture.

Bone destruction alters bone strength, and even osteoblastic lesions can alter the response of the bone to load and increase the risk of fracture. Imminent fracture is also painful on loading of the pathological bone. The use of prophylactic fixation of long bones in this situation can stabilize the bone in the face of continuing destruction and allow load bearing through the implant despite loss of skeletal support.

The most widely used scoring system to assess the need for prophylactic fixation is that of Mirels [49] (Table 15.6). This assesses location, type of metastasis (blastic or lytic), amount of pain and the amount of cortex destroyed. A score of eight or more indicates the need for fixation. The standard implant for a midshaft lesion is a statically locked intramedullary nail. Lesions in the proximal femur may be addressed by an arthroplasty, either a standard hip replacement or a modular proximal femoral replacement. Acetabular disease can also be reconstructed using joint replacement technology, although the addition of Steinmann pins driven through from the iliac crest to the periacetabular region acting to distribute the load more widely throughout the pelvis may well be indicated [50]. Any cavitary defects can be filled with cement or prosthesis as necessary. If arthroplasty is undertaken, the components must be well fixed with cement to allow immediate stability for mobilization and greater protection against implant failure as a result of loss of structural support from disease

Table 15.6 Mirels' scoring system for metastatic bone disease [49]

Variable	Score		
	1	2	3
Site	Upper limb	Lower limb	Peritrochanteric
Pain	Mild	Moderate	Functional
Lesion	Blastic	Mixed	Lytic
Size[1]	< 1/3	1/3–2/3	> 2/3

[1]As seen on plain X-ray, maximum destruction of cortex in any view. Maximum possible score is 12. If lesion scores 8 or above then prophylactic fixation is recommended prior to radiotherapy.

progression. An added benefit is the sterilizing effect to any residual tumour cells in the intramedullary canal from the exothermic reaction of the cement as it hardens.

In the presence of a fracture, the reconstructive options are very much the same as for the impending fracture, using load-bearing intramedullary nails or cemented arthroplasty depending on location.

Adjuvant therapy is indicated for both the impending and subsequently fixed lesion and the fixed fracture. This is usually in the form of a course of radiotherapy. It is worth noting that there is an increasing incidence of osteoporotic non-metastatic fractures following androgen deprivation therapy [51], and these fractures need to be considered in the context of the underlying bone disease. The presentation of a fracture or a patient with bone pain who is known to have metastasis must be assumed to be secondary to metastatic disease initially; this must also be borne in mind as the management may well alter.

REFERENCES

1. Jaffe WL. *Tumours and Tumourous Conditions of the Bones and Joints*. Lea & Febiger, Philadelphia, 1958.
2. Soresen PS, Helweg-Larsen S, Mouridsen H *et al*. Effect of high dose dexamethasone in carcinomatous metastatic spinal cord compression treated with radiotherapy: a randomised trial. *Eur J Cancer* 1994; 30A:22–27.
3. Franks LM. Latent carcinoma of the prostate *J Pathol Bacteriol* 1954; 68:603.
4. Abrams HL, Spiro R, Goldstein N. Metastases in carcinoma; analysis of 1000 autopsied cases. *Cancer* 1950; 3:74–85.
5. Elkin M, Mueller HP. Metastases from cancer of the prostate; autopsy and roentgenological findings. *Cancer* 1954; 7:1246–1248.
6. Turner JW, Jaffe HL. Metastatic neoplasms. A clinical and roentgenological study of the involvement of the skeleton and lungs. *Am J Roentgenol* 1940; 43:479.
7. Willis RA. Secondary tumours of bones. In: *The Spread of Tumours in the Human Body*, Third edn. Butterworth, London, 1973, p. 229.
8. Flynn DF, Shipley WU. Management of spinal cord compression secondary to metastatic prostatic carcinoma. *Urol Clin North Am* 1991; 18:145.
9. Zelefsky MJ, Scher HI, Krol G *et al*. Spinal epidural tumour in patients with prostate cancer: Clinical and radiographic predictors of response to radiation therapy. *Cancer* 1992; 70:2319–2325.
10. Cook GB, Watson FR. Events in the natural history of prostate cancer: using salvage curves, mean age distributions and contingency coefficients. *J Urol* 1968; 99:87.
11. Liskow A, Chang CH, DeSanctis P *et al*. Epidural cord compression in association with genitourinary neoplasms. *Cancer* 1986; 59:949–954.
12. British Orthopaedic Association and British Orthopaedic Oncology Society. *Metastatic Bone Disease. A Guide to Good Practice*. Available at www.boa.ac.uk.
13. Osborn JL, Getzenberg RH *et al*. Spinal cord compression in prostate cancer. *J Neurooncol* 1995; 23: 135–147.
14. Gilbert RW, Kim JH *et al*. Epidural spinal cord compression from metastatic tumor: diagnosis and treatment. *Ann Neurol* 1978; 3:40–51.

15. Cereceda LE, Flechon A et al. Management of vertebral metastases in prostate cancer: a retrospective analysis in 119 patients. *Clin Prostate Cancer* 2003; 2:34–40.
16. Smith EM, Hampel N et al. Spinal cord compression secondary to prostate carcinoma: treatment and prognosis. *J Urol* 1993; 149:330–333.
17. Rosenthal MA, Rosen D et al. Spinal cord compression in prostate cancer. A 10-year experience. *Br J Urol* 1992; 69:530–583.
18. Schaberg J, Gainor BJ. A profile of metastatic carcinoma of the spine. *Spine* 1985; 10:19–20.
19. Grant R, Papadopoulos SM et al. Metastatic epidural spinal cord compression. *Neurol Clin* 1991; 9:825–841.
20. Stark RJ, Henson JA et al. Spinal metastases. A retrospective survey from a general hospital. *Brain* 1982; 105(Pt 1):189–213.
21. Chen TC. Prostate cancer and spinal cord compression. *Oncology (Huntingt)* 2001; 15:841–861.
22. Godersky JC, Smoker WR , Knutson R. Use of magnetic resonance imaging in the evaluation of metastatic spinal disease. *Neurosurgery* 1987; 21:676–680.
23. Carmody RF, Yang PJ et al. Spinal cord compression due to metastatic disease: diagnosis with MR imaging versus myelography. *Radiology* 1989; 173:225–259.
24. Li KC, Poon PY. Sensitivity and specificity of MRI in detecting malignant spinal cord compression and in distinguishing malignant from benign compression fractures of vertebrae. *Magn Reson Imaging* 1988; 6:547–556.
25. Portenoy RK, Galer BS et al. Identification of epidural neoplasm. Radiography and bone scintigraphy in the symptomatic and asymptomatic spine. *Cancer* 1989; 64:2207–2213.
26. Pollen JJ, Gerber K, Ashburn WL et al. The value of nuclear bone imaging in advanced prostate cancer. *J Urol* 1981; 125:222–223.
27. Merrick MV, Stone AR, Chisolm GD. Prostatic cancer. Nuclear medicine. *Recent Res Cancer Res* 1981; 78:108–118.
28. Weissman DE, Gilbert M, Wong H et al. The use of computed tomography of the spine to identify patients at high risk of epidural metastases. *J Clin Oncol* 1985; 3:1541–1544.
29. Tomita K, Kawahara N, Kobayashi T et al. Surgical strategy for spinal metastases. *Spine* 2001; 26:298–306.
30. Tokuhashi Y, Matsuzaki H, Toriyama S et al. Scoring system for the preoperative evaluation of metastatic spine tumor prognosis. *Spine.* 1990; 15:1110–1113.
31. Martenson JA, Evans RG et al. Treatment outcome and complications in patients treated for malignant epidural spinal cord compression (SCC). *J Neurooncol* 1985; 3:77–84.
32. Greenberg HS, Kim JH et al. Epidural spinal cord compression from metastatic tumor: results with a new treatment protocol. *Ann Neurol* 1980; 8:361–366.
33. World Health Organization. Cancer pain relief and palliative care. Report of a WHO Expert Committee. *World Health Organization Technical Report Series, 804.* World Health Organization, Geneva, 1990, pp. 1–75.
34. Patchell RA, Tibbs PA et al. Direct decompressive surgical resection in the treatment of spinal cord compression caused by metastatic cancer: a randomised trial. *Lancet* 2005; 366:643–648.
35. Tong D, Gillick L et al. The palliation of symptomatic osseous metastases: final results of the study by the Radiation Therapy Oncology Group. *Cancer* 1982; 50:893–899.
36. Findlay GF. The role of vertebral body collapse in the management of malignant spinal cord compression. *J Neurol Neurosurg Psychiatry* 1987; 50:151–154.
37. Tomita TJ, Galicich H et al. Radiation therapy for spinal epidural metastases with complete block. *Acta Radiol Oncol* 1983; 22:135–143.
38. Helweg-Larsen S Johnsen A et al. Radiologic features compared to clinical findings in a prospective study of 153 patients with metastatic spinal cord compression treated by radiotherapy. *Acta Neurochir (Wien)* 1997; 139:105–111.
39. Sasagawa I, Gotoh H et al. Hormonal treatment of symptomatic spinal cord compression in advanced prostatic cancer. *Int Urol Nephrol* 1991; 23:351–356.
40. McLain RF, Bell GF. Newer management options in patients with spinal metastasis. *Cleve Clin J Med* 1998; 65:359–366.
41. Aebi M. Spinal metastasis in the elderly. *Eur Spine J* 2003; Suppl. 2:S202–213
42. Soresen PS, Helweg-Larsen S, Mouridsen H et al. Effect of high dose dexamethasone in carcinomatous metastatic spinal cord compression treated with radiotherapy: a randomised trial. *Eur J Cancer* 1994; 30A:22–27.

43. Heimdal K, Hirschberg H *et al*. High incidence of serious side-effects of high-dose dexamethasone treatment in patients with epidural spinal cord compression. *J Neurooncol* 1992; 12:141–144.
44. Tillman R. Metastatic disease of the appendicular skeleton. *JBJS* 1999; 81B:1–2.
45. Hartsell WF, Scott CB *et al*. Randomised control trial of short versus long course radiotherapy for palliation of painful bone metastases. *J Natl Cancer Inst* 2005; 97:798–804.
46. Capanna R, Campanacci DA. The treatment of metastases in the appendicular skeleton. *JBJS* 2001; 83B:471–481.
47. Aaron AD. Treatment of metastatic adenocarcinoma of the pelvis and extremities. *JBJS* 1997; 79A:917–932.
48. Hipp JA, Rosenburg AE *et al*. Mechanical properties of trabecular bone within and adjacent to osseous metastasis. *J Bone Min Res* 1992; 7:1165–1171.
49. Mirels H. Metastatic disease in long bones. A proposed scoring system for diagnosing impending pathological fractures. *CORR* 2003; 415 S:S148–157.
50. Harrington KD. Orthopaedic management of extremity and pelvic lesions. *Clin Orthop* 1995; 312:136–147.
51. Shahinian VB, Yong- Fang Kuo *et al*. Risk of fracture after androgen deprivation for prostate cancer. *NEJM* 2005; 352:154–164.

16

Treatment strategies for urinary obstruction

Roger S. Kirby

INTRODUCTION

The term 'obstructive uropathy' encompasses patients with bladder outflow obstruction and those with hydronephrosis, and can be caused by local extension and/or lymphatic spread of prostate cancer. Obstructive uropathy is a relatively common occurrence in patients with advanced, metastatic prostate cancer; reported incidence rates vary between 3.3% and 16% [1–6]. The first step in management is to accurately establish the diagnosis. Treatment strategies depend on whether the underlying cause is from hormone-naive prostate cancer or whether it is hormone resistant prostate cancer; the prognosis for the latter is significantly worse. Close liaison between urologist, oncologist and radiologist is essential to manage optimally patients with these conditions.

LOWER URINARY TRACT SYMPTOMS AND OBSTRUCTIVE UROPATHY

Lower urinary tract symptoms (LUTS) are common among men suffering from locally advanced prostate cancer [7]. Classical symptoms are similar to non-malignant obstruction and commonly include poor flow and frequency, as well as the sensation of incomplete bladder emptying. Other problems may include haematuria, anorexia and weight loss, which may indicate incipient renal failure. The presence of a palpable bladder indicates urinary retention, this occurs in approximately 13% of men with locally advanced prostate cancer [8].

PRESENTATION/DIAGNOSIS

It is essential to determine whether one is dealing with malignant or non-malignant uropathy. A digital rectal examination (DRE) is essential, and any prostate asymmetry, a palpable nodule or an irregular hardening, requires further investigation. On examination of a non-malignant prostate gland, the median sulcus is usually identifiable and the seminal vesicles are impalpable; loss of the sulcus or irregularity in the seminal vesicles indicates malignant involvement. If there is any suspicion of malignancy in a patient who does not have a diagnosis of prostate cancer, it is necessary to perform a transrectal ultrasound and biopsy. The first-line assessment of the urinary tract should be with ultrasound, which should include a measurement of residual urine volume, imaging of the kidneys and, in addition, a flow rate is often useful. A computed tomography (CT) or magnetic resonance imaging (MRI) scan may be indicated if more detail is needed, specifically to determine the extent and location of any metastases.

Roger S. Kirby, MA MD FRCS (Urol) The Prostate Centre, London, UK

MANAGEMENT AND TREATMENT OPTIONS

There are a number of treatment options available for men with LUTS and bladder out-flow obstruction (BOO). These include long-term bladder catheterization, medical or surgical therapy and systemic treatment for the underlying cancer including hormone therapy. Obviously, the most appropriate treatment for this condition will depend on whether previous definitive primary treatment has been undertaken as well as past systemic therapies for prostate cancer.

In an attempt to predict the likelihood of outflow obstruction after different treatment modalities for prostate cancer, Oefelein studied a population of 260 patients with advanced metastatic prostate cancer over a median of 12 years [9]. Results showed that disease progression causing BOO after radical prostatectomy is extremely rare at 2.8% (1/36 patients); however, disease progression causing BOO was relatively common for both external beam radiotherapy at 17.8% (8/45 patients) and androgen deprivation 18.1% (26/144 patients) [9].

In hormone-naive patients presenting with severe LUTS, hormone treatment is usually recommended. Bilateral orchidectomy was traditionally undertaken to improve voiding function, but luteinizing hormone releasing hormone (LHRH) agonists may be equally effective. In patients with urinary retention (acute or chronic), androgen ablation may facilitate voiding with temporary bladder catheterization [10]. In an early study by Fleischman and Catalona, 35 patients with prostate cancer presenting in acute urinary retention were studied: 68% of patients were able to void after orchidectomy alone [11]. Original work by Huggins *et al.* in 1941 suggested that maximum decrease in prostatic volume occurred at 3 months [12]. In practice, if voiding is unsuccessful after 8 weeks of androgen ablation then consideration for transurethral resection of the prostate (TURP) is necessary [13].

PALLIATIVE TURP (PTURP)

Palliative TURP (pTURP) or 'channel' TURP is usually performed because of refractory urinary retention, BOO with high post-void residual urinary volume, bladder stones or haematuria. It is sometimes suggested that pTURP may have a negative oncological impact with tumour dissemination at the time of surgery owing to high irrigation pressures resulting in intravascular dissemination through open venous sinuses [14, 15]. Certainly, Moreno *et al.* have detected prostate cancer cells in the peripheral circulating blood in all cases undergoing pTURP [14]. In principle, incision through malignant tumour is generally to be avoided. The exact significance of this in the context of pTURP is unclear. A number of studies have attempted to define the oncological outcomes of patients undergoing pTURP. In a surgical series of 490 stage C patients, Nativ *et al.* reported no unfavourable outcome in those who were diagnosed following TURP compared with those who were diagnosed by needle biopsy [16]. Some of these concerns are still not completely resolved but they contrast with the negative impact of long-term catheterization, acute urinary retention or bladder stones on quality of life. pTURP also has a higher perioperative morbidity and mortality (mortality can be ~2% [17] with a risk of stress incontinence of 5–10% [17, 18]), and this needs to be fully explained to the patient. In one study of 89 palliative TURPs, it was noted that 79% of men voided spontaneously after this type of surgery but a repeat TURP was necessary in 25% of patients [17]. Heavy bleeding following pTURP can sometimes be problematic; however, preoperative androgen ablation may reduce tumour volume and tumour vascularity. Alpha-1-adrenoceptor antagonists are less effective in malignant obstruction than in benign prostatic hypertrophy (BPH). External beam radiotherapy to the prostate may be considered for local control and may reduce a tendency to haemorrhage.

PROSTATIC STENTING

Prostatic stents have been inserted in men with BOO for locally advanced prostate cancer for many years. The rationale for stent insertion is that it avoids the morbidity and mortality of pTURP. Prostatic stenting may also be of use in those patients unfit for general anaesthesia as insertion may be performed under local anaesthesia. Anson *et al.* were some of the first to use a temporary urospiral stent, in combination with androgen suppression, to treat acute urinary retention. All patients (10/10) voided spontaneously immediately postoperatively, with one patient needing early removal of the stent due to irritative voiding symptoms [19]. Removal of stents at 3 months reduces the potential long-term complications of stent encrustation, urinary tract infection and chronic pain [20]. In patients who are hormone resistant, long-term stents are more appropriate. Guazzoni *et al.* inserted the UroLume® stent in 11 patients with advanced prostate cancer who were in urinary retention and had a high surgical risk. All patients voided after the procedure and urodynamic follow-up at 1 year revealed relief of BOO. Another study examined the use of the same stent for refractory retention following brachytherapy [21]: all patients voided spontaneously immediately after insertion, but two patients suffered stent-related symptoms necessitating subsequent removal. Preliminary data look promising for the use of prostatic stents, but large-scale trials are needed to further evaluate their use. At present, prostatic stents appear to have a role in patients unfit for surgery who have BOO or in those patients with refractory retention post brachytherapy. In future, there may also be a role for laser vaporization in view of its low surgical morbidity.

UPPER URINARY TRACT OBSTRUCTION AND OBSTRUCTIVE UROPATHY

Prostate cancer can cause upper urinary tract obstruction due to local extension of prostatic tissue compressing the vesicoureteric junction, invasion of tumour into the ureteric orifice or by metastatic spread to lymph nodes involving the intramural ureter. Urinary tract obstruction is a common finding at diagnosis and at the later stages of this disease [3]. If left untreated it may lead to renal impairment and subsequent kidney failure. Patients presenting with urinary tract obstruction typically have a poor prognosis [22] with troublesome complications causing significant morbidity. While lower urinary tract obstruction (BOO), does not appear to be of prognostic value in predicting response to androgen blockade, the same is not true of upper tract obstruction [3]. Hydronephrosis has been shown to have an independent prognostic value for progression after hormonal treatment and correlates also with time to death from prostate cancer [3]. Furthermore, persistent or newly developed hydronephrosis during treatment also predicts a shorter time to progression.

PRESENTATION/DIAGNOSIS

Presentation is classically insidious with deranged blood biochemistry or the incidental finding of ureteric dilatation or renal cortical atrophy on ultrasound imaging [22]. Occasionally patients may present acutely with renal colic [23]. Bilateral ureteric obstruction (acute or chronic) is associated with a decreased urine output and uraemia, which progresses to renal failure. Urinary retention as a cause for bilateral hydronephrosis must be excluded clinically or sonographically and, if found, should be immediately treated with bladder catheterization. Indications for emergency decompression of the upper urinary tract by percutaneous nephrostomy include deteriorating renal function and renal sepsis.

INVESTIGATION OF OBSTRUCTIVE UROPATHY

In patients with previously confirmed prostate cancer, possible urinary tract obstruction should be anticipated and the patient monitored accordingly [3]. Investigation of the patient with an elevated serum creatinine and suspected obstructive uropathy should include a urinary tract ultrasound. Further investigation with a non-contrast CT or MRI scan may be necessary to assess the level of obstruction, and the extent of local or nodal disease. In patients with adequate renal function, intravenous urography (IVU) and radionucleotide renography may be useful.

Ultrasound

This is the most common form of imaging for the urinary tract when obstruction is suspected. Ultrasound will diagnose hydronephrosis and hydroureter and will also give an assessment of renal cortical thickness and possible level of obstruction. One disadvantage of ultrasound is the inability to visualize the mid- and lower-thirds of the ureter. If such information is necessary then CT scanning may be more appropriate and this can also assesses any concurrent lymphadenopathy.

Computed Tomography

CT scanning is a useful imaging tool when ultrasound and other modalities have proved inconclusive. CT is particularly useful for providing more detailed information on any potential obstructing lesion. Ideally, intravenous contrast should be used, but this may not be possible in patients with uraemia. A prospective study of 36 patients with hydronephrosis secondary to obstructive nephropathy of uncertain aetiology revealed that abdominal CT scan proved useful in 92% of cases. In addition extrinsic masses were demonstrated in 20 patients with metastatic disease [24].

MRI

Recent advances in MRI, in particular excretion MR urography, have made this modality a useful adjunct in assessing renal tract obstruction. MR urography has the advantage over ultrasound and CT in providing a detailed picture of the obstructing lesion while avoiding ionizing radiation and nephrotoxic contrast media. In a study of 45 patients with obstructive uropathy due to both benign and malignant pathology, it was established that MR urography was able to provide high quality images for diagnosing and determining the cause of urinary obstruction, defining the position and severity of dilatations and showing localization of the pathology [25]. In another study of obstructive uropathy involving groups of patients with calculi, strictures of the pelvi-ureteric junction, benign or malignancy-induced ureterostenosis, it was noted that MR urography was able to detect the degree and level of ureterohydronephrosis in 100% of cases of malignancy-induced ureterostenosis. In fact MR urography appears to be more useful in the setting of non-calculus urinary obstruction [26]. While MRI may not be the first choice of imaging for obstructive uropathy, it does have a role for patients with contrast allergies or those with contraindications to ionizing radiation. It also provides high-quality images of the primary prostatic lesion.

Radionuclide Renography

Dynamic radionuclide renography scanning may be suited to evaluate renal obstruction and differential renal function. Radionuclides that may be used include technetium-99m-labelled MAG-3 (mercaptoacetyltriglycine) or technetium-99m-DTPA (diethylenetriamine pentaacetic acid) [27]. In general, radionuclides evaluate renal function at the time of examination and not the potential for renal recovery.

MANAGEMENT AND TREATMENT OPTIONS

Deciding on the optimum treatment for obstructive uropathy is dependent on the level of obstruction present and the hormonal status of the patient. Patients with ureteric obstruction due to hormone-naive locally advanced prostate cancer are suitable for treatment with androgen blockade or orchidectomy [4]. However, the majority of patients are hormone insensitive and these patients may need some form of urinary diversion procedure. This usually takes place by percutaneous nephrostomy followed by antegrade or retrograde stenting. In patients with low-grade obstruction or partial chronic obstruction, intervention may be delayed [28]. However, bilateral obstruction or unilateral obstruction with progressive renal impairment or symptoms of pyonephrosis requires immediate management and drainage to prevent irreversible renal damage. Uraemia as a result of malignant ureteric obstruction is a recognized event and if left untreated is rapidly terminal.

The treatment of renal obstruction in patients with advanced prostate cancer (particularly hormone-resistant prostate cancer, HRPC) may raise an ethical dilemma for the treating physicians. While urinary decompression may be technically feasible it does not mean that this is always the correct treatment decision where the procedure is subsequently regretted or further intervention may be required. Where further treatment is feasible (see Chapter 12), the temporizing measure of urinary drainage may be worthwhile. However, where end-stage HRPC exists, it may not be in the patient's best interest to prolong life, particularly when suffering may be prolonged. Needless to say, a full and frank discussion is needed with the patient and relatives present. An individually tailored management plan is necessary for each person.

Intervention

Historically, patients with malignant obstruction would be treated by open surgical urinary diversion or open ureteral stent placement [29, 30]. However, minimally invasive technologies including percutaneous needle nephrostomy (PCNN), long-term ureteric stenting (antegrade or retrograde) and endoscopic ureteroneocystotomy have largely replaced open surgical procedures [4, 31]. If conventional ureteric stenting is not possible, extra-anatomical stenting may be indicated [32]. The decision on which primary treatment is best is complex and may involve discussion between radiology and urology departments. The role of TURP is only indicated to achieve improved voiding or LUTS. It does not have a principal role in the management of prostate cancer or the management of upper urinary tract obstruction [13].

In general, insertion of a retrograde ureteric stent would not be the first choice for patients with acute ureteric obstruction secondary to locally advanced prostate cancer. PCNN as a primary treatment has a number of benefits over retrograde ureteric stenting. The nephrostomy tube may be left as a long-term drainage tube or, alternatively, this can be converted to an antegrade stent once serum electrolytes have normalized. This also has the advantage of being able to perform a nephrostogram prior to nephrostomy tube removal to confirm that the stent is draining.

Percutaneous Needle Nephrostomy

PCNN is a commonly performed procedure for benign and malignant obstructive uropathy. While the indications for PCNN are very similar to those for retrograde ureteric stenting, there are a number of clinical indicators which favour one over the other. In most patients with ureteric obstruction the collecting system and ureter are dilated allowing for the, relatively, easy insertion of a percutaneous nephrostomy tube. Nephrostomy tubes may be left in as a long-term urinary diversion; however, they are not well tolerated causing discomfort and urine infection, and they can become dislodged. Therefore, it may be appropriate to convert to an antegrade stent at a convenient time when the kidney has decompressed and the emergency has been dealt with. Antegrade stenting following nephrostomy can be quite complicated when one is dealing with proximal obstructing lesions, particularly those involving the renal pelvis. In some cases, insertion of a retrograde ureteric stent may be more appropriate.

PCNN is an extremely well-tolerated procedure with a good chance of renal function improvement. In one study of 206 PCNNs [33] for benign ($n = 30$) and malignant ($n = 125$) obstruction, 66% of patients noted a return to normal renal function, 28% noted an improvement in renal function, therefore avoiding the need for dialysis, and only 6% noted no significant improvement. This was achieved with a 99% success rate and no serious complications [33]. PCNN allows the subsequent insertion of antegrade ureteric stenting, which approaches 80% success rate. However, this same study noted advanced age and prostate cancer to be negative predictive factors for renal improvement. Therefore, whether PCNN should be utilized in advanced prostate cancer patients is subject to debate. In a study of 22 patients with advanced pelvic cancer, 24 nephrostomies were performed (bilateral in two patients) for malignant ureteric obstructions. Indications for nephrostomy in this group included renal failure, urosepsis or pretreatment before chemotherapy. Sixty-eight per cent of patients were able to achieve a useful lifestyle after the procedure, with a survival time ranging from 3 months to 2 years [34]. Similarly, in a study of 77 patients with obstructive uropathy secondary to pelvic malignant disease, a successful nephrostomy insertion rate resulted in an overall median patient survival of over 6 months [35].

Although percutaneous drainage of the kidney provides a reliable method of allowing renal recovery, the impact of treatment on patient quality of life remains controversial. While the two previous studies [34, 35] show an improvement in survival, these have included various primary tumour types: the situation in advanced HRPC is less clear. One study of 22 HRPC patients studied the impact of PCNN intervention on overall survival [5]. They noted that, on average, patients spent 41% of their remaining life in hospital with the vast majority ($n = 18$) not surviving more than 3 months. The conclusions from this study were that PCNN did not improve the quality of life for these patients.

In those patients who are hormone naive, urinary tract decompression may be worthwhile. One study of 36 patients with bilateral ureteric obstruction and renal failure showed a median survival of 21 months following ureteric decompression and subsequent hormone therapy [4]. The same study also examined those patients with HRPC and noted a significantly worse prognosis with median survival of 2.7 months. The authors concluded that in patients with bilateral ureteric obstruction secondary to prostate cancer who have not undergone hormone manipulation, there should be little hesitation in the use of upper tract decompression in either short- or long-term disease management. In another study of 15 hormone-naive prostate cancer patients, including unilateral and bilateral ureteric obstruction, survival rates were reported as even longer. Chiou *et al.* noted a 73% and 47% 1-year and 2-year survival rate respectively [6]. In those patients who had undergone hormone therapy the figures fell to 48% and 19%. The authors did not advocate withholding PCNN in HRPC patients due to the high number of patients who survive longer than 1 year.

Ureteric Stenting

Endoscopic procedures for treating malignant strictures tend to be less successful with endoureterotomy having a dismal outcome for treating this condition [36]. Byun *et al.* performed balloon dilatation on malignant strictures with a similarly disappointing result: success rates at 12 and 36 months were 18% and 14% respectively [37]. Therefore, the use of long-term ureteric stents changed periodically may be the best option.

Retrograde ureteric stenting is a recognized technique in the case of obstructive uropathy; however, it may not be technically feasible in all circumstances. Locally advanced prostate cancers often invade the trigone and occlude or distort the ureteric orifices (UOs). This makes cannulation of the UOs a difficult, if not impossible, task at times. Secondly, the requirement for formal anaesthesia in persons with deranged renal function may make this a high-risk procedure. Finally, urinary drainage via stenting occurs through the stent lumen in malignant disease, therefore any blockage of the lumen results in stent failure; as reflected by the high failure rates for ureteric stents [38].

In an attempt to decrease the chance of single stents becoming obstructed due to tumour progression, a number of groups have suggested the placement of two ipsilateral ureteral stents [39, 40]. Two stents theoretically create a potential space along the ureter between the grooves of the stent. In a small group of seven patients with malignant obstruction, who had previously failed single-stent management, two double-J stents were inserted in all patients and proved to be safe and well tolerated [39]. Other groups have investigated the role of metallic stents as a more viable solution to malignant occlusion [41, 42]. Pauer and Lugmayr report a 55% primary patency rate in 58 malignant ureteric strictures treated by self-expanding endoluminal stents [42]. Others have attempted to coat stents in non-reactive Dacron [43] or Nitinol [44] in order to try and reduce the degree of tissue ingrowth, which compromises ureteral patency. However, these studies have met with very mixed results: Barbalias et al. reported a 81% failure rate using a Nitinol stent with stent migration into the bladder [44]. Clearly, malignant ureteric obstruction is a difficult problem.

Endoscopic Ureteroneocystostomy

Endoscopic ureteroneocystostomy can restore ureterovesical continuity through the resection of the ureteric meatus following either PCNN or ureteric stent placement. Chefchaouni et al. performed endoscopic ureteroneocystostomy in 31 patients with renal failure from advanced unilateral ($n = 12$) or bilateral ($n = 18$) obstructive uropathy secondary to prostate cancer, in an attempt to restore continuity of the ureteric orifice [45]. Eleven patients were hormone naive, whilst 18 had HRPC. All patients underwent PCNN prior to ureteroneocystostomy. Under fluoroscopic guidance, the position of the obstruction was then determined, and deep resection of the lateral part of the trigone was performed, enabling the reopening of the ureteric lumen. The nephrostomy tube was removed after normalization or stabilization of renal function. Continuity of the ureteric orifice was achieved in 76% of patients, and a median survival after surgery of 8 months was achieved. Additionally, the average time in hospital was reduced from 27.5 days to 6.8 days following ureteroneocystostomy. The hormonal status of patients had no effect on survival. The authors concluded that ureteroneocystostomy provided an attractive option for patients with obstructive uropathy, due to the short hospital stay and high success rate of this treatment.

CONCLUSIONS

Malignant obstruction to the urinary tract encompasses a broad range of clinical conditions, for which the correct management differs for each individual patient. A number of important factors need to be addressed in deciding on the best course of action and these must include an assessment of the tumour itself, its hormone responsiveness, potential for further therapies and overall prognosis. Treatment decisions are best made with involvement of the individual patient, his family, and a multidisciplinary medical team including urologists, radiologists, oncologists and palliative care specialists.

REFERENCES

1. Michigan S, Catalona W. Ureteral obstruction from prostatic carcinoma: response to endocrine and radiation therapy. *J Urol* 1977; 118:733–738.
2. Sandhu D, Mayor P, Sambrook P et al. Outcome and prognostic factors in patients with advanced prostate cancer and obstructive uropathy. *Br J Urol* 1992; 70:412–416.
3. Colombel M, Mallame W, Abbou C. Influence of urological complications on the prognosis of prostate cancer. *Eur Urol* 1997; 31(Suppl 3):21–24.
4. Paul A, Love C, Chisholm. The management of bilateral ureteric obstruction and renal failure in advanced prostate cancer. *Br J Urol* 1994; 74:642–645.
5. Dowling R, Carrasco C et al. Percutaneous urinary diversion in patients with hormone-refractory prostate cancer. *Urology* 1991; 37:89–91.

6.   Chiou R, Chang W, Horan J. Ureteral obstruction associated with prostate cancer: the outcome after percutaneous nephrostomy. *J Urol* 1990; 143:957–959.

7.   Hamilton W, Sharp D. Symptomatic diagnosis of prostate cancer in primary care: a structured review. *Br J Gen Prac* 2004; 54:617–621.

8.   Moul J, Davis R, Vaccaro J, Sihelnik S, Belville W, McLeod D. Acute urinary retention associated with prostatic carcinoma. *J Urol* 1989; 141:1357–1377.

9.   Oefelein M. Prognostic significance of obstructive uropathy in advanced prostate cancer. *Urology* 2004; 63:1117–1121.

10. Thomas D, Balaji V, Coptcoat M, Abercrombie G. Acute urinary retention secondary to carcinoma of the prostate. Initial channel TURP beneficial? *J Roy Soc Med* 1992; 853:318–319.

11. Fleischmann J, Catalona W. Endocrine therapy for bladder outlet obstruction from carcinoma of the prostate. *J Urol* 1985; 134:498–500.

12. Huggins C, Stevens R Jr, Hodges C. Studies on prostatic cancers 2. The effects of castration on advanced carcinoma of the prostate. *Arch Surg* 1941; 43:209.

13. Kirby R. Managing the complications of advanced prostate cancer. *Prostate Cancer: Principles and Practice.* Taylor and Francis, 2006, pp. 1031–1042.

14. Moreno J, O'Hara S, Long J *et al.* Transrectal ultrasound-guided biopsy causes haematogenous dissemination of prostate cells as determined by RT-PCR. *Urology* 1997; 49:515–520.

15. Hanks G, Leibel S, Kramer S. The dissemination of cancer by transurethral resection of locally advanced prostate cancer. *J Urol* 1983; 129:309–311.

16. Nativ O, Bergstralh E, Boyle EJ, Zincke H. Transurethral resection versus needle biopsy prior to radical prostatectomy for stage C prostate cancer. *Urology* 1991; 37:22–27.

17. Marszalek M, Ponholzer A, Rauchenwald M, Madersbacher S. Palliative transurethral resection of the prostate; functional outcome and impact on survival. *BJU Int* 2007; 991:56–59.

18. Mazur A, Thompson I. Efficacy and morbidity of 'channel' TURP. *Urology* 1991; 386:526–528.

19. Anson K, Barnes D, Briggs T, Watson G, Miller R. Temporary prostatic stenting and androgen suppression: a new minimally invasive approach to malignant prostatic retention. *J Roy Soc Med* 1993; 86:634–636.

20. Madersbacher S. Stents for prostatic diseases: any progress after 25 years. *Eur Urol* 2006; 49:212–214.

21. Konety B, Phelan M, O'Donnell W, Antiles L, Chancellor M. Urolume stent placement for the treatment of postbrachytherapy bladder outlet obstruction. *Urology* 2000; 55:721–724.

22. Russo P. Urologic emergencies in the cancer patient. *Semin Oncol* 2000; 27:284–298.

23. Villavicencio H. Quality of life of patients with advanced metastatic prostatic carcinoma. *Eur Urol* 1993; 27:118–121.

24. Bosniak M, Megibow A, Ambos M *et al.* Computed tomography of ureteral obstruction. *Am J Roentgenol* 1982; 138:1107–1113.

25. Karabacakoglu A, Karakose S, Ince O, Cobankara O, Karalezi G. Diagnostic value of diuretic-enhanced excretory MR urography in patients with obstructive uropathy. *Eur J Rad* 2004; 52:320–327.

26. Zielonko J, Studniarek M, Markuszewski M. MR urography of obstructive uropathy: diagnostic value of the method in selected clinical groups. *Eur Radiol* 2003; 134:802–809.

27. Thomsen H, Hvid-Jacobsen K, Meyhoff H *et al.* Combination of DMSA-scintigraphy and hippuran renography in unilateral obstructive nephropathy. Improved prediction of recovery after intervention. *Acta Radiol* 1987; 28:653–655.

28. Chevalier R, Klahr S. Therapeutic approaches in obstructive uropathy. *Semin Oncol* 1998; 18:652–658.

29. Rose P. Operative retroperitoneal ureteral catheterization for obstructive uropathy in primary locally advanced carcinoma of the cervix: description of a technique and experience. *Gynecol Oncol* 1996; 61:79–82.

30. Holden S, McPhee M, Grabstald H. The rationale of urinary diversion in cancer patients. *J Urol* 1979; 121:19–21.

31. Lang E. Antegrade ureteric stenting for dehiscence, strictures, and fistulae. *Am J Roentgenol* 1984; 143:795–801.

32. Minhas S, Irving H, Lloyd S *et al.* Extra-anatomic stents in ureteric obstruction: experience and complications. *BJU Int* 1999; 84:762–764.

33. Pappas P, Stravodimos K, Mitropoulos D *et al.* Role of percutaneous urinary diversion in malignant and benign obstructive uropathy. *J Endourol* 2000; 145:401–405.

34. Hoe J, Tung K, Tan E. Re-evaluation of indications for percutaneous nephrostomy and interventional uroradiological procedures in pelvic malignancy. *Br J Urol* 1993; 71:469–472.

35. Lau M, Temperley D, Mehta S *et al.* Urinary tract obstruction and nephrostomy drainage in pelvic malignant disease. *Br J Urol* 1993; 71:469–472.

36. Lu D, Papanicolaou N, Girard M, Lee M, Yoder I. Percutaneous internal ureteral stent placement: Review of technical issues and solutions in 50 consecutive cases. *Clin Radiol* 1994; 49:256–261.

37. Byun S, Kim J, Oh S, Kim H. Simple retrograde dilatation for treatment of ureteral strictures: etiology-based analysis. *Yonsei Med J* 2003; 44:273–278.

38. Docimo S, DeWolf W. High failure rate of indwelling ureteral stents in patients with extrinsic obstruction. *J Urol* 1989; 142:277–279.

39. Rotariu P, Yohannes P, Alexianu M *et al.* Management of malignant extrinsic compression of the ureter by simultaneous placement of two ipsilateral ureteral stents. *J Endourol* 2001; 1510:979–983.

40. Liu J, Hrebinko R. The use of 2 ipsilateral ureteral stents for relief of ureteral obstruction from extrinsic compression. *J Urol* 1998; 159:179–181.

41. Lugmayr H, Pauer W. Self-expanding stents for palliative treatment of malignant ureteral obstruction. *Am J Roentgenol* 1992; 159:1091–1094.

42. Pauer W, Lugmayr H. Self-expanding permanent endoluminal stents in the ureter. 5 years results and critical evaluation. *Urology A* 1996; 35:485–489.

43. Tekin M, Aytekin C, Aygun C. Covered metallic ureteral stent in the management of malignant ureteral obstruction: preliminary results. *Urology* 2001; 58:919–923.

44. Barbalias G, Liatsikos E, Kalogeropoulou C. Externally coated ureteral metallic stents: an unfavourable clinical experience. *Eur Urol* 2002; 42:276–280.

45. Chefchaouni M, Flam T, Pacha K *et al.* Endoscopic ureteroneocystostomy: palliative urinary diversion in advanced prostate cancer. *Tech Urol* 1998; 4:46–50.

17

Treatment strategies for erectile dysfunction

Arthur L. Burnett

INTRODUCTION

In recent years, prostate cancer has emerged from an often trivialized medical condition, relegated to older men and thought to exert little lifetime consequence, to a disease state of major importance. The significance of the disease has increased in large part because of its dramatic stage migration in the modern prostate-specific antigen (PSA) era, and this is typified by increasingly early clinical stage diagnoses and diagnoses made increasingly in young men. As a result, the need exists for improved disease control via effective oncological control while maximally preserving functional outcomes. This matter is most noteworthy in the area of erectile function, particularly as it is viewed that other historical complications of treatment, such as urinary incontinence following radical prostatectomy, have greatly been reduced [1]. Indeed, as patients currently consider the impact of various treatment approaches for prostate cancer on their quality of life, many place paramount importance on the opportunity for retaining natural erectile function [2].

This chapter provides an assessment of the current literature on the subject of erectile dysfunction following treatment for prostate cancer. It includes a review of the significance and impact of the problem, its causes and associations, and both current and future approaches in its clinical management. Emphasis is appropriately given to the consequences of radical prostatectomy, in which this matter has been most intensively studied. However, it is recognized that all interventions for prostate cancer, including external beam radiotherapy, brachytherapy and hormonal ablation, have the potential to affect penile erections.

SIGNIFICANCE OF THE PROBLEM

Erectile dysfunction has long been known to be a potential consequence of treating prostate cancer, perhaps best associated with radical prostatectomy. Historically, erectile dysfunction was a universal outcome of undergoing this surgery. However, in the past 20 years, with the advent of cavernous nerve-sparing modifications of the surgery, postoperative erectile function rates have improved [3]. The initial descriptions of the course of the cavernous nerves surrounding the prostate and supplying the penis represented a major historical advance [4]. As it is currently understood, anatomic radical prostatectomy refers to an improved understanding of the surgical anatomy of the prostate and its surrounding surgical structures in the deep pelvis, and the implementation of a rational plan for surgical dissection based on circumstances of the oncological presentation [3]. In the current era of nerve-sparing radical prostatectomy, the rates of erectile function recovery satisfactory for sexual intercourse following the surgery as reported at major academic centres staffed by highly experienced

Arthur L. Burnett, MD, Department of Urology, Johns Hopkins Hospital, Baltimore, Maryland, USA

surgeons range between 60% and 85%, a dramatic improvement over historical rates [5–7]. Contemporary results generated elsewhere may differ. However, in support of these figures, a subset analysis from the cohort study of Cancer of the Prostate Strategic Urologic Research Endeavor (CaPSURE), representing 29 academic and community-based sites across the USA, recently found a 75% potency rate in men younger than 65 years after radical prostatectomy [8].

Notwithstanding these developments, the recovery of erectile function following radical prostatectomy remains problematic for many men undergoing the surgery. Recovery delay remains profound for this functional outcome after surgery, and erections suitable for intercourse may not be achieved in many men for as much as 2 years postoperatively, even when nerve-sparing technique is performed [5, 6]. In addition, current clinical surveys show that among patients eventually recovering erectile function, the quality of erections is frequently inferior to that of those achieved preoperatively [6]. Thus, for many men, delayed or incomplete recovery of erectile function after surgery is common, even with current refinements in surgical technique.

It is reasonable to wonder whether erectile function status following radical prostatectomy differs from that of other interventions for clinically localized prostate cancer. A growing interest in pelvic radiation including brachytherapy is supported by the conjecture that erections are better preserved with this treatment modality than with surgery. Clearly, surgery is associated with an immediately precipitous and extensive loss of erectile function although recovery is frequently observed given sufficient follow-up [5, 6]. Radiation therapy yields a distinct pattern of erectile function loss, which indeed can be fairly significant over time following treatment. This intervention definitely is associated with a steady decline in erectile function after some delay [9–11]. According to the Prostate Cancer Outcomes Study, a retrospective survey of community-based men diagnosed and treated without randomization to treatment options for prostate cancer in the mid-1990s, substantial erectile dysfunction rates in radical prostatectomy and external beam radiation therapy groups were similarly observed (79% and 63% respectively) at 5 years postintervention [11]. However, considerations as to whether and how well nerve-sparing surgery was performed remain unclear in this analysis, and the results may not be representative of the highest level performance of this technique. In another community-based study, which did specify performance of nerve-sparing technique at radical prostatectomy, sexual function score was equivalent in men receiving this modification of the surgery and men having undergone pelvic radiation by 2-year follow-up [12].

Brachytherapy also carries a significant rate of erectile dysfunction, and this problem is compounded with adjuvant therapies. In one study, 5-year actuarial potency rates were 76% for men treated with brachytherapy as monotherapy, 56% for those treated with a combination of brachytherapy and external beam radiotherapy, 52% for those treated with neoadjuvant androgen deprivation and brachytherapy and 29% for those treated with neoadjuvant androgen deprivation in combination with brachytherapy and external beam radiotherapy [13].

Conceivably, the loss of erectile function only seems much more significant for men undergoing surgery given the precipitousness and extent of the loss as well as its immediacy following treatment. For pelvic radiation, patients may perceive the erection loss to occur with a lesser likelihood of life-changing circumstances while they may gradually adapt to the loss over time.

ERECTILE DYSFUNCTION RISK ASSESSMENT

Factors confounding precise determinations of erectile function status following surgery include failure to document preoperative erection ability in patients undergoing the surgery, widely disparate definitions of erectile function used by many investigators, biases in the ascertainment of this functional outcome following the surgery and failure to stratify functional outcome results based on comorbid risk factors associated with erectile dysfunction [14]. Similar issues predictably apply to assessments of this functional outcome in the face of other prostate cancer treatments. A trend towards applying rigorous clinical investigation methodology may lead to improved knowledge of erectile function recovery following treatment. Basic principles for studying and reporting this outcome include prospective study design, which includes the assessment of preoperative erectile function and serial monitoring over a sufficient duration of time (at least 18 months). This approach would then provide a determination consistent with function that has achieved a constant level, either maximal recovery in the context of radical prostatectomy or maximal preservation in the context of pelvic radiation. The application of standardized definitions of erectile function, e.g. erectile ability sufficient to perform satisfactory sexual intercourse, and standardized tools for erection assessment would also assist greatly in assessing this outcome. In the latter regard, objective tests or subjectively based instruments, e.g. erectile function questionnaires or inventories of sexual activity, may be used alternatively, although subjective instruments are perceived to be advantageous since they are generally less expensive and invasive and are more easily administered, particularly for repeated assessments.

Efforts to identify and correlate clinical risk factors for erectile dysfunction in the setting of prostate cancer treatment have taken central importance in evaluating post-treatment erectile function outcomes. For radical prostatectomy, surgeon experience and the volume of surgeries performed are conceivably dominant factors influencing this outcome [15, 16]. However, other relevant risk factors may also govern this outcome following surgery (Table 17.1). Walsh and colleagues originally described the relevance of patient age, clinical and pathological disease stage, and surgical technique as primary prognostic variables [17]. Recent analyses have confirmed the importance of patient preoperative erectile function status and surgical technique as predominant prognostic factors [18–20]. From the CaPSURE database, certain variables such as race/ethnicity, education and relationship status were affirmed to exert no influence on erectile function outcome following surgery [8]. This same database did affirm, however, that the condition of fewer health comorbidities such as cardiovascular disease, diabetes and cigarette smoking, which alone constitute risk factors for erectile dysfunction, was associated with a higher rate of return to baseline erectile function status [8]. This database also produced a less instinctive result that a household income of more than US$30 000 is associated with a greater likelihood of returning to baseline sexual function [8].

Table 17.1 Factors favouring erectile function recovery after radical prostatectomy

Related to the surgeon
Surgical experience
Volume of surgeries
Focus on perfecting techniques

Related to the prostate cancer/surgery
Stage (≤T2)
Nerve-sparing (bilateral > unilateral > none)

Related to the patient
Preoperatively intact erectile function status
Age (≤60 years)
Absence of health comorbidities
Household income (> US $30,000)

MECHANISMS OF TREATMENT-ASSOCIATED ERECTILE DYSFUNCTION

The loss of erectile function after treatment for prostate cancer would reasonably be evaluated in the context of variables associated with normal erection physiology. Penile erection is a neurovascular biological process modulated by hormonal, local biochemical and biomechanical/structural factors of the penis. Among these elements, specific factors implicated in radical prostatectomy are understood to be neurogenic and to a lesser extent vasculogenic [14, 19]. A neurogenic basis is widely accepted when surgery involves deliberately wide excision of the cavernous nerves. However, it also applies to nerve-sparing surgery. Plausible mechanisms in support of this proposal are that nerve injury may nonetheless occur during surgery from unintentional direct severance of nerve tissue, mechanically induced nerve traction injury, thermal damage to nerve tissue if electrocoagulative instruments are used adjacent to the cavernous nerves, ischaemic effects on nerve tissue resulting from attempts to control surgical bleeding and local inflammatory effects occurring simply because of the surgical trauma [14].

The clinical observation that many preoperatively potent men experience a temporary deficit in erectile function but do eventually recover this function suggests a 'neuropraxia' phenomenon. Erection recovery over time after the surgery then coincides with a biological sequence of peripheral nerve regeneration after initial nerve injury. Considerations of vascular injury have been proposed as a possible basis for postoperative erectile dysfunction [21]. In fact, penile blood flow studies in patients having undergone radical prostatectomy document substantial penile blood flow abnormalities, including decreased arterial inflow and veno-occlusive dysfunction [22, 23]. One hypothesis proposed to explain these objective phenomena is that injury is sustained by accessory pudendal arteries during the surgery [24]. It is more than likely that functional or structural damage of the penile nerve supply results in subsequent deterioration of cavernosal tissue physiology, consistent with the induction of 'penile neuropathy' [14]. Atrophic and fibrotic changes of the penis have been documented in men undergoing radical prostatectomy [25, 26]. These changes are consistent with the process of Wallerian degeneration with loss of normal nerve terminations and associated neuroregulatory function and homeostasis in the penis. In turn, corporal smooth muscle deteriorates and becomes infiltrated with collagen [27, 28]. This tissue destruction alters the biophysical compliance required for maintenance of erection and predisposes the development of veno-occlusive dysfunction [29]. The pathophysiological basis for these changes is believed to be associated with corporal smooth muscle apoptosis, programmed cell death [30, 31], as well as hypoxaemic tissue effects and oxidative stress mechanisms [32].

The pathophysiology of erectile dysfunction following pelvic radiation involves derangements of both structural and functional components of the erection response. Even when conformal radiation therapy techniques are performed, radiation is dispersed to the proximal aspect of the penis in the region of the bulb, where the cavernosal vessels and nerves are known to enter the penis [33, 34]. Nerve tissue is particularly sensitive to radiation suggesting that a neurogenic aetiology is also a major aetiological factor for erectile dysfunction when pelvic radiation is performed [35]. Hormonal ablation for prostate cancer is associated with multiple levels of tissue damage including pathophysiological changes of penile vasculature, cavernous nerves and cavernosal tissue [36].

Non-somatic pathogenic factors may also play roles in sexual function impairment after treatment for prostate cancer. Psychological factors related to the stress of being diagnosed and undergoing treatment, the uncertainty of cancer control, interference with intimacy because of physical weakness or impaired urinary or bowel function and other psychodynamic issues may well affect the readiness of the patient and partner to resume sexual activity [37].

CLINICAL MANAGEMENT

It is clear that erectile dysfunction may be a consequence of any intervention used today for the treatment of prostate cancer. Indeed, some extent of erection loss is demonstrable for all interventions despite techniques applied to optimize their use. As exemplified in men undergoing radical prostatectomy, major importance is assigned to the resumption of sexual activity postoperatively and interest is strong to use erectile aids to be functional [38–40]. One recent population-based study of prostate cancer survivors treated by various approaches for clinically localized prostate cancer found that approximately half pursued erectile dysfunction treatment [41]. Factors positively associated with erectile dysfunction treatment were younger patient age, availability of a sexual partner and baseline sexual activity. In another recent report, the investigators explored the extent of erectile dysfunction management among men treated for prostate cancer who were bothered by their post-treatment erectile dysfunction, finding that erectile dysfunction treatment was sought by 77% of those who had undergone radical prostatectomy in contrast with 52% of those who had undergone brachytherapy and 39% of those who had undergone three-dimensional conformal external beam radiotherapy [42].

A host of conventional treatment approaches are currently available for treating erectile dysfunction in prostate cancer survivors (Table 17.2). These range from pharmacotherapeutic treatments, e.g. oral pills, intraurethral suppositories and intracavernosal injections, to non-pharmacotherapeutic treatments, e.g. mechanical vacuum constriction devices and penile prosthetic surgery. The treatment algorithm generally adheres to the stepwise process of care model, developed by several consensus bodies [43, 44]. Principles of this process include application of options initially that are least invasive, easily administered and generally less expensive while subsequently escalating management as needed. Additional considerations are the reliability, efficacy and safety of different treatment approaches in different clinical practices, and the inclinations of both patient and partner to use one or another approach.

ORAL THERAPY

Oral medications ordinarily constitute first-line management for erectile dysfunction in the prostate cancer survivor. This option refers to phosphodiesterase type-5 (PDE-5) inhibitors, e.g. sidenafil (Viagra, Pfizer, New York, New York), tadalafil (Cialis, Eli Lilly, Indianapolis, IN, USA) and vardenafil (Levitra, Bayer-GSK, Pittsburgh, PA, USA), which have been demonstrated to be a most effective intervention for erectile dysfunction of any aetiology or severity. These medications as a class have shown a success rate of approximately 70% for 'on-demand' use in achieving erections useful for sexual intercourse [45]. In the radical prostatectomy population, it was shown early that approximately 40% of men who had undergone radical prostatectomy responded to sildenafil [46]. Further investigation into this area revealed that the extent of nerve-sparing affected medication response. Patients who underwent bilateral cavernous nerve-sparing surgery had a better response (72%) than patients who underwent unilateral (50%) or non-nerve-sparing (15%) surgery [47]. Additionally, it was shown that a time dependency-governed responsiveness to this therapy with successful outcomes occurred most dramatically at an interval of at least 6 months after surgery [48, 49]. These observations are consistent with the concept that success with PDE-5 inhibitor therapy hinges on the functional release of the erection chemical mediator nitric oxide from the cavernous nerves, which is reduced if these nerves are damaged or incompletely recovered. At this time, additional investigations have been carried out for sildenafil as well as for tadalafil and vardenafil in this population, finding comparable statistically significant efficacy rates above placebo rates [50–52].

The use of PDE-5 inhibitor therapy has also been studied in patients undergoing radiation therapy for localized prostate cancer. An early report documented a 71% erection response

Table 17.2 Pharmacological and non-pharmacological interventions for erectile dysfunction

Treatment option	Role	Efficacy (RP) %	Efficacy (RT) %	Comment
Oral PDE-5 inhibitors	First line	70–80 (nerve-sparing, after 18 months) 0–15 (non-nerve-sparing)	70 (early) 40–50 (after 24 months)	Function of 'nitric oxide-producing' penile nerves essential; sexual stimulation required
Intraurethral alprostadil	Second line	20–55	20–40	In-office instruction and titration recommended
Intracavernosal injections	Second line	70–85	70–90	In-office instruction and titration recommended
Vacuum constriction devices	Second line	60–95	60–95	Basic instruction sufficient
Penile implants (malleable and inflatable)	Third line	95–100	95–100	Surgical expertise required

PDE-5, phosphodiesterase type-5; RP, radical prostatectomy; RT, radiation therapy (inclusive of external beam irradiation and brachytherapy).

Efficacy refers to percentage approximations of men having successful intercourse.

rate with erections sufficient for vaginal intercourse in a small group of men at approximately 2 years after prostate cancer treatment [53]. Efficacy has been confirmed in additional studies as well [54, 55]. In another more recent study, patient responses to sildenafil were found to decline progressively over time after radiation therapy, and rates were 44% and 38% for brachytherapy and external beam irradiation, respectively, at an interval 3 years following treatment [56]. The addition of androgen deprivation to radiation therapy significantly lessens sildenafil response rates from that of radiation therapy alone [13]. These data point to the efficacy of PDE-5 inhibitor therapy again relating to integrity of cavernous nerve function and conceivably overall cavernosal tissue function.

OTHER MEDICAL TREATMENTS

In patients who do not respond to, or who are unable to use, PDE-5 inhibitors because of contraindications, second- and third-line treatment options may be pursued. Intraurethral alprostadil, also known as MUSE (Medicated Urethral System for Erection, Vivus, Mountain View, CA, USA), has been successfully used in the treatment of erectile dysfunction [57]. The technique relies on the absorption of medication through the urethral mucosal lining into the surrounding corpus spongiosum, with passage via small vascular channels into the corpora cavernosa. Known overall efficacy rates for MUSE in eliciting responses sufficient for sexual intercourse for various aetiologies of erectile dysfunction have been documented to be 20–40% [58]. In men having erectile dysfunction after radical prostatectomy, a 55% efficacy rate was reported in one series [59]. Equivalent responses were noted independent of nerve-sparing performance and irrespective of medication dose. Intraurethral alprostadil applied in combination with oral sildenafil has been reported to salvage sildenafil failures in the radical prostatectomy population [60, 61]. Long-term treatment is hampered by inefficacy and side-effects such as local urogenital pain and minor urethral bleeding [59].

Intracavernosal injection of vasoactive agents, conventionally consisting of prostaglandin E_1 [(alprostadil (Prostin VR, Caverject, Edex)], papaverine and phentolamine, has been used very successfully for the treatment of a broad range of causes of erectile dysfunction. Efficacy rates commonly range between 70% and 90% [58]. In the radical prostatectomy population, success rates in achieving erection rigidity were reported to range between 70% and 85% [62, 63]. Intracavernous injection therapy may facilitate the switch to oral therapy in men following radical prostatectomy [64]. Of note, long-term compliance appears to be a major limitation with this treatment [63].

Vacuum constrictive device therapy has long provided a feasible option for diverse causes of erectile dysfunction. The fundamental concept underlying this therapy is that an erection can be induced by placing the penis in a vacuum chamber or cylinder which draws blood into the corpora cavernosa; the placement of a constriction ring around the base of the penis allows the erection to be maintained. Success rates reported in the literature vary from 60% to 80% [65]. Patient reports of dissatisfaction because of unnaturalness and discomfort recognizably contribute to a less than maximal success rate with this therapy [58]. In the radical prostatectomy population, up to a 92% rate of success has been reported [66]. The combination of sildenafil and vacuum constrictive device therapy in the setting of radical prostatectomy improved sexual satisfaction with rigidity to 77% of users from the rate of 58% associated with vacuum constrictive device therapy alone [67].

Penile implants have served to treat erectile dysfunction utilizing a device surgically placed within the corporal bodies to replace natural penile rigidity. Successful implantation rates reported in the literature generally approximate 95%, although patient satisfaction rates are generally somewhat less at about 85% [68]. These rates conceivably apply to erectile dysfunction resulting from any cause including treatments for prostate cancer. The idea to immediately place a penile prosthesis simultaneous with radical prostatectomy has been investigated, with a 96% successful sexual intercourse rate assessed at 3 months postoperatively [69].

Psychotherapy is identified to have a role in the management of erectile dysfunction and may be a useful adjunct even when a primary somatic basis underlies the presentation of erectile dysfunction. The benefits of counselling intervention for prostate cancer survivors and their partners were demonstrated in a recent study [37]. At 3 months after initiation of therapy, improvements were achieved in male overall distress, male global sexual function and female global sexual function.

NEW DIRECTIONS

New directions to manage erectile dysfunction in association with prostate cancer treatment would seemingly aim to surpass the limitations of conventional management options (erectile aids), which afford only temporary, repetitive means for an erectile response or are unnatural. In keeping with the notion that ideal therapy achieves spontaneous, natural erections, the ultimate goal in managing erectile dysfunction in the setting of treating prostate cancer as for any circumstance of erectile dysfunction is to recover this exact level of functional ability. Proposals for this concept include rehabilitation therapy and tissue regenerative or reconstitutive strategies.

POSTOPERATIVE REHABILITATION

In the modern era of cavernous nerve-sparing radical prostatectomy, a reality of erection recovery is that a timeline of as much as 2 years is often required for the majority of men to achieve this functional outcome [1]. The psychological distress of this requirement for natural recovery has prompted the application of a host of therapies, including standard erectile aids, early penile prosthesis surgery and therapeutic counselling. A relatively recent alternative strategy is erection rehabilitation, referring to a concept that early postoperative sexual stimulation and induced blood flow in the penis may facilitate the return of natural erectile function and resumption of medically unassisted sexual activity. Besides helping advance the return of an aspect of quality of life, this strategy has been theorized to afford healthful effects on the penis by inhibiting corporal hypoxia and mechanisms associated with penile atrophy and fibrosis. In this mode, pharmacological approaches including intracavernous injection [70, 71] and oral pharmacotherapy [72–74] have taken centre stage in this effort. While early results are promising, more investigations applying controlled clinical trial methodology are needed to affirm the validity and efficacy of these approaches. Additionally, no current consensus exists with regard to the specific protocol to be used in implementing pharmacological rehabilitation programmes, including the initiation time, the frequency of application, and the type, dose and delivery of vasoactive agents. Whether early and regular vacuum constrictive device use after surgery yields an earlier and better erectile functional outcome also remains empirical at this time.

CAVERNOUS NERVE RECONSTITUTIVE STRATEGIES

Consistent with the knowledge that a neuropathic basis probably accounts for many presentations of erectile dysfunction following radical prostatectomy as well as other treatments for prostate cancer, it seems relevant to develop strategies directed towards this concern. A therapeutic prospect in this direction is neuromodulatory therapy. This intervention encompasses the basic science of neurotrophic growth factors, neural development, neuroprotection, neural regeneration and the prevention of neuronal cell death referable to the nerve supply of the penis. Neurogenic approaches conceivably range from the exogenous supply of trophic factors that may improve axonal regeneration and accelerate target reinnervation to technologies that protect the penile nerve supply in the face of cavernous nerve injury (Table 17.3).

Neuropharmacotherapeutic prospects have gained great interest for this purpose. One such option is the use of corticosteroids, conjectured to have a counteractive effect on the inflammatory basis for tissue injury. Two reports have appeared in the literature demonstrating their investigation at the clinical level in the setting of radical prostatectomy. One study involved the administration of corticosteroid methylprednisolone for a short course immediately following surgery [75] and the other involved the local application of betamethasone cream 0.1% to the cavernous nerves at the time of radical prostatectomy [76]. Neither study demonstrated appreciable improvement in erection recovery compared with the absence of treatment up to 12 months postoperatively. While there were no complications associated with either of these treatments, support for this option seems lacking at this time. Neurotrophins have also garnered interest because of their perceived involvement in penile neurogenesis and their description in the biology of peripheral nerve injury. Preclinical investigation has been carried out for such effectors as nerve growth factor, brain-derived neurotrophic factor, and vascular endothelial growth factor, all showing impressive neuroregenerative effects [77]. Great interest exists to bring these neurotrophins to the clinical arena. However, early investigations for other disease states such as diabetic polyneuropathy and HIV-related neuropathy have not demonstrated efficacy, and painful side-effects were noted [77]. At the present time, the utility of neurotrophins for facilitating erectile function recovery after radical prostatectomy or other prostate cancer treatments is uncertain.

Immunophilin ligands have received a great deal of interest lately following significant preclinical investigation in support of this therapy for cavernous nerve injury [77]. Such agents as the immunosuppressant drug tacrolimus (FK506) and related non-immunosuppressant drugs have been shown to decrease the extent of cavernous nerve degeneration and promote erectile function recovery in animal models of cavernous nerve injury. Although the mechanism of action of immunophilin ligands remains elusive, it is believed that they target specific binding proteins for these ligands and target only injured nerves. Alternative hypotheses have centred on antioxidant abilities of these drugs and their role in glutathione up-regulation. At this time, clinical trials are under way to evaluate the potential role of immunophilin ligands in the setting of radical prostatectomy. Additional neurotrophic agents including poly-(ADP-ribose) polymerase-1 inhibitors, atypical neurotrophic factors and nerve guides are receiving attention with preclinical work showing their potential applications for radical prostatectomy [77].

Additionally, concepts of tissue reconstruction have been applied to neural components of the erection apparatus with the supposition that tissue engineering or stem cell therapy may have roles in the face of cavernous nerve injury [77]. While this application has caused enormous excitement, much more scientific investigation is required to establish therapeutic

Table 17.3 Potential cavernous nerve reconstitutive therapies

Neuropharmacotherapy
Corticosteroids
Neurotrophins
Immunophilin ligands
PARP-1 inhibitors
Atypical neurotrophic factors
Nerve guides
Tissue engineering/stem cell therapy
Gene therapy
Electrical stimulation
Cavernous nerve interposition grafting
PARP, poly(ADP-ribose) polymerase.

utility. Similarly, gene therapy, the genetic modification of differentiated target cells, as it is applied to the penis for the promotion of penile erection has offered another neuromodulatory therapeutic strategy [77]. Early preclinical studies have been carried out with gene constructs for neuronal nitric oxide synthase and neurotrophic growth factors suggestive of this purpose clinically. However, it is acknowledged that major safety concerns, as well as issues regarding the controlled delivery of gene therapies and elicitation of a conditional response, must be addressed prior to bringing this application to the clinical level.

Surgical techniques have also been advanced in the realm of cavernous nerve reconstitution. A recent resurgence in interest has gone towards electrical stimulation of the cavernous nerves, beyond applications intra-operatively to assist in cavernous nerve localizations when performing nerve-sparing surgery [77]. Based on preliminary work that has shown efficacy of electrical current delivered to the penis which causes smooth muscle functional recovery after partial cavernous nerve denervation clinically, additional clinical work is under way to evaluate the feasibility of an implantable electrical stimulator in patients undergoing radical prostatectomy. Cavernous nerve interposition grafting has been promoted as an option to facilitate the recovery of erectile function in men undergoing radical prostatectomy [78]. The rationale is consistent with nerve grafting performed elsewhere for other indications to enable the reconnection of nerve tissue with appropriate targets that mediate erectile function. Studies have been carried out extensively in animal models and then subsequently in several clinical studies stimulating this interest. Donor nerve grafts have consisted of the sural nerve and genitofemoral nerve predominantly, reportedly retrievable with minimal morbidity. Enthusiasm for this intervention has been restrained because of uncertainty as to whether it confers benefit [79]. Men with more advanced disease locally who would require a non-nerve-sparing procedure would seem to be ideal candidates to receive this intervention, but there is the additional concern that many of these patients will require adjuvant local or systemic therapies that will probably devitalize the graft. Further clinical trials will be most helpful to establish the optimal role of cavernous nerve grafting after radical prostatectomy.

OTHER STRATEGIES

The very best performance of nerve-sparing techniques remains critical for the best surgical approach towards preserving erectile function following radical prostatectomy. In this mode, intense focus has been given in recent years to gaining an improved understanding of the course of the cavernous nerve fibres surrounding the prostate and supplying the penis, from which to perform the surgery with maximal cavernous nerve preservation [80, 81]. Recent reports suggest that improved erectile function outcomes may occur with innovative techniques for cavernous nerve preservation [82, 83]. Nevertheless, even with these refinements, cavernous nerve trauma to some degree remains a feature of radical prostatectomy, and it is probable that some degree of delayed or incomplete erectile function recovery persists in spite of these refinements. Despite their attractiveness, current revisions of cavernous nerve-sparing are likely to have finite levels of success consistent with current outcomes of erection recovery, and they are unlikely to produce prompt, full erection recovery on a regular basis following radical prostatectomy. Considerations should be given to developing perioperative interventions adjunctively, such as erection rehabilitation and neuromodulation, to improve functional outcomes even further.

CONCLUSION

Because of the prevalence of prostate cancer, many men will undergo various interventions for disease control or cure. In so doing, many will also experience potential complications including consequences with regard to erectile function. It is clear that matters of sexual function loss are critical aspects influencing considerations for prostate cancer treatment in many men. Major objectives exist today to preserve sexual function outcomes while meeting oncological management goals. In moving forward at this time, it is important to understand risk factors for erectile dysfunction and pathogenic mechanisms associated with this condition following treatments for prostate cancer. Management consists of current standard interventions, typically offered according to a stepwise treatment algorithm, while it is also understood that novel treatments currently under study, such as erection rehabilitation and neuromodulatory therapies, may best achieve the ideal outcome of rapidly restored or preserved natural erectile function. Efforts to employ optimization techniques with treatments for prostate cancer, which lessen adverse effects on sexual function, also remain meritorious. Effective erectile dysfunction management in administering prostate cancer treatments offers an opportunity for maximally preserving quality of life.

REFERENCES

1. Burnett AL. Erectile dysfunction following radical prostatectomy. *JAMA* 2005; 293:2648–2653.
2. Cooperberg MR, Broering JM, Litwin MS *et al.* The contemporary management of prostate cancer in the United States: lessons from the Cancer of the Prostate Strategic Urologic Research Endeavor (CaPSURE), a national disease registry. *J Urol* 2004; 171:1393–1401.
3. Walsh PC. Anatomic radical prostatectomy: evolution of the surgical technique. *J Urol* 1998; 160:2418–2424.
4. Walsh PC, Donker PJ. Impotence following radical prostatectomy: insight into etiology and prevention. *J Urol* 1982; 128:492–497.
5. Walsh PC, Marschke P, Ricker D *et al.* Patient-reported urinary continence and sexual function after anatomic radical prostatectomy. *Urology* 2000; 55:58–61.
6. Rabbani F, Stapleton Am, Kattan NW *et al.* Factors predicting recovery of erections after radical prostatectomy. *J Urol* 2000; 164:1929–1934.
7. Kundu SD, Roehl KA, Eggener SE *et al.* Potency, continence and complications in 3,377 consecutive radical retopubic prostatectomies. *J Urol* 2004; 172:2227–2231.
8. Hu JC, Elkin EP, Pasta DJ *et al.* Predicting quality of life after radical prostatectomy: results from CaPSURE. *J Urol* 2004; 171:703–707.
9. Mantz CA, Song P, Farhangi E *et al.* Potency probability following conformal megavoltage radiotherapy using conventional doses for localized prostate cancer. *Int J Radiat Oncol Biol Phys* 1997; 37:551–557.
10. Sanchez-Ortiz RF, Broderick GA, Rovner ES *et al.* Erectile function and quality of life after interstitial radiation therapy for prostate cancer. *Int J Impot Res* 2000; 12(Suppl 3):S18-S24.
11. Potosky AL, Davis WW, Hoffman RM *et al.* Five-year outcomes after prostatectomy or radiotherapy for prostate cancer: the prostate cancer outcomes study. *J Natl Cancer Inst* 2004; 96:1358–1367.
12. Litwin MS, Flanders SC, Pasta DJ *et al.* Sexual function and bother after radical prostatectomy or radiation for prostate cancer: multivariate quality-of-life analysis from CaPSURE. Cancer of the Prostate Strategic Urologic Research Endeavor. *Urology* 1999; 54:503–508.
13. Potters L, Torre T, Fearn PA *et al.* Potency after permanent prostate brachytherapy for localized prostate cancer. *Int J Radiat Oncol Biol Phys* 2001; 50:1235–1242.
14. Burnett AL. Rationale for cavernous nerve restorative therapy to preserve erectile function after radical prostatectomy. *Urology* 2003; 61:491–497.
15. Han M, Partin AW, Pound CR *et al.* Long-term biochemical disease-free and cancer-specific survival following anatomic radical retropubic prostatectomy. The 15-year Johns Hopkins experience. *Urol Clin North Am* 2001; 28:555–565.
16. Begg CB, Riedel ER, Bach PB *et al.* Variations in morbidity after radical prostatectomy. *N Engl J Med* 2002; 346:1138–1144.
17. Quinlan DM, Epstein JI, Carter BS *et al.* Sexual function following radical prostatectomy: influence of preservation of neurovascular bundles. *J Urol* 1991; 145:998–1002.
18. Montorsi F, Burnett AL. Erectile dysfunction after radical prostatectomy. *BJU Int* 2004; 93:1–2.
19. Dubbelman YD, Dohle GR, Schroder FH. Sexual function before and after radical retropubic prostatectomy: a systematic review of prognostic indicators for a successful outcome. *Eur Urol* 2006; 50:711–720.
20. Michl UH, Friedrich MG, Graefen M *et al.* Prediction of postoperative sexual function after nerve sparing radical retropubic prostatectomy. *J Urol* 2006; 176:227–231.

21. Bahnson RR, Catalona WJ. Papaverine testing of impotent patients following nerve-sparing radical prostatectomy. *J Urol* 1988; 139:773–774.
22. Mulhall JP, Slovick R, Hotaling J et al. Erectile dysfunction after radical prostatectomy: hemodynamic profiles and their correlation with the recovery of erectile dysfunction. *J Urol* 2002; 167:1371–1375.
23. Gontero P, Pontana F, Bagnasacco A et al. Is there an optimal time for intracavernous prostaglandin E1 rehabilitation following nonnerve sparing radical prostatectomy? Results from a hemodynamic prospective study. *J Urol* 2003; 169:2166–2169.
24. Aboseif S, Shinohara K, Breza J et al. Role of penile vascular injury in erectile dysfunction after radical prostatectomy. *Br J Urol* 1994; 73:75–82.
25. Fraiman MC, Lepor H, McCullough AR. Changes in penile morphometrics in men with erectile dysfunction after nerve-sparing radical retropubic prostatectomy. *Mol Urol* 1999; 3:109–115.
26. Savoie M, Kim SS, Soloway MS. A prospective study measuring penile length in men treated with radical prostatectomy for prostate cancer. *J Urol* 2003; 169:1462–1464.
27. Podlasek CA, Gonzalez CM, Zeiner DJ et al. Analysis of NOS isoform changes in a post radical prostatectomy model of erectile dysfunction. *Int J Impot Res* 2001; 13(Suppl 5):S1–S15.
28. Iacono F, Giannella R, Somma P et al. Histological alterations in cavernous tissue after radical prostatectomy. *J Urol* 2005; 173:1673–1676.
29. Nehra A, Goldstein I, Pabby A et al. Mechanisms of venous leakage: a prospective clinicopathological correlation of corporeal function and structure. *J Urol* 1996; 156:1320–1329.
30. Klein LT, Miller MI, Buttyan R et al. Apoptosis in the rat penis after penile denervation. *J Urol* 1997; 158:626–630.
31. User HM, Hairston JH, Zeiner DJ et al. Penile weight and cell subtype specific changes in a post-radical prostatectomy model of erectile dysfunction. *J Urol* 2003; 169:1175–1179.
32. Leungwattanakij S, Bivalacqua TJ, Usta MF et al. Cavernous neurotomy causes hypoxia and fibrosis in rat corpus cavernosum. *J Androl* 2003; 24:239–245.
33. Merrick GS, Butler WM, Wallner KE et al. Erectile function after prostate brachytherapy. *Int J Radiat Oncol Biol Phys* 2005; 62:437–447.
34. Mulhall JP, Yonover P, Sethi A et al. Radiation exposure to the corporeal bodies during 3-dimensional conformal radiation therapy for prostate cancer. *J Urol* 2002; 167:539–542.
35. Carrier S, Hricak H, Lee SS et al. Radiation-induced decrease in nitric oxide synthase-containing nerves in the rat penis. *Radiology* 1995; 195:95–99.
36. Traish AM, Guay AT. Are androgens critical for penile erections in humans? Examining the clinical and preclinical evidence. *J Sex Med* 2006; 3:382–404.
37. Canada AL, Neese LE, Sui D et al. Pilot intervention to enhance sexual rehabilitation for couples after treatment for localized prostate carcinoma. *Cancer* 2005; 104:2689–2700.
38. Lim AJ, Brandon AH, Fiedler J et al. Quality of life: radical prostatectomy versus radiation therapy for prostate cancer. *J Urol* 1995; 154:1420–1425.
39. McCammon KA, Kolm P, Main B et al. Comparative quality-of-life analysis after radical prostatectomy or external beam radiation for localized prostate cancer. *Urology* 1999; 54:509–516.
40. Gralnek D, Wessells H, Cui H et al. Differences in sexual function and quality of life after nerve sparing and non-nerve sparing radical retropubic prostatectomy. *J Urol* 2000; 163:1169–1170.
41. Stephenson RA, Mori M, Hsieh YC et al. Treatment of erectile dysfunction following therapy for clinically localized prostate cancer: patient reported use and outcomes from the Surveillance, Epidemiology, and End Results Prostate Cancer Outcomes Study. *J Urol* 2005; 174:646–650.
42. Miller DC, Wei TJ, Dunn RL et al. Use of medications or devices for erectile dysfunction among long-term prostate cancer treatment survivors: potential influence of sexual motivation and/or indifference. *Urology* 2006; 68:166–171.
43. No authors listed. The process of care model for evaluation and treatment of erectile dysfunction. The Process of Care Consensus Panel. *Int J Impot Res* 1999; 11:59–70.
44. Lue TF, Giuliano F, Montorsi F et al. Summary of the recommendations on sexual dysfunctions in men. *J Sex Med* 2004; 1:6–23.
45. Burnett AL. Phosphodiesterase 5 mechanisms and therapeutic applications. *Am J Cardiol* 2005; 96:29M–31M.
46. Goldstein I, Lue TF, Padma-Nathan H et al. Oral sildenafil in the treatment of erectile dysfunction. Sildenafil Study Group. *N Engl J Med* 1998; 338:1397–1404.
47. Zippe CD, Jhaveri FM, Klein EA et al. Role of Viagra after radical prostatectomy. *Urology* 2000; 55:241–245.

48. Hong EK, Lepor H, McCullough AR. Time dependent patient satisfaction with sildenafil for erectile dysfunction (ED) after nerve-sparing radical retropubic prostatectomy (RRP). *Int J Impot Res* 1999; 11(Suppl 1):S15–S22.

49. Raina R, Lakin MM, Agarwal A *et al.* Efficacy and factors associated with successful outcome of sildenafil citrate use for erectile dysfunction after radical prostatectomy. *Urology* 2004; 63:960–966.

50. Montorsi F, McCullough A. Efficacy of sildenafil citrate in men with erectile dysfunction following radical prostatectomy: a systematic review of clinical data. *J Sex Med* 2005; 2:658–667.

51. Montorsi F, Nathan HP, McCullough A *et al.* Tadalafil in the treatment of erectile dysfunction following bilateral nerve sparing radical retropubic prostatectomy: a randomized, double-blind, placebo controlled trial. *J Urol* 2004; 172:1036–1041.

52. Brock G, Nehra A, Lipshultz LI *et al.* Safety and efficacy of vardenafil for the treatment of men with erectile dysfunction after radical retropubic prostatectomy. *J Urol* 2003; 170:1278–1283.

53. Kedia S, Zippe CD, Agarwal A *et al.* Treatment of erectile dysfunction with sildenafil citrate (Viagra) after radiation therapy for prostate cancer. *Urology* 1999; 54:308–312.

54. Valicenti RK, Choi E, Chen C *et al.* Sildenafil citrate effectively reverses sexual dysfunction induced by three-dimensional conformal radiation therapy. *Urology* 2001; 57:769–773.

55. Incrocci L, Hop WC, Slob AK. Efficacy of sildenafil in an open-label study as a continuation of a double-blind study in the treatment of erectile dysfunction after radiotherapy for prostate cancer. *Urology* 2003; 62:116–120.

56. Ohebshalom M, Parker M, Guhring P *et al.* The efficacy of sildenafil citrate following radiation therapy for prostate cancer: temporal considerations. *J Urol* 2005; 174:258–262.

57. Hellstrom WJ, Bennett AH, Gesundheit N *et al.* A double-blind, placebo-controlled evaluation of the erectile response to transurethral alprostadil. *Urology* 1996; 48:851–856.

58. Rowland DL, Burnett AL. Pharmacotherapy in the treatment of male sexual dysfunction. *J Sex Res* 2000; 37:226–243.

59. Raina R, Agarwal A, Ausmundson S *et al.* Long-term efficacy and compliance of MUSE for erectile dysfunction following radical prostatectomy: SHIM (IIEF-5) analysis. *Int J Impot Res* 2005; 17:86–90.

60. Nehra A, Blute ML, Barrett DM *et al.* Rationale for combination therapy of intraurethral prostaglandin E(1) and sildenafil in the salvage of erectile dysfunction patients desiring noninvasive therapy. *Int J Impot Res* 2002; 14(Suppl 1):S38–S42.

61. Raina R, AGarwal A, Zippe CD. Management of erectile dysfunction after radical prostatectomy. *Urology* 2005; 66:923–929.

62. Dennis RL, McDougal WS. Pharmacological treatment of erectile dysfunction after radical prostatectomy. *J Urol* 1998; 139:775–776.

63. Raina R, Lakin MM, Thukral M *et al.* Long-term efficacy and compliance of intracorporeal (IC) injection for erectile dysfunction following radical prostatectomy: SHIM (IIEF-5) analysis. *Int J Impot Res* 2003; 15:318–322.

64. Raina R, Lakin MM, Agarwal A *et al.* Long-term intracavernous therapy responders can potentially switch to sildenafil citrate after radical prostatectomy. *Urology* 2004; 63:532–537.

65. Sidi AA, Becher EF, Zhang G *et al.* Patient acceptance of and satisfaction with an external negative pressure device for impotence. *J Urol* 1990; 144:1154–1156.

66. Baniel J, Israilov S, Segenreich E *et al.* Comparative evaluation of treatments for erectile dysfunction in patients with prostate cancer after radical retropubic prostatectomy. *BJU Int* 2001; 88:58–62.

67. Raina R, Agarwal A, Allamaneni SS *et al.* Sildenafil citrate and vacuum constriction device combinatioin enhances sexual satisfaction in erectile dysfunction after radical prostatectomy. *Urology* 2005; 65:360–364.

68. Lewis RW. Long-term results of penile prosthetic implants. *Urol Clin North Am* 1995; 22:847–856.

69. Khoudary KP, DeWolf WC, Bruning CO III *et al.* Immediate sexual rehabilitation by simultaneous placement of penile prosthesis in patients undergoing radical prostatectomy: initial results in 50 patients. *Urology* 1997; 50:395–399.

70. Montorsi F, Guazzoni G, Strambi LF *et al.* Recovery of spontaneous erectile function after nerve-sparing radical retropubic prostatectomy with and without early intracavernous injections of alprostadil: results of a prospective, randomized trial. *J Urol* 1997; 158:1408–1410.

71. Brock G, Tu LM, Linet OI. Return of spontaneous erection during long-term intracavernosal alprostadil (Caverject) treatment. *Urology* 2001; 57:536–541.

72. Padma-Nathan H, McCullough A, Forest C. Erectile dysfunction secondary to nerve-sparing radical retropubic prostatectomy: comparative phosphodiesterase-5 inhibitor efficacy for therapy and novel prevention strategies. *Curr Urol Rep* 2004; 5:467–471.

73. Gallo L, Perdona S, Auitorino R *et al.* Recovery of erection after pelvic urologic surgery: our experience. *Int J Impot Res* 2005; 17:484–493.

74. Mulhall J, Land S, Parker M *et al.* The use of an erectogenic pharmacotherapy regimen following radical prostatectomy improves recovery of spontaneous erectile function. *J Sex Med* 2005; 2:532–540.

75. Parsons JK, Marschke P, Maples P *et al.* Effect of methylprednisolone on return of sexual function after nerve-sparing radical retropubic prostatectomy. *Urology* 2004; 64:987–990.

76. Deliveliotis C, Delis A, Papatsoris A *et al.* Local steroid application during nerve-sparing radical retropubic prostatectomy. *BJU Int* 2005; 96:533–535.

77. Burnett AL, Lue TF. Neuromodulatory therapy to improve erectile function recovery outcomes after pelvic surgery. *J Urol* 2006; 176:882–887.

78. Kim ED, Scardino PT, Hampel O *et al.* Interposition of sural nerve restores function of cavernous nerves resected during radical prostatectomy. *J Urol* 1999; 161:188–192.

79. Nelson BA, Chang SS, Cookson MS *et al.* Morbidity and efficacy of genitofemoral nerve grafts with radical retropubic prostatectomy. *Urology* 2006; 67:789–792.

80. Costello AJ, Brooks M, Cole OJ. Anatomical studies of the neurovascular bundle and cavernosal nerves. *BJU Int* 2004; 94:1071–1076.

81. Takenaka A, Murakami G, Matsubara A *et al.* Variation in course of cavernous nerve with special reference to details of topographic relationships near prostatic apex: histologic study using male cadavers. *Urology* 2005; 65:136–142.

82. Menon M, Kaul S, Bhandari A *et al.* Potency following robotic radical prostatectomy: a questionnaire based analysis of outcomes after conventional nerve sparing and prostatic fascia sparing techniques. *J Urol* 2005; 174:2291–2296.

83. Montorsi F, Salonia A, Suardi N *et al.* Improving the preservation of the urethral sphincter and neurovascular bundles during open radical retropubic prostatectomy. *Eur Urol* 2005; 48:938–945.

18

Therapeutic strategies for pain

Colin Purcell, Joe O'Sullivan

INTRODUCTION

Advanced and metastatic prostate cancer is associated with a number of pain syndromes. The principal source of pain in metastatic prostate cancer results from skeletal involvement. As many as 50% of men with skeletal metastases from prostate cancer will have uncontrolled pain [1]. Pain in advanced disease can also result from local invasion of pelvic structures, in particular the rectum, bladder and nerve plexi. This chapter will focus on pain management strategies for skeletal metastases. Pain management strategies discussed will include external beam radiotherapy, bone-seeking radionuclide therapy and bisphosphonate therapy. The use of other systemic therapies including cytotoxic chemotherapy is described elsewhere in this book.

EXTERNAL BEAM RADIOTHERAPY

Radiation therapy has been used to control pain from bone metastases for almost 100 years. In the initial years of this modality, the dose of radiation delivered to bone was limited by the tolerance of the normal structures irradiated in the field. For bone metastases this included the overlying skin and soft tissues; however, with the advent of cobalt-60 machines and subsequently megavoltage linear accelerators (Figure 18.1), it became feasible to deliver larger doses of ionizing radiation to areas deep within the body with skin-sparing effects. Irradiation of bony metastatic disease is now one of the most common uses of external beam radiotherapy.

INDICATIONS AND EFFICACY

External beam radiotherapy (EBRT) is effective in the palliation of painful bone metastases from most solid tumours with published response rates of the order of 40–70% [2, 3]. In some patients the onset of pain relief can be within 2 days; however, in others it may take up to 6 weeks for the full benefit of the treatment to be realized [4]. The onset of pain relief and the likelihood of a clinically useful response will depend a lot on the aetiology of the pain. Nerve or soft tissue compression caused by collapse of a vertebra or pathological fracture of a long bone will be unlikely to respond well to external beam radiotherapy, whereas pain secondary to soft tissue tumour growth will generally have a better outcome. EBRT also has an important role in the treatment of pain caused by pelvic and para-aortic nodal metastases.

Colin Purcell, MB MRCP, Specialist Registrar in Medical Oncology, The Northern Ireland Cancer Centre, Centre for Cancer Research and Cell Biology, Queen's University Belfast, Belfast City Hospital, Belfast, UK
Joe O'Sullivan, MD FRCPI FFRRCSI, Consultant/Senior Lecturer in Oncology, The Northern Ireland Cancer Centre, Centre for Cancer Research and Cell Biology, Queen's University Belfast, Belfast City Hospital, Belfast, UK

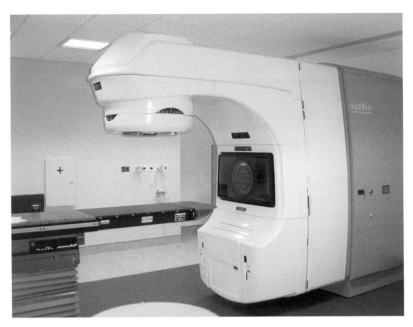

Figure 18.1   A modern linear accelerator.

EBRT carries a risk of toxicity. Early or acute toxicity, occurring within 3 months of palliative EBRT depends on the region of the body and the surrounding normal tissues being
irradiated. The most common side-effects are tiredness, nausea and vomiting and diarrhoea.
Patients receiving large single fractions of radiotherapy who are at risk of nausea and vomiting should receive prophylactic antiemetics such as a 5-hydroxytryptamine (5HT) antagonist
prior to radiation. In general the toxicity associated with palliative radiotherapy to bone is
minimal and most patients will tolerate this treatment very well. Late toxicities can occur
months or years after radiotherapy and again depend on the surrounding normal tissues
in the radiation field. The late toxicities associated with the palliative irradiation of bone
secondaries can include nerve damage and permanent bowel injury. However, in view of
the relatively short prognosis of men with symptomatic androgen-independent metastatic
prostate cancer, late toxicity of palliative radiotherapy is generally not a major consideration and must be balanced against the benefits of treatment for each individual patient.
However, particularly in men who have had previous EBRT treatment, care must be taken
not to exceed normal tissue tolerance of critical structures such as spinal cord [5].

TECHNIQUE

EBRT is delivered using megavoltage linear accelerators or cobalt machines. Common techniques employed include direct single fields and parallel-opposed radiation fields. The treatment is designed using simple conventional treatment planning. The treatment fields are
mapped using information from the clinical history, physical examination and radiological
assessment using isotope bone scans, plain X-rays, or cross-sectional imaging. Treatment
fields are planned with the help of a simulator (Figure 18.2). This machine has many of the
same characteristics as the treatment machine (linear accelerator) as well as a diagnostic
X-ray unit. It is designed to 'simulate' a radiotherapy treatment machine and can provide
live fluoroscopic images of the patient, as well as a record of the treated area for future reference. Using the simulator, a field encompassing the bone metastases can be designed. It is

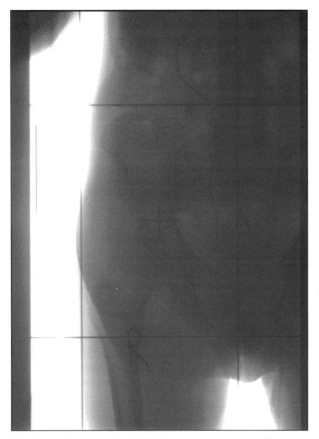

Figure 18.2   A simulator image of a pelvic field in the treatment of symptomatic metastatic prostate cancer.

also possible to identify any areas of normal tissue within the field that can be shielded using lead blocks and this can help reduce toxicity.

There are a wide range of dose-fractionation schedules in use for the palliation of bone pain with EBRT for metastatic prostate cancer, and controversy exists with regard to the optimum. Single fractions of 8 Gy are most commonly given for palliation of bone pain in the UK, while in the USA more prolonged fractionation schedules are often used. Single fractionation schedules reduce the number of hospital visits required by patients and help free up linear accelerator time, thus allowing more patients to be treated. There have been several randomized studies of dose fractionation in the treatment of bone pain secondary to metastatic disease, most of which have included large numbers of men with prostate cancer.

A Dutch multicentre study published by Steenland *et al.* reported on 1171 patients (of whom 23% had prostate cancer) who were randomized to receive either a single fraction of 8 Gy, or six fractions of 4 Gy [6] for the treatment of bone pain secondary to skeletal metastases. The primary endpoint was pain response, as judged by a two-point decrease on a 10-point pain scale. There was no difference in outcome seen, with 71% overall response rate. Retreatment was four times more common in the single fraction group; however, it was postulated that there may have been a lower threshold for retreatment in this group. Price *et al.* performed a prospective randomized trial of 288 patients with bone metastases (30% of whom had prostate cancer) comparing a single fraction of 8 Gy with 30 Gy in 10 daily fractions [7]. There was no statistically significant difference in the speed of onset or duration of pain relief between the two treatment regimes. In another study, Gaze *et al.* randomized 280 patients (54 with prostate cancer) to receive either a single 10 Gy treatment or a course of 22.5 Gy in five daily fractions for the relief of metastatic bone pain [8]. There was no statistically significant difference seen in response rates between the two arms, with complete response rates of 38.8% for single treatment and 42.3% for patients receiving five fractions. Quality of life parameters were the same for both groups. A further study published by Nielsen *et al.* randomized 241 patients with bone pain secondary to metastatic disease to receive either a single fraction of 8 Gy or 20 Gy in five fractions [9]. Prostate cancer was the primary site in 34% of patients. No difference in the degree or duration of pain relief, the number of new painful sites or the need for re-irradiation was observed between the two treatment groups.

The choice of dose for single fraction schedules has been the subject of a randomized trial carried out in the UK. Hoskin and colleagues randomized 270 patients with painful bone metastases to receive single fractions of 4 Gy or 8 Gy [10]. Pain was assessed by patients on a four-point graded scale using pain charts. Response was defined as an improved rating compared with the pretreatment value. There was a statistically significant difference in response rates in favour of 8 Gy at 4 weeks (69% vs. 44%). There was no difference in complete response rates at 4 weeks, or duration of response between the two arms. The authors conclude that 8 Gy gives a higher probability of pain relief than 4 Gy, but that 4 Gy can be an effective alternative in situations of reduced tolerance.

A multicentre trial by the Radiation Therapy Oncology Group (RTOG) studied pain relief in 759 patients randomly assigned to a variety of dose-fractionation schedules: 2.7 Gy×15 fractions, 3 Gy×10, 3 Gy×5, 4 Gy×5, and 5 Gy×5 [4]. Initially the low-dose, short-course schedules were shown to be as effective as the high-dose protracted programmes. However, subsequent reanalysis claimed that the protracted schedules were more effective in terms of complete combined relief, i.e. absence of pain and cessation of the use of narcotics [11].

The Trans-Tasman Radiation Oncology Group (TROG) have recently reported the results of a randomized trial of two radiotherapy fractionation schemes in patients with neuropathic pain secondary to bone metastases [12]. In total, 272 patients were randomized to receive either 20 Gy in five fractions in 1 week or 8 Gy in one fraction. Seventy-nine (29%) of the patients had prostate cancer. The trial was powered as an equivalence study with primary endpoints of pain response within 2 months and time to treatment failure (TTF). The intention-to-treat overall response rates (95% CI) for 8 Gy/one fraction vs. 20 Gy/five fractions were 53% (45–62%) vs. 61% (53–70%) (P = 0.18). Complete response rates were 26% (18–34%) vs. 27% (19–35%), P = 0.89. There were no statistically significant differences in the median TTFs. The authors conclude that there were no statistically significant differences in the rates of retreatment, cord compression or pathological fracture by arm. This was the first randomized trial to look specifically at the problem of neuropathic pain secondary to bone metastases and it appears to suggest a trend towards better outcome for fractionated schemes.

The use of multiple fractions for palliation of bone metastases is more common in North America and Australia than in Europe [13, 14]. However, within Europe there are wide variations in practice. Lievens *et al.* performed a survey of palliative radiotherapy practice for bone metastases, covering 565 radiotherapy centres in 19 western European countries [15]. Perhaps surprisingly, the most frequently used schedule was 30 Gy in 10 daily fractions (50%), and single large fractions were used in just 11% of centres.

HEMI-BODY IRRADIATION

In patients with large areas of the skeleton involved with prostate cancer, hemi-body irradiation (HBI) is a therapeutic option. After steroid premedication, men receive either 6 Gy for the upper half of the body, or 8 Gy for the lower half. Potential toxicities include nausea, vomiting, lethargy and myelosuppression. Pain relief is achieved in 71–89% of patients, and maintained until death in approximately two-thirds [16–18]. Dearnaley *et al.* performed a retrospective analysis comparing the results of treatment using HBI with isotope therapy using the bone-seeking isotope strontium-89 (^{89}Sr) in patients with prostate cancer metastatic to bone [18]. There was no statistically significant difference in pain response between the two groups at 3 months. Transfusion requirements were higher for the HBI group than for the matched ^{89}Sr group but other bone marrow toxicity was similar. Despite routine anti-emetic therapy, 37% of patients treated with HBI had some nausea or vomiting.

In summary, EBRT is a cost-effective and well-tolerated method of improving pain control for bone metastases in metastatic prostate cancer. Single-fraction treatments appear to be as effective as the more prolonged schedules.

BONE-SEEKING RADIONUCLIDES

Bone-seeking radionuclides including ^{89}Sr, rhenium-186-hydroxyethylene diphosphonate ([186]Re-HEDP) and samarium-153 ([153]Sm) have been used for many years in the palliation of bone metastases in prostate cancer [19, 20]. The characteristics of the most commonly used radionuclides are shown in Table 18.1. There are two principal ways in which radioisotopes can be attracted to areas of osteoblastic reaction in bone. Firstly, the isotope may have an inherent chemical affinity for bone, as is the case for the calcium analogue [89]SrCl. The second mechanism is to chemically bind the radioisotope to another chemical with affinity for reactive bone, such as a bisphosphonate hydroxyethylene diphosphonate (e.g. [186]Re-HEDP). Pain responses in the order of 70% have been reported with the most commonly used isotopes, [89]SrCl, [153]Sm and [186]Re-HEDP [21].

Despite level 1 evidence of effectiveness, bone-seeking radionuclides are underutilized in the treatment of painful bone metastases. The reasons for the relative underuseage of these agents are complex but include a perceived lack of cost effectiveness, limited availability and limited clinical experience [19]. The cost-effectiveness of radionuclides in prostate cancer has been studied by a number of investigators. McEwan *et al.* compared the costs of those receiving ^{89}Sr with those receiving placebo in a Canadian randomized controlled trial of ^{89}Sr-chloride as adjunctive therapy in patients with prostate cancer metastatic to bone [22]. The study suggested that treatment with ^{89}Sr-chloride could bring about meaningful reductions in lifetime management costs in patients with advanced prostate cancer. Malberg *et al.* used data from the same trial to assess the cost effectiveness of ^{89}Sr in a Swedish setting [23]. This retrospective analysis used data from the actual care consumption information of 79 consecutive patients who received EBRT for skeletal pain due to bone metastases from prostate cancer. They estimated the average cost of a relapse treated with EBRT alone. The authors concluded that ^{89}Sr, as a supplement to EBRT for palliation of pain in androgen-independent metastatic disease was beneficial with regard to lifetime health service costs.

Table 18.1 Characteristics of the commonly used bone-seeking radionuclides

Radionuclide	Pharmaceutical	Half-life (days)	β_{max} energy (MeV)	Max range in tissue (mm)	γ-photon (keV)
Rhenium-186	HEDP	3.8	1.07	4.7	137
Samarium-153	EDTMP	1.95	0.8	3.4	103
Strontium-89	Chloride	50.5	1.46	6.7	0

EDTMP, ethylene-diamine-tetra-methylene-phosphonate; HEDP, hydroxyethylene diphosphonate.

STRONTIUM-89

Strontium-89 (^{89}Sr, Metastron[TM]) is an analogue of calcium, which concentrates in osteoblastic bone metastases. The isotope may remain in bone for 100 days and is almost exclusively excreted in the urine. Strontium is a pure beta-emitter with a mean range in tissue of 2.4 mm and a physical half-life of 50.5 days. Normal bone takes up a very small proportion of administered activity and bone marrow depression is transient with a nadir occurring at approximately 4–6 weeks. An administered activity of 150 MBq is the standard regimen. Treatment is usually administered in a Nuclear Medicine Department under the supervision of a trained radionuclide physicist. An isolation room is not necessary and treatment is given as an outpatient by intravenous infusion. The major contraindications to treatment with ^{89}Sr are bone marrow suppression and uncontrolled urinary incontinence (because the isotope is excreted in urine and may cause contamination). Significant side-effects are uncommon apart from transient thrombocytopenia. Patients may experience facial flushing or nausea during the infusion but this is usually short-lived. A proportion of patients may experience a flare in bone pain in the days following treatment with strontium.

The use of ^{89}Sr in the treatment of bone pain secondary to metastatic prostate cancer has been investigated in several randomized studies. Lewington et al. performed a double-blind crossover study in 32 patients with prostate cancer and painful bone metastases. The men were randomized between ^{89}Sr-chloride or non-radioactive strontium which was used as a placebo [24]. Only patients receiving the active compound experienced complete pain relief. There was a statistically significant improvement in pain control between the two groups. Quilty et al. randomized 284 patients with prostate cancer and painful bone metastases to receive either EBRT or 200 MBq of [89]Sr [25]. There was no significant difference in median survival and both treatments provided effective pain relief. However, there were statistically significantly fewer patients reporting new pain sites after ^{89}Sr than after local or hemi-body radiotherapy. A Canadian phase III trial randomized 126 patients with androgen-independent metastatic prostate cancer to receive local field radiotherapy and either ^{89}Sr as a single injection or placebo [22, 26]. No significant differences in survival or in relief of pain at the index site were observed, although there was a significant benefit for the use of ^{89}Sr in terms of analgesic intake, new sites of pain, need for further radiotherapy and physical activity. The authors concluded that the addition of ^{89}Sr is an effective adjuvant therapy to local field radiotherapy, reducing progression of disease and improving quality of life in this group of patients.

SAMARIUM-153 EDTMP

Samarium-153-labelled ethylene-diamine-tetra-methylene-phosphonate ([153]Sm-EDTMP, Quadramet[TM]) is the other commonly used bone-seeking radionuclide. It has been licensed for the treatment of bone metastases for almost 10 years and is also commonly used to treat painful metastases secondary to breast cancer. The distribution of [153]Sm mirrors that seen with ^{99m}Tc-methylene diphosphonate (MDP) when it is injected for bone scintigraphy. Use of [153]Sm combined with EDTMP was first described in 1987 [27]. The maximum emitted beta energy is 0.81 MeV. The isotope also emits a gamma ray with an energy of 103 keV. The average beta particle energy is 233 keV with a mean penetration of 3.1 mm in soft tissue and 1.0 mm in cortical bone. The physical half-life is 46.3 h.

In a clinical study, Resche et al. randomized 114 patients with painful bone metastases to receive varying activities of [153]Sm-EDTMP [28]. Fifty-five patients received single doses of 18.5 MBq/kg (0.5 mCi/kg) and 59 patients received single doses of 37 MBq/kg (1.0 mCi/kg). The physicians judged that approximately half of the patients in each dose group were experiencing some degree of pain relief by week 2. This value increased to 55% for the 18.5 MBq/kg group and 70% for the 37 MBq/kg group at week 4. The results suggest that the 1.0 mCi/kg dose of ^{153}Sm-EDTMP is safe and effective for the treatment of painful bone metastases. In a double-blind, placebo-controlled study, 118 patients with painful bone metastases secondary to a variety of primary malignancies were randomized to receive ^{153}Sm-EDTMP 18.5/37 MBq, or placebo. Pain relief was observed in 62–72% of those who received the 18.5 MBq/kg dose during the first 4 weeks, with marked or complete relief noted in 31% by week 4. A significant correlation was observed between reductions in opioid analgesic use and of pain scores only for those patients who received 37 MBq/kg^{153}Sm-EDTMP.

RHENIUM-186 HEDP

Rhenium-186 (ReBone™) is licensed for the treatment of osteoblastic bone metastases in a number of European countries and is less well established than ^{89}Sr and ^{153}Sm. Like ^{153}Sm, ^{186}Re-HEDP emits both gamma and beta rays. The beta rays deliver the therapy while the gamma rays allow for scintigraphic imaging of the isotope distribution (Figure 18.3). The usual administered activity of ^{186}Re-HEDP is between 1100 and 2500 MBq. The excretion of this drug is renal and the dose-limiting toxicity is thrombocytopenia. A benefit over placebo has been shown in a randomized trial of 20 patients with prostate cancer metastatic to bone, using a double-blind crossover design with ^{99m}Tc-MDP as placebo [29]. A single intravenous administration of 1110–1295 MBq was associated with prompt pain relief in 80% of patients receiving the active isotope. We have conducted a phase I activity-escalation study using high activities of ^{186}Re-HEDP with peripheral blood stem cell support in patients with prostate cancer metastatic to bone. In this study, we demonstrated an activity response with regard to prostate-specific antigen (PSA) reduction using activities above 3500 MBq [30, 31]. Phase III studies are needed to fully evaluate the potential of this radionuclide.

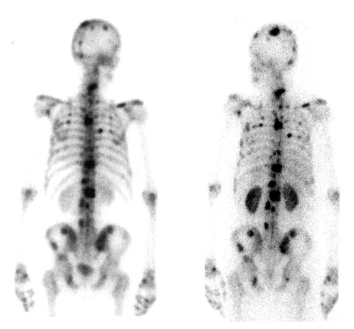

Figure 18.3 Scintigram of patient with metastatic prostate cancer following injection of ^{99m}Tc (left) and the same patient post-treatment with rhenium-186 HEDP demonstrating almost identical distribution of radioisotope.

OTHER RADIONUCLIDES

A number of other radionuclides are currently being assessed in the treatment of metastatic prostate cancer. Rhenium-188-HEDP is a generator-produced radionuclide with a physical half-life of 17 h. It emits both therapeutic beta rays and imageable gamma rays.

One of the most exciting new radionuclides is the alpha emitting agent radium-223. This agent is a calcium analogue which emits powerful alpha rays over a very short distance. One of the major advantages of this type of agent is the low bone marrow toxicity thus allowing the potential for retreatment. Several clinical trials are currently under way to determine the optimum schedule for this agent.

RADIONUCLIDES PLUS CHEMOTHERAPY

Attempts have been made to enhance the effect of ^{89}SrCl by using concomitant chemotherapy as a putative radiosensitizer. Cisplatin at low doses has been shown to improve pain palliation in patients treated with ^{89}SrCl in a randomized trial [32]. Seventy patients with metastatic androgen-independent prostate cancer were randomized to 148 MBq ^{89}Sr plus either 50 mg/m^2 cisplatin or placebo. Overall pain relief occurred in 91% of patients receiving ^{89}Sr + cisplatin compared to 63% of patients receiving ^{89}Sr + placebo ($P < 0.01$). Significantly less bone disease progression was observed in the experimental arm (27% versus 64%), with no clinically significant difference in toxicity between the arms.

Tu *et al.* have also studied the addition of ^{89}Sr to chemotherapy [33]. Seventy-two patients with androgen-independent prostate cancer responding to an induction regimen of keto-conazole and doxorubicin alternating with estramustine and vinblastine, were randomized to receive further doxorubicin with or without ^{89}Sr. There was a statistically significant difference in median survival for the group receiving ^{89}Sr [27.7 vs. 16.8 months ($P = 0.0014$)]. While this strategy may not be applicable to the majority of men with metastatic prostate cancer, it is encouraging to note that this is one of the few randomized trials in this setting to report a survival advantage.

A number of ongoing studies are addressing the potential for improved outcomes by combining bone-seeking radionuclides with cytotoxic chemotherapy including the TRAPEZE study (Birmingham, UK) and the Rhenium-Taxotere Study (Belfast, UK, and Amersfoort, Holland).

In summary, bone-seeking radionuclides are a very useful, if underutilized treatment option in the management of symptomatic bone metastases from prostate cancer. Ongoing clinical trials may lead to the incorporation of these agents earlier in the history of the disease.

BISPHOSPHONATES

Healthy bone undergoes a constant controlled regeneration by a process termed 'remodelling'. This process requires a balanced activity of osteoclasts, which are responsible for bone resorption, and osteoblasts, which form new bone tissue, as well as a controlled release of growth factors that regulate the process. Although bone metastases in prostate cancer usually appear osteoblastic or osteosclerotic on radiological imaging, they are characterized at a cellular level by increased osteoclast activity as well as increased osteoblast activity [34]. This results in disorganized bone remodelling which underlies many of the skeletal symptoms associated with this disease. Bisphosphonates are a class of drugs that can inhibit bone resorption and influence calcium metabolism. Indications for their use in clinical practice include the management of conditions that are associated with increased bone resorption such as Paget's disease, hypercalcaemia of malignancy and osteoporosis. They have also become an important treatment for patients with advanced malignancies involving bone including multiple myeloma, breast cancer and prostate cancer as well as other solid tumour types.

Bisphosphonates are analogues of pyrophosphate that contain a phosphorus–carbon–phosphorus (P-C-P) backbone. Many of their pharmacological properties are influenced by variation of the R1 and R2 side chains [35]. The P-C-P backbone confers a high affinity for hydroxyapetite and this is enhanced by the presence of a hydroxyl group (–OH) at the R1 position. The structure of the R2 side chain determines the antiresorptive potency of the drug. Compounds that contain a primary amino group at the R2 position are more potent than non-amino-containing compounds and modification of this amino group can significantly increase the potency further. Thus, zoledronate, a heterocyclic imidazole containing third-generation bisphosphonate, has potency approximately 10 000 times that of etidronate, a non-amino-containing bisphosphonate.

The antiresorptive effects of the bisphosphonates are primarily mediated by their inhibitory effect on osteoclasts; however, the exact mechanisms by which this occurs are not well characterized. Due to their high affinity for calcium, bisphosphonates bind to areas of exposed bone mineral such as those that occur around resorbing osteoclasts. They are then internalized by the osteoclasts and directly inhibit key cellular mechanisms including attachment and differentiation as well as promoting osteoclast apoptosis. This results in inhibition of osteoclast activity and reduced bone resorption. It has also been suggested that bisphosphonates may inhibit osteoclasts indirectly by an effect on osteoblast function.

A number of the currently available bisphosphonates including etidronate, clodronate, pamidronate and ibandronate have been assessed in non-randomized trials in the treatment of men with hormone-refractory prostate cancer (HRPC) and bone metastases [36–40]. These small studies have demonstrated that these agents are associated with a reduction in bone pain or analgesia requirements in this group of patients; however, the results of these studies have failed to be replicated or have not yet been evaluated in larger trials. Recently, three reports have presented results of randomized controlled trials of bisphosphonates in metastatic HRPC. Studies of pamidronate [41] and clodronate [42] failed to demonstrate clear evidence of benefit. However, a large study of zoledronate [43] in this group of patients has reported a significant reduction in bone pain when compared with placebo as well as a delayed time to skeletal-related morbidity. As a result, zoledronate has received approval for use in men with HRPC metastatic to bone.

PAMIDRONATE

The effect of intravenous pamidronate on pain secondary to bone metastases in prostate cancer has been evaluated in the combined analysis of two separate randomized placebo-controlled trials (trials INT-05 and CGP 032), which were conducted concurrently [41].

Patients with progressive HRPC metastatic to bone and associated bone pain were enrolled in the studies. They were randomized to receive pamidronate 90 mg by intravenous infusion over 2 h every 3 weeks for a total of 27 weeks, or placebo. The primary endpoint was to determine if there was a reduction in pain or analgesic use associated with intravenous pamidronate compared with placebo. Pain was assessed using the self-administered Brief Pain Inventory (BPI) and daily analgesia use was recorded in a diary and allocated oral morphine equivalents (OME). The primary assessment for pain was the difference between worst pain score at baseline and at week 9. A secondary analysis was completed at week 27. In total, 374 patients received study treatment, 180 patients in the pamidronate group and 194 in the placebo group. The majority of patients received all planned study infusions. There was no significant change from baseline BPI scores between pamidronate and placebo groups at week 9 or week 27. BPI scores decreased in both groups but these changes were not clinically relevant. Similarly, no significant changes in analgesia requirements were seen between the groups.

Secondary endpoints included the proportion of patients experiencing at least one skeletal-related event (SRE) at weeks 9 and 27. An SRE was defined as hypercalcaemia, pathological fracture (vertebral or non-vertebral), need for radiotherapy to bone for pain control or to prevent fracture or spinal cord compression, surgery to treat or prevent fractures, spinal cord compression or, in the case of one of the protocols, the need for a spinal orthotic brace. No difference between treatment groups in the proportion of patients with an SRE was observed. The skeletal morbidity rate (SMR), defined as the ratio of the number of SREs divided by the time on the trial, was also similar between the groups.

CLODRONATE

A multicentre Canadian study was designed to determine the incidence of palliative response in patients with HRPC treated with mitoxantrone and prednisolone (MP) plus clodronate compared to that of patients treated with MP alone [42]. A previous study reported a 38% palliative response rate in HRPC for the combination of mitoxantrone and prednisolone compared to a 21% response rate for prednisolone alone. Patients were eligible for the clodronate study if they had HRPC with symptomatic bone involvement. In this study, pain was assessed using the six-point present pain intensity (PPI) scale of the McGill–Melzack Pain Questionnaire. Patients required a score of at least 1, indicating mild pain, prior to inclusion. A stable analgesic score, based on an analgesic diary was also required prior to inclusion.

All patients in the study received prednisolone 5 mg twice daily and mitoxantrone 12 mg/ m^2 every 3 weeks. In addition they were randomly assigned to receive clodronate 1500 mg intravenously over 3 h every 3 weeks or placebo. The primary endpoint of palliative response was defined as either a 2-point reduction in PPI score (or a fall to 0) without an increase in analgesia score or disease progression or a greater than 50% reduction in analgesia score without an increase in PPI score. Secondary endpoints included symptomatic progression-free survival and overall survival.

A total of 227 patients were randomized, 115 to the clodronate arm and 112 to the placebo arm. Fifty per cent of the clodronate patients and 44% of the placebo patients received at least seven cycles of therapy. A greater palliative response rate was seen in the clodronate group than in the placebo group (45% vs. 39%) although this was not statistically significant ($P = 0.54$). No significant difference in symptomatic progression-free survival or overall survival was seen between the groups.

ZOLEDRONATE

In a randomized phase III study, 643 men with HRPC and bone metastases were randomized to receive intravenous infusions of zoledronate 4 mg, zoledronate 8 mg or placebo every 3 weeks. The primary endpoint of the study was the proportion of patients having at least one SRE (pathological fracture, spinal cord compression, surgery or radiation therapy to bone or change in antineoplastic therapy to treat bone pain). Secondary endpoints included change in pain scores assessed by BPI. Initial reported analysis was at 15 months [43] with a further analysis carried out at 24 months [44]. There were some concerns regarding renal toxicity and, because of this, protocol amendments were implemented during the study to increase the infusion time of zoledronate from 5 min to 15 min and also to reduce the zoledronate 8 mg dose to 4 mg. Zoledronate 4 mg by 15-min infusion did not have a significant adverse effect on renal function when compared with placebo and other toxicity observed in the study was mild.

The percentage of patients who had an SRE was significantly reduced in the zoledronate 4 mg group compared with the placebo group (33.2% vs. 44.2% at 15 months, $P = 0.021$, and 38% vs. 49% at 24 months, $P = 0.028$). The time to first SRE was significantly longer in the zoledronate 4 mg group compared with placebo (448 days vs. 321 days, $P = 0.009$).

Of note, patients who received zoledronate 4 mg reported significantly smaller increases in pain scores over the duration of the trial with significant differences in pain scores observed at 3 months ($P = 0.003$), 9 months ($P = 0.03$), 21 months ($P = 0.014$) and 24 months ($P = 0.024$)

[44]. This provides the first evidence from a large randomized controlled trial that bisphosphonate therapy can provide significant and durable reductions in bone pain associated with metastatic prostate cancer.

On the basis of this study zoledronate 4 mg, intravenously over 15 min every 3–4 weeks has become a recognized treatment for men with HRPC and bone metastases. Due to observed renal toxicity in clinical trials, it is recommended that prior to initiation of treatment, serum creatinine and creatinine clearance should be determined. A dose reduction is required for patients with a calculated creatinine clearance less than 60 ml/min.

Recently, a connection between bisphosphonate treatment, particularly with zoledronate and pamidronate, and osteonecrosis of the jaw has been established. This complication is most often seen in patients who have been receiving concurrent treatment with chemotherapy or corticosteroids or in those who have undergone dental procedures. Characteristically it presents as an area of exposed and painful jaw bone often at the site of a previous dental extraction. It is recommended that all patients should have a dental examination and any required preventative dental procedures carried out prior to starting treatment with either of these drugs.

CONCLUSIONS

Advanced prostate cancer is a devastating illness characterized by deteriorating mobility, increasing pain and impaired quality of life. This chapter has outlined the evidence for EBRT, bone-seeking radionuclide therapy and bisphosphonates in the management of pain from the disease. Importantly, the overall management of such patients needs to involve the multidisciplinary team and will include a variety of systemic therapeutic manoeuvres, and appropriate palliative care as well as addressing the individual psychosocial needs of the patient.

REFERENCES

1. Bonica JJ. Importance of effective pain control. *Acta Anaesthesiol Scand Suppl* 1987; 85:1–16.
2. Arcangeli G, Micheli A, Arcangeli G et al. The responsiveness of bone metastases to radiotherapy: the effect of site, histology and radiation dose on pain relief. *Radiother Oncol* 1989; 14:95–101.
3. McQuay HJ, Collins SL, Carroll D, Moore RA. Radiotherapy for the palliation of painful bone metastases. *Cochrane Database Syst Rev* 2000; 2:CD001793.
4. Tong D, Gillick L, Hendrickson FR. The palliation of symptomatic osseous metastases: final results of the study by the Radiation Therapy Oncology Group. *Cancer* 1982; 50:893–899.
5. Schultheiss TE. Spinal cord radiation tolerance. *Int J Radiat Oncol Biol Phys* 1994; 30:735–736.
6. Steenland E, Leer JW, van Houwelingen H et al. The effect of a single fraction compared to multiple fractions on painful bone metastases: a global analysis of the Dutch Bone Metastasis Study. *Radiother Oncol* 1999; 52:101–109.
7. Price P, Hoskin PJ, Easton D, Austin D, Palmer SG, Yarnold JR. Prospective randomised trial of single and multifraction radiotherapy schedules in the treatment of painful bony metastases. *Radiother Oncol* 1986; 6:247–255.
8. Gaze MN, Kelly CG, Kerr GR et al. Pain relief and quality of life following radiotherapy for bone metastases: a randomised trial of two fractionation schedules. *Radiother Oncol* 1997; 45:109–116.
9. Nielsen OS, Bentzen SM, Sandberg E, Gadeberg CC, Timothy AR. Randomized trial of single dose versus fractionated palliative radiotherapy of bone metastases. *Radiother Oncol* 1998; 47:233–240.
10. Hoskin PJ, Price P, Easton D et al. A prospective randomised trial of 4 Gy or 8 Gy single doses in the treatment of metastatic bone pain. *Radiother Oncol* 1992; 23:74–78.
11. Blitzer PH. Reanalysis of the RTOG study of the palliation of symptomatic osseous metastasis. *Cancer* 1985; 55:1468–1472.
12. Roos DE, Turner SL, O'Brien PC et al. Randomized trial of 8 Gy in 1 versus 20 Gy in 5 fractions of radiotherapy for neuropathic pain due to bone metastases (Trans-Tasman Radiation Oncology Group, TROG 96.05). *Radiother Oncol* 2005; 75:54–63.

13. Chow E, Danjoux C, Wong R et al. Palliation of bone metastases: a survey of patterns of practice among Canadian radiation oncologists. *Radiother Oncol* 2000; 56:305–314.

14. Roos DE. Continuing reluctance to use single fractions of radiotherapy for metastatic bone pain: an Australian and New Zealand practice survey and literature review. *Radiother Oncol* 2000; 56:315–322.

15. Lievens Y, Kesteloot K, Rijnders A, Kutcher G, Van den Bogaert W. Differences in palliative radiotherapy for bone metastases within Western European countries. *Radiother Oncol* 2000; 56:297–303.

16. Salazar OM, Rubin P, Hendrickson FR et al. Single-dose half-body irradiation for the palliation of multiple bone metastases from solid tumors: a preliminary report. *Int J Radiat Oncol Biol Phys* 1981; 7:773–781.

17. Hoskin PJ, Ford HT, Harmer CL. Hemibody irradiation HBI for metastatic bone pain in two histologically distinct groups of patients. *Clin Oncol R Coll Radiol* 1989; 1:67–69.

18. Dearnaley DP, Bayly RJ, A'Hern RP, Gadd J, Zivanovic MM, Lewington VJ. Palliation of bone metastases in prostate cancer. Hemibody irradiation or strontium-89? *Clin Oncol R Coll Radiol* 1992; 4:101–107.

19. Lewington VJ. Cancer therapy using bone-seeking isotopes. *Phys Med Biol* 1996; 4110:2027–2042.

20. Porter AT, Davis LP. Systemic radionuclide therapy of bone metastases with strontium-89. *Oncology Williston Park* 1994; 8:93–6; discussion 96, 99–101.

21. Mertens WC, Stitt L, Porter AT. Strontium 89 therapy and relief of pain in patients with prostatic carcinoma metastatic to bone: a dose response relationship? *Am J Clin Oncol* 1993; 16:238–242.

22. McEwan AJ, Amyotte GA, McGowan DG, MacGillivray JA, Porter AT. A retrospective analysis of the cost effectiveness of treatment with Metastron 89Sr-chloride in patients with prostate cancer metastatic to bone. *Nucl Med Commun* 1994; 15:499–504.

23. Malmberg I, Persson U, Ask A, Tennvall J, Abrahamsson PA. Painful bone metastases in hormone-refractory prostate cancer: economic costs of strontium-89 and/or external radiotherapy. *Urology* 1997; 50:747–753.

24. Lewington VJ, McEwan AJ, Ackery DM et al. A prospective, randomised double-blind crossover study to examine the efficacy of strontium-89 in pain palliation in patients with advanced prostate cancer metastatic to bone. *Eur J Cancer* 1991; 27:954–958.

25. Quilty PM, Kirk D, Bolger JJ et al. A comparison of the palliative effects of strontium-89 and external beam radiotherapy in metastatic prostate cancer. *Radiother Oncol* 1994; 31:33–40.

26. Porter AT, McEwan AJ, Powe JE et al. Results of a randomized phase-III trial to evaluate the efficacy of strontium-89 adjuvant to local field external beam irradiation in the management of endocrine resistant metastatic prostate cancer. *Int J Radiat Oncol Biol Phys* 1993; 25:805–813.

27. Goeckeler WF, Edwards B, Volkert WA, Holmes RA, Simon J, Wilson D. Skeletal localization of samarium-153 chelates: potential therapeutic bone agents. *J Nucl Med* 1987; 28:495–504.

28. Resche I, Chatal JF, Pecking A et al. A dose-controlled study of 153Sm-ethylenediaminetetramethylenephosphonate EDTMP in the treatment of patients with painful bone metastases. *Eur J Cancer* 1997; 3310:1583–1591.

29. Maxon HR III, Schroder LE, Hertzberg VS et al. Rhenium-186SnHEDP for treatment of painful osseous metastases: results of a double-blind crossover comparison with placebo. *J Nucl Med* 1991; 3210:1877–1881.

30. O'Sullivan JM, McCready VR, Flux G et al. High activity Rhenium-186 HEDP with autologous peripheral blood stem cell rescue: a phase I study in progressive hormone refractory prostate cancer metastatic to bone. *Br J Cancer* 2002; 8611:1715–1720.

31. O'Sullivan JM, Norman AR, McCready VR et al. A phase 2 study of high-activity 186Re-HEDP with autologous peripheral blood stem cell transplant in progressive hormone-refractory prostate cancer metastatic to bone. *Eur J Nucl Med Mol Imaging* 2006; Mar 30.

32. Sciuto R, Festa A, Rea S et al. Effects of low-dose cisplatin on 89Sr therapy for painful bone metastases from prostate cancer: a randomized clinical trial. *J Nucl Med* 2002; 43:79–86.

33. Tu SM, Millikan RE, Mengistu B et al. Bone-targeted therapy for advanced androgen-independent carcinoma of the prostate: a randomised phase II trial. *Lancet* 2001; 3579253:336–341.

34. Clarke NW, McClure J, George NJ. Morphometric evidence for bone resorption and replacement in prostate cancer. *Br J Urol* 1991; 68:74–80.

35. Rogers MJ, Watts DJ, Russell RG. Overview of bisphosphonates. *Cancer* 1997; 808 (Suppl):1652–1660.

36. Carey PO, Lippert MC. Treatment of painful prostatic bone metastases with oral etidronate disodium. *Urology* 1988; 32:403–407.

37. Cresswell SM, English PJ, Hall RR, Roberts JT, Marsh MM. Pain relief and quality-of-life assessment following intravenous and oral clodronate in hormone-escaped metastatic prostate cancer. *Br J Urol* 1995; 76:360–365.

38. Kylmala T, Tammela TL, Lindholm TS, Seppanen J. The effect of combined intravenous and oral clodronate treatment on bone pain in patients with metastatic prostate cancer. *Ann Chir Gynaecol* 1994; 83:316–319.

39. Lipton A, Glover D, Harvey H *et al.* Pamidronate in the treatment of bone metastases: results of 2 dose-ranging trials in patients with breast or prostate cancer. *Ann Oncol* 1994; 5(Suppl 7):S31–35.

40. Heidenreich A, Elert A, Hofmann R. Ibandronate in the treatment of prostate cancer associated painful osseous metastases. *Prostate Cancer Prostatic Dis* 2002; 5:231–235.

41. Small EJ, Smith MR, Seaman JJ, Petrone S, Kowalski MO. Combined analysis of two multicenter, randomized, placebo-controlled studies of pamidronate disodium for the palliation of bone pain in men with metastatic prostate cancer. *J Clin Oncol* 2003; 2123:4277–4284.

42. Ernst DS, Tannock IF, Winquist EW *et al.* Randomized, double-blind, controlled trial of mitoxantrone/prednisone and clodronate versus mitoxantrone/prednisone and placebo in patients with hormone-refractory prostate cancer and pain. *J Clin Oncol* 2003; 2117:3335–3342.

43. Saad F, Gleason DM, Murray R *et al.* A randomized, placebo-controlled trial of zoledronic acid in patients with hormone-refractory metastatic prostate carcinoma. *J Natl Cancer Inst* 2002; 9419:1458–1468.

44. Saad F, Gleason DM, Murray R *et al.* Long-term efficacy of zoledronic acid for the prevention of skeletal complications in patients with metastatic hormone-refractory prostate cancer. *J Natl Cancer Inst* 2004; 9611:879–882.

Abbreviations

2-D	two-dimensional
3-D	three-dimensional
3-D-CRT	three-dimensional conformal radiotherapy
5HT	5-hydroxytryptamine
5FU	5-fluorouracil
AA	anti-androgen
ADT	androgen deprivation therapy
AIPC	androgen-independent prostate cancer
AMACR	Alpha-methylacyl coenzyme A racemace
ANN	artificial neural networks
AR	androgen receptor
ASCENT	AIPC Study of Calcitriol Enhancing Taxotere
ASAP	atypical small acinar proliferation suspicious for but not diagnostic of malignancy
ASAPB	atypical small acinar proliferation suspicious for but not diagnostic of malignancy, favour benign
ASAPH	atypical small acinar proliferation highly suspicious for but not diagnostic of malignancy
ASAPS	atypical small acinar proliferation suspicious for but not diagnostic of malignancy
ASTRO	American Society for Therapeutic Radiology and Oncology
ATBC	Alpha-Tocopherol, Beta-Carotene Cancer Prevention Trial
AUC	area under the curve
BAP	bone-specific alkaline phosphatase
BED	biological effective dose
bNED	biochemical no evidence of disease
BMI	body mass index
BPH	benign prostatic hyperplasia
BPI	Brief Pain Inventory
BFS	biochemical free survival
BOO	bladder outflow obstruction
BRFS	biochemical recurrence free survival
CALGB	Cancer and Leukemia Group B
CARET	beta-Carotene and Retinol Efficacy Trial
CART	classification and regression trees

CaPSURE	Cancer of the Prostate Strategic Urologic Research Endeavor
CIS	carcinoma *in situ*
CPA	cyproterone acetate
CT	computed tomography
CTLA4	cytotoxic T lymphocyte-associated protein 4
CTX	cross-linked C-terminal
DEXA	dual energy X-ray absorptiometry
DHA	docosahexaenoic acid
DHT	dihydrotestosterone
DRE	digital rectal examination
DTPA	diethylenetriamine pentaacetic acid
DVT	deep vein thrombosis
EBRT	external beam radiation therapy
EDTMP	ethylene-diamine-tetra-methylene-phosphonate
EGF	epidermal growth factor
ECOG	Eastern Cooperative Oncology Group
EGFR	epidermal growth factor receptor
EORTC	European Organisation for Research and Treatment of Cancer
EORTC QLQ	European Organisation for Research and Treatment of Cancer Quality-of-Life Questionnaire
EPA	eicosapentaenoic acid
EPC	Early Prostate Cancer study
EPCA	Early Prostate Cancer Antigen
ERSPC	European Randomized Study of Screening for Prostate Cancer study
ESCC	epidural and spinal cord compression
ET	endothelin
EZH2	enhancer of zeste homolog 2
FA	fatty acids
FACT–P	Functional Assessment of Cancer Therapy – Prostate
FFF	freedom from failure
GMCSF	granulocyte–macrophage colony-stimulating factor
GnRHa	gonadotrophin-releasing hormone agonists
GTCs	green tea catechins
HBI	hemi-body irradiation
HCAs	heterocyclic amines

HDAC	histone deacetylase	PDGFR	platelet-derived growth factor receptor
HDR	high dose rate		
H&E	haematoxylin and eosin	PFA	polyunsaturated fatty acids
HEDP	hydroxyethylene diphosphonate	PIN	prostatic intraepithelial neoplasia
HER	human epidermal growth factor receptor	PLCO	Prostate, Lung, Colon and Ovary study
HIFU	high-intensity focused ultrasonography	PPI	present pain intensity
		PSA	prostate-specific antigen
HR	hazard ratio	PSADT	prostate specific-antigen doubling time
HRPC	hormone-refractory prostate cancer		
HRQOL	health-related quality of life	PSMA	prostate-specific membrane antigen
ICU	intensive care unit	PTH	parathyroid hormone
IGF	insulin-like growth factor	pTURP	palliative transurethral resection of the prostate
IGFBP	insulin-like growth factor-binding proteins		
		QOL	quality of life
IHT	intermittent hormonal therapy	RADICALS	Radiotherapy and Androgen Deprivation In Combination After Local Surgery
IL	interleukin		
IMRT	intensity-modulated radiotherapy		
IVU	intravenous urography	RECIST	Response Evaluation Criteria in Solid Tumors
LDH	lactate dehydrogenase		
LHRH	luteinizing hormone releasing-hormone	RR	relative risk
		RRP	radical retropubic prostatectomy
LHRHa	luteinizing hormone-releasing hormone agonist	RTOG	Radiation Therapy Oncology Group
		SAHA	suberoylanilide hydroxamic acid
LMN	lower motor neurone	SARD	selective androgen receptor down-regulator
LNI	lymph node invasion		
LUTS	lower urinary tract symptoms	SEARCH	Shared Equal Access Regional Cancer Centre Hospital
MAB	maximal androgen blockade		
MAG	mercaptoacetyltriglycine	SEER	Surveillance Epidemiology and End Results study
MARS	multiple adaptive regression splines		
MCM-5	minichromosome maintenance 5	SELDI TOF	surface-enhanced laser desorption/ionization time-of-flight
MDP	methylene diphosphonate		
MFA	monounsaturated fatty acids	SELECT	Selenium and Vitamin E Cancer Prevention Trial
MP	mitoxantrone and prednisolone		
MRC	Medical Research Council	SFA	saturated fatty acids
MRI	magnetic resonance imaging	SHBG	sex hormone-binding globulin
MRP	multidrug-resistant protein	SMR	skeletal morbidity rate
MUSE	Medicated Urethral System for Erection	SPARC	Satraplatin and Prednisolone Against Refractory Cancer study
NHT	neoadjuvant hormonal therapy	SRE	skeletal-related event
NICE	National Institute for Clinical Excellence	SSRIs	selective serotonin re-uptake inhibitors
NNT	number needed to treat	SWOG	Southwest Oncology Group Protocol
NPC	Nutritional Prevention of Cancer trial	TAP	tartrate-resistant acid phosphatase
		TGF	transforming growth factor
NTX	cross-linked N-terminal	TIL	tumour-infiltrating lymphocyte
OBD	optimal biological dose	TNF	tumour necrosis factor
OME	oral morphine equivalents	TRAP	telomeric repeat amplification protocol
OPG	osteoprotegerin		
OR	odds ratio	TROG	Trans-Tasman Radiation Oncology Group
PAHs	polycyclic aromatic hydrocarbons		
PAP	prostate acid phosphatase	TRUS	transrectal ultrasonography
PAP-GMCSF	prostate acid phosphatase–granulocyte-macrophage colony-stimulating factor	TRUSP	transrectal ultrasound of the prostate
		TTF	time to treatment failure
		TTP	time to progression
PCNN	percutaneous needle nephrostomy	TURP	transurethral resection of the prostate
PCPT	Prostate Cancer Prevention Trial		
PCSD	prostate cancer-specific death	UMN	upper motor neurone
PCTCG	Prostate Cancer Trialists Collaborative Group	UO	ureteric orifice
		VEGF	vascular endothelial growth factor
PDE-5	phosphodiesterase type-5	WHO	World Health Organization
PDGF	platelet-derived growth factor		

Index

Note: page numbers in *italic* refer to figures and/or tables